The Methamphetamine Crisis

STRATEGIES TO SAVE ADDICTS, FAMILIES, AND COMMUNITIES

Edited by
Herbert C. Covey

Foreword by
Commander Lori Moriarty

D0209815

PRAEGER

Westport, Connecticut
London

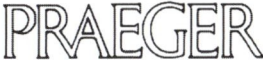

Library of Congress Cataloging-in-Publication Data

The methamphetamine crisis : strategies to save addicts, families, and communities / edited by Herbert C. Covey ; foreword by Commander Lt. Lori Moriarty.

    p. cm.

  Includes bibliographical references and index.

  ISBN 0-275-99322-1 (alk. paper)

  1. Methamphetamine abuse—United States. 2. Methamphetamine—United States. 3. Drug addicts—Rehabilitation—United States. 4. Children of drug addicts—United States. I. Covey, Herbert C.

  HV5825.M397   2007

  362.29'9—dc22   2006025913

British Library Cataloguing in Publication Data is available.

Library of Congress Catalog Card Number: 2006025913

ISBN: 0–275–99322–1

First published in 2007

Praeger Publishers, 88 Post Road West, Westport, CT 06881

An imprint of Greenwood Publishing Group, Inc.

www.praeger.com

Printed in the United States of America

The paper used in this book complies with the Permanent Paper Standard issued by the National Information Standards Organization (Z39.48–1984).

10 9 8 7 6 5 4 3 2 1

This book is dedicated to all those individuals, first responders, child protection workers, therapists, and addicts in recovery who are committed to addressing the methamphetamine crisis and helping children and families. Special thanks to Dwight Eisnach, who reviewed early versions of this manuscript; Marty Covey, who helped with the library searches; and Debora Carvalko of Greenwood Publishing, who was a hardworking driving force behind this book's publication.

Contents

Foreword

On April 4, 2002, during the investigation and seizure of a methamphetamine lab, members of the North Metro Task Force and the Thornton/Northglenn, Colorado SWAT team discovered a 14-month-old child living in the dangerous drug environment. There were no broken bones, no blood or signs of violence; the toxins left behind were invisible, but the picture was clear. The child, wearing only a diaper, had not only been neglected and emotionally and psychologically abused by his mother, but those sworn to serve and protect had also forgotten him.

I've watched the video a hundred times, and the painful impact it has on me never diminishes. The camera follows the SWAT officers as they round the corner to a bedroom looking for suspects. The moment is caught forever. An innocent child sits on the floor with no emotion, ignoring the outreached hand of his mother, who is making a gesture to comfort him. Moments later, the child shows little fear as SWAT officers wearing protective clothing and self-contained breathing apparatus carry him down the stairs and out the door.

This incident changed my life and left me questioning how we ever missed this abuse in the first place. Should it have been obvious? I've been a police officer for 18 years, and the toughest part of the job is seeing innocent children abused. Why didn't we recognize the problem of drug-endangered children? These children suffer physical or psychological harm or neglect as a result of exposure to illegal drugs and exposure to persons under the influence of illegal drugs. Additionally, they are exposed to dangerous environments where drugs are being manufactured. So why had I missed the same thing six months earlier when we responded to another methamphetamine lab where we found a 10-year-old? Looking back now, I can honestly say we had tunnel vision and that our response, like every other discipline's response, was specific. We were working in a vacuum.

Our primary focus was the investigation of an illegal drug lab, and the presence of the 10-year-old child was just a minor inconvenience. It was actually the first time since I had been assigned to the unit that we found a child in a drug lab during the raid. So exactly how many children have we left behind? What about the children who came home from school to an empty house after we left? That was obviously the case for this 10-year-old, because we had raided his house four times previously and never even knew about him. Needless to say, we were not prepared during raid number five. Standard protocol called for decontamination of anyone inside the residence because of the toxic byproducts and methamphetamine left behind from the manufacturing process. Unfortunately, we had no clean clothes for the 10-year-old, so we had to dress him in a prison jump suit. Not only had we missed the child abuse, but I felt that we were now contributing to it. The entire situation was horrible. During decontamination the child told the firefighters that this was a "crappy" day. When the fire captain agreed, the child looked up at him and said, "It's not the shower in the street that's the bad part. The bad part is, it's my birthday." A day to remember, and when it was over, without even thinking twice, the task force found a neighbor to take custody of the child, and social services was never even notified.

Fast-forward 12 months to the early morning of October 23, 2002. The street was empty and the house was dark where undercover detectives were conducting surveillance, preparing for the execution of a search warrant on another drug lab. The traffic on the police radio had been silent. As SWAT officers began their initial approach from several blocks away, one of the detectives watching the house keyed his radio and alerted everyone to stop. He advised that someone was coming out the front door and added, "It's a skeleton." He went on to explain that the skeleton figure appeared to be the four-year-old child social services had told us about. Calling social services was now standard practice, and they had also advised us that a nine-month-old female was also living in the house. The detective went on to describe how the boy was on the front porch looking up and down the street. A few minutes later the boy came back out and began looking up and down the street again. Being undercover detectives, we decided that the child was countersurveillance and was acting as a lookout for his parents. We revised our tactics and told the SWAT officers to execute the search warrant, using extreme caution.

After the raid was over, the SWAT team placed several adults into custody and removed the four-year-old boy. I interviewed the child and explained that I was curious why he was dressed in a skeleton outfit, standing on his front porch, looking up and down the street so early in the morning. His eyes lit up with excitement as he explained that today was his Halloween costume party at school. His shoulders then slumped when he went on to tell me that he really wanted to go but he could not wake his mom up and he didn't know where the bus stop was. The young boy said he got up early and put his costume on, thinking that he could watch the street and catch the bus as it drove by.

Later in the interview, I asked the young boy if he could count. He immediately shouted he could count to "one hundred," but seemed embarrassed when he couldn't get past seven. As if trying to prove how smart he really was, he shifted his focus and told me he knew why I was there. I listened without interruption as he told me that he knew I was a police officer and that I was there because his mom made oil. Understanding a child's perspective and knowing that the manufacturing process of making methamphetamine looks like making oil, I agreed. He corrected me, demonstrating the full extent of his knowledge, and told me his mom was actually making drugs. He then told me he could draw a picture of it if I wanted him to. I located a pen and paper and the boy drew in detail a picture of an entire methamphetamine drug lab. He explained the condenser tube that was used to cool down the cooking process and pointed out a bag that trapped the gases.

Immediately after drawing the lab, he took his pen and pointed to a spot on the paper. He explained, "If we are sitting here in my front yard and you drive down to the end of my block," he drew a line on the piece of paper detailing what he meant. "Then take a right and go down to a white car parked in the street," he continued, drawing another line on the paper. "That is where my mom's boyfriend makes his oil." We followed his directions and found another meth lab and realized that the small boy who we originally thought was countersurveillance was actually our youngest confidential informant reaching out for help. After all of this, I want to point out that the nine-month-old was not on scene when we raided the house, and we would have left without even knowing she existed if we had not developed a close working relationship with social services. Within one hour after raiding the house we were able to locate the little girl and place her into protective custody as well.

I share these stories because the problem of drug endangered children has gone unrecognized for years. Drug endangered children are part of a very large and growing population of children whose lives have been seriously and negatively impacted by dangerous drugs. Thousands of these children across our state go unnoticed and do not receive the necessary care and treatment to heal from these abusive environments. If ignored and left unmonitored, these children continue to be victims caught in a cycle of drug abuse.

After the incident on April 4, 2002, I presented my concerns to the Colorado Drug Unit Commanders at a quarterly meeting held at Rocky Mountain High-Intensity Drug Traffic Area (HIDTA). Everyone agreed that efforts should be made to identify and protect these children. Within a few months the Colorado Alliance for Drug Endangered Children was formed, and professionals from different disciplines across the state came together and began collaborating on the efforts to protect children from the harms associated with the dangerous drug environments in which they live. Parents and caregivers who use illicit drugs such as methamphetamine, cocaine, and heroin create these dangerous and abusive environments for their children. These harms may include injury from explosion, fire, or exposure to toxic chemicals found at clandestine lab sites; physical abuse; sexual abuse; medical neglect; and lack of basic care including failure to provide meals, sanitary and safe living conditions, or schooling.

Early community responses have been challenged to address the complex causes and vulnerabilities of children exposed to these environments. Compounding the challenge is the growing number of children discovered in these circumstances in our communities. In July 2003, Colorado Drug Endangered Children, Inc. (doing business as the Colorado Alliance for DEC) was established as a not-for-profit corporation in an effort to bring disciplines together to focus our response on what is in the best interest of the child.

Our approach focuses on the formation of community-based partnerships that take advantage of existing agency personnel, resources, and responsibilities and coordinate their mutual interests and duties to meet the specific needs of these children. A multifaceted strategy that includes prevention, law enforcement, prosecution, courts, probation, social services, and treatment, and mental health, medical, child welfare, education, public health, nonprofit organizations and the community is required to fight this crisis. The focus is on these children's needs throughout the entire process until the child is in a permanent, safe, and positive functioning environment. We seek the long-term goal of providing supportive and drug-free environments that permit children to prosper. We advocate intervention on behalf of these children and support our state services and local communities by helping to build efficient and effective strategies, tools, and resources that better leverage existing resources that assist and interface with these child victims.

The time has arrived when the general public, communities, and the agencies that serve them must join together to address the crises of methamphetamine use and manufacture. This book will open the eyes of public to the insidious problems associated with meth. How meth is spreading across the country and destroying the lives of users, their children, and families, as well as the communities where it is present, will be revealed in this book.

I join with the authors of this volume in making the plea that we must all address meth collaboratively and proactively. All of the authors have brought their own experiences and expertise to the public dialogue and response to meth. We can learn from what they have to say. There are positive steps that can be taken to deal with drug endangered children, meth treatment, and community safety. Many of these steps or strategies are suggested by the authors in this book. For example, contrary to the opinion of some, the authors of this book show that meth addiction can be treated effectively. We cannot be silent but must bring all dimensions of this drug to the forefront of public attention. It is only through working together that we can protect our children and build safer communities. The problems of methamphetamine are complex and require balancing the interests of the child, family, and community and agencies working together as integrated systems to achieve common and disparate objectives; creating integrated planning and response capacities in local communities; equipping systems with the evidence-based orientation, knowledge, and skills to provide effective responses; and balancing the short- and long-term fiscal challenges to ensure sustainable solutions.

This book, written by those who care a lot about substance abuse and particularly methamphetamine, represents a significant contribution to our thinking and working together to address the meth crisis, especially for drug-endangered children.

Lori Moriarty, Commander, North Metro Task Force

Preface

THE PURPOSE OF THIS BOOK

This book is a resource for professionals working with methamphetamine users, addicts in recovery, and families who have members involved with meth. Its emphasis is on the families and children affected by meth use and manufacture. Many child protection caseworkers and other professionals currently have little guidance on how to work with persons using or making meth. The book provides information on what to expect and how to handle a variety of situations when meth is involved. It also provides viewpoints on the destructive impact of meth from child welfare caseworkers, public health officers, the parent of an ex-user, addicts in recovery, substance abuse specialists, substance abuse therapists, a physician, a chemist, law enforcement officers, an epidemiologist, and a social scientist. All of these individuals bring different perspectives to the issue of meth, but are unanimous in their agreement that its use is the single most concerning, and potentially dangerous, drug abuse problem facing the nation today.

Many of the contributors to this book have direct experience with meth as users in recovery, family members, or professionals. It taps into the experiences of professionals directly involved in meth including substance abuse treatment, case management, investigation, decontamination, child welfare, and other related services, and it also features firsthand accounts of users and those closest to them. The book includes an extensive review of much of the current literature and research on meth and shares discoveries on what we know about its use, manufacture, addiction, health risks, recovery, treatment, and case management.

WHO SHOULD READ THIS BOOK?

One only has to glance at the mass media to find case after case of meth abuse and its impact on children and families. Meth use, while not pervasive, can have devastating affects on all those involved. Of particular concern are the impacts of use and manufacture on families and children. Children pay a particularly heavy social and emotional price when parents or guardians are using, selling, and or cooking meth. When child protection, law enforcement, and other service agencies arrest their parents or caretakers, take away their toys, make them leave home, and decontaminate them, the children are further victimized by this drug. They also have problems understanding and coping with all of the negative things that happen to them when meth is present. Their health is also at risk when their parents or guardians are manufacturing or using heavily. Many professionals are currently working on their own without important information addressing these issues.

The subculture of meth use and manufacture is difficult for outsiders to understand. The insights of experienced professionals, addicts in recovery, and people who have had direct contact with the meth subculture can be valuable in understanding this powerful stimulant. More importantly, we should all be concerned with how it affects entire communities. Meth manufacturing, sales, and use are becoming major concerns for many law enforcement, human service, public health, substance abuse treatment, mental health, employment, correctional, and judicial agencies.

PART I

The Basics
of Methamphetamine

The chapters in this part provide a general introduction to meth—its abuse, its dramatic impact on users and those around them, its prevalence, and why we should be concerned. Chapter 1 covers the basics of meth as a substance, its short- and long-term effects on the user, its addictive properties, and its unique character, which makes it a significant problem for communities and professionals charged with working with meth users and their children.

Chapter 2 provides information on the prevalence and incidence of meth use, treatment, and other indicators in the United States. While alcohol, marijuana, and other drugs may be more prevalent, meth touches users, families, children, and communities in a powerful way. Trend data are presented to give a sense of whether meth use, manufacture, and treatment are increasing, decreasing, or staying steady.

CHAPTER 1

What Is Methamphetamine and How and Why Is It Used?

Herbert C. Covey, Ph.D.

WHAT IS METHAMPHETAMINE?

Methamphetamine, also known as "speed," "crystal," "ice," "crank," or "chalk," is a powerfully addictive stimulant that chemically affects the central nervous system by producing intoxication through the increased stimulation of the dopamine and norepinephrine receptors in the brain. Dopamine is associated with pain suppression, appetite control, and the brain's self-reward center. Norepinephrine activates the body's fight-or-flight response in emergencies. Meth acts on the brain reward pathway by increasing the release of the neurotransmitters noradrenaline, dopamine, and serotonin and reducing the reuptake of dopamine. These neurotransmitters carry messages from one nerve to another and are critical to the individual's sense of pleasure. Meth provides the user, at least initially, with a tremendous sense of pleasure.

Meth is a synthetic stimulant commonly used as a recreational drug. Physicians legally prescribe the drug as a treatment for attention deficit disorder (ADD) under the brand name Desoxyn, for both children and adults. The illegal from of the drug is made easily in clandestine labs with over-the-counter ingredients. For addicts, it is relatively inexpensive to purchase and has desired effects that last for hours. Some users find it appealing because it causes decreased appetite (resulting in weight loss), heightens energy levels, enhances attention, enables people to be physically (sexually) active for long periods, and provides a general sense of well-being and euphoria similar to that of cocaine. The desired effects of meth use can last between six and eight hours, which are then followed by a coming-down period when the user becomes agitated and potentially violent. It is particularly addictive for females because of the "benefit" of its corresponding weight loss.

Meth is a Schedule II stimulant in the United States, meaning that it is illegal to buy, sell, or possess without a prescription. Outside of the United States, it is legally controlled in most countries and is only available by prescription. The federal government classifies methamphetamine as a controlled substance. The 1970 Controlled Substances Act placed strict limitations on the importing, manufacture, and retail availability of amphetamine-related drugs.

The 2000 Methamphetamine Anti-Proliferation Act applied further limits on the sale of precursor ingredients used in other products.

Criminal sentencing for crystal meth is determined by U.S. sentencing guidelines, which are based on the statutory sentences, including quantity-based mandatory minimum sentences, in the Controlled Substances Act. For meth, the statute and guidelines both set forth alternative formulations for determining quantity-based sentences, because "actual" or "pure" meth is distinguished from "a mixture or substance containing" meth. Under federal law, meth trafficking carries a minimum of five years in prison and fines of $2 million for individuals or $4 million for more than one individual for first offenses involving 50 grams or less. Life imprisonment is the maximum penalty for trafficking with two or more prior offenses. U.S. sentencing guidelines should be consulted for specific penalties for trafficking, purity, quantity, forms, and other legal considerations. Unprescribed meth is illegal in every state.

HISTORY OF METHAMPHETAMINE AND ITS USE

Closely related to meth is the drug amphetamine. Amphetamine was first synthesized in 1887 in Germany by a scientist named L. Edeleano, who named it phenylisopropylamine. Initially, amphetamine had no known medical application. During the 1920s, researchers investigated it as a treatment for depression, as a decongestant, and for other medical purposes. By the 1930s, retailers marketed amphetamine as Benzedrine, which was an over-the-counter inhaler used to treat nasal congestion. By the late 1930s, physicians prescribed amphetamine for narcolepsy, attention-deficit/hyperactivity disorder, and depression. During WWII, military organizations used amphetamines (and methamphetamine) to keep soldiers ready and available for duty. As use of amphetamines spread, so did their abuse. To some, amphetamines became a cure-all for such things as weight control and treating mild depression.

In 1919, a Japanese chemist named A. Ogata produced the first meth. In contrast to amphetamine, meth is more powerful and easier to manufacture. Meth's progenitor is ephedrine, which is naturally found in Mahuang, a Chinese plant whose stimulant properties have been documented for over 5,100 years (Holthouse and Rubin 1997, 1997a). During WWII, the Japanese military used meth to improve military performance. It was also sold over the counter in Japan to increase work performance and endurance during the war (Anglin and Burke et al. 2000). Following the war, its use, including intravenously, became epidemic in Japan, as supplies were readily available (Wermuth 2000). It has been suggested that Adolf Hitler may have been a heavy user.

Following the war, Dexedrine (dextroamphetamine) and Methedrine became readily available in the United States. College students, truck drivers, motorcycle gangs, and athletes used the drug to stay awake and to improve concentration and performance.

In the mid-1960s, people were using meth in San Francisco and parts of the West Coast. In 1967, the first meth lab bust occurred in Santa Cruz, California (Holthouse and Rubin 1997a). By 1970, use of the drug declined following the 1970 Controlled Substances Act, which restricted the production of injectable meth (Wermuth 2000). However, meth made inroads in the gay community by the late 1970s (Bonné 2004) and spread in popularity in California during the late 1980s (Leinwand 2003). Hawaii, California, and Arizona were some of the earliest and hardest impacted states. California was hit particularly hard because of the smuggling of ephedrine, a critical ingredient in the production of meth, across the Mexican border. With tighter federal controls over ephedrine, pseudoephedrine became a replacement ingredient. In 1996, Congress passed the Methamphetamine Control Act of 1996. This Act doubled the maximum penalties for possession of the drug and increased the penalty for the possession of equipment used to manufacture meth from 4 to 10 years. The Act cracked down on large purchases of the ingredients, such as red phosphorous and iodine, and increased civil penalties for companies that sell precursor chemicals to people that manufacture meth. It did not, however, stop the flow of ephedrine into the United States.

By the 1990s, some young adults found methamphetamine to be a popular alternative to cocaine and heroin. White motorcycle gangs controlled production and distribution of meth before the 1990s (Gibson et al. 2002). Small home labs and Mexican-based criminal organizations eventually took over production and distribution of meth. Mexican-based criminal organizations established "superlabs" in California and Mexico that were capable of producing large amounts of highly pure meth. In congressional testimony to the Senate Judiciary Committee, authority Donnie R. Marshall reported that about 85 percent of all methamphetamine used in the United States in 2000 was produced by these superlabs (Marshall 2000). During the 1990s and up to the present day, another shift occurred as cooks started to produce meth in small, home-based clandestine labs.

The meth on the streets today is often more powerful than that available in earlier years. Today, meth cooks have refined recipes to the point that some batches have as much as six times the potency of meth cooked in the 1960s (Mills 1999). This meth is not always sold on the street, but rather cooks circulate (give or sell) it among friends and acquaintances.

Today, meth is a Schedule II drug that is available only through a highly restricted prescription procedure. Physicians have used meth to treat overeating disorders, depression, Parkinson's disease, obesity, attention deficit disorder, and narcolepsy (see chapter 4).

STREET AND SLANG TERMS FOR METHAMPHETAMINE

Users and others have developed a set of terms for meth and its related behaviors similar to those used with other street drugs. These terms can be divided into street terms for the drug itself, the behaviors associated with its use, and the types of users. The following terms are an extensive compilation of words used to refer to meth (Mills 1999; Office of National Drug Control Policy 2003). The most commonly used terms are boldfaced in Figure 1.1.

STREET AND SLANG TERMS FOR METHAMPHETAMINE ADDICTS

Just as there are different terms for meth, there are terms for its addicts. Many street terms have evolved to describe or refer to meth addicts: Basehead, Battery Bender, Cluckers, Chicken-Headed Clucks, Crack Heads, Crackies, Crankster, Cranker, Doorknobbers, Fienda, Fiends, Fiendz, Gacked, Geek(ers), Geekin, Geeter, Go Go Loser, Jibby, Jibby Bear, Jibbhead, Krista, Loker or Lokers, neck Creature, Shadow people (due to an aversion of users to light), Sketchpad or Schetchers, Skitzers, Sketch Cookie, Sketch Monster, Speed Freak, Spin Doctor, Spinsters, Tweakers, Tweekin/the Go, or Wiggers.

STREET AND SLANG TERMS FOR BEHAVIORS/ FEELINGS

Meth addicts have developed a number of terms they use to describe their state of mind when using meth: Ampin, Amped, Awake, Bache Knock 2 Rock, Bachin, "Bob" (as in discombobulated), Buzzed, Cranked Up, Crank Whore Jamie, Feelin Shity, Foiled, Fried, Gakked, Gassing, Gear or Gear-up, Geeked, Geekin, Gurped, Heated, High, Jacked, Lit, Peaking, Pissed, Pumped, Psychosis, Ring Dang Doo, Riped, Rollin or Rollin Hard, Scattered, Schlep Heads, Sketching, Spin-Jo, Speeding, Sparked, Spracked, Spun, Spun Monkey or Spun Turkey, Stoked, Talkie, Trippin, Twacked, Tweaking, Tweeked, Twisted, Wide Open, Wired, Worked, Woop Chicken, Zipper, and Zoomin. When the user is experiencing the initial rush from using meth, they are "amping." Amping refers to the "amplified" euphoria they are feeling during the rush.

MISCELLANEOUS METH-RELATED TERMS

The meth drug trade has its own set of terms, including those used by meth addicts and distributors for the sales and distribution of the drug. An eightball refers to $1/8$ of an ounce of meth. A teenager, Tina, or Teena refers to $1/16$ of an ounce, and a paper is a term for a quarter gram of meth.

Paraphernalia is a general term for medical supplies or equipment used to make or use meth. Addicts refer to needles as points, rigs, or slammers. They sometimes call a straw or device used to snort meth a "tooter." Those involved in making it need to shop or otherwise acquire the precursors (materials) needed

Figure 1.1
Slang Terms for Methamphetamine

Albino Poo, Alffy, All Weekend Long, All Tweakend Long, Amp, Anny, Anything Going On, Bache Knock, Bache Rock, Bag Chasers, Baggers, Barney Dope, Batak (Philippine), Bato ((Philippine), Batu Kilat (Philippine), Batu or Batunas (Hawaii), Batuwhore, Beegokes, Bianca, Bikerdope, Bikers Coffee, Billy (Great Britain) Bitch, Biznack, Blanco, Blizzard, Blue Acid, Blue Belly, Blue Funk, Blue Meth, Bomb, Booger, Boorit-Cebuano (Filipino), Boo-Yah, Brian Ed, Buff Stick, Buggar Sugar, Buggs, Bumps, Buzzard Dust, Caca, Candy, Cankinstien, CC, Chach, Cha Cha Cha, Chalk, Chalk Dust, Chank, Cheebah, Cheese, Chicken Feed, Chicken Flippin, Chikin or Chicken, Chicken Feed, Chingadera, Chittle, Chizel, Chiznad, Choad, Cinnamon, Clavo, Coco, Coffee, Cookies, Crack Whore, Crank, Cri Cri (Mexican border), Criddler, Cringe, Crink, Critty, Cristy, Crizzy, Croch Dope, CR (California), Crow, Crunk, Crypto, Crystal, Crystal Meth, Crystalight, Cube, Debbie, Tina, and Crissy, Desocsins, Devil Dust, Devil's Dandruff, Devil's Drug, Dingles, Dirt, Dirty, Dizzy D, D-monic or D, Do Da, Doody, Doo-My-Lau, Dope, Drano, Dummy Dust, Dyno, Epimethrine, Epod, Ersar Dust, Ethyl-M, Evil Yellow, Fatch, Fedrin, Fil-Layed, Fizz Whizz, Gackle-a Fackle-a, Gak, Gas, Geep, Gemni, Glass, Go Speed, Glass, Go Fast, Go-ey, Go-Go, Go-Go Juice, Gonzales, Goop, Got Anything, Granulated Orange, Grit, Gumption, Gyp, Hawaiian Salt, Hank, Hanyak, High Speed Chicken Feed, Highten, Hillbilly Crack, Hippy Crack, Homework, Hoo, Horse Mumpy, Hot Ice, Hydro, Hypes, Ice, Ice Cream, Icee, Ish, Izice, Jab, Jasmine, Jenny Crank Program, Jet Fuel, Jib, Jib Nugget, Jinga, Juddha, Juice, Junk, Kaksonjac, Kibble, Killer, KooLAID, Kryptonite, L.A., L.A. Glass, Lamer, Laundry Detergent, Lemon Drop, Life, Lily, Linda, Lost Weekend, Love, Low, Lucille, M Man, Magic, Meth, Meth Monsters, Methaine, Methandfriend, Methandfriendsofmine, Methanfelony, Methatrim, methmood, Method, Motivation (Colorado), Nazi Dope, Ned, Newday, No Doze, Nose Candy, On a Good One, OZs, Patsie, Peaking, Peanut Butter, Peel Dope, Pepsi (means meth), Pepsi One (Crystal meth), Phazers, Phets, Philopon (East Asia), Pieta, Pink, Poison, Poop, Poo'd Out, Poor Man's Cocaine, Pootanany, Powder, Power Monkeys, Powder Point, Project Propellant, Puddle, Pump, Q'd , Quartz, Quick (Canada), Quill, Racket jaw, Rails, Rank, Redneck Heroin, Richie Rich, Rip, Rock, Rocket Fuel, Rocky Mountain High, Rosebud, Rudy's Rumdumb, Running Pizo, Sack, Sam's Sniff, Sarahs, Satan Dust, Scante, Scap, Schlep Rock, Scooby Snax, Scud, Scwadge, Shab, Shabu, Sha-bang, Shabs, Shabu, Shards, Shit, Shiznack, Shiznac, Sciznac, Shiznastica, Shiznit, Shiznitty, Shizzo, Shnizzie Snort, Agua, Shwack, Skeech, Sketch, Ski, Skitz, Sky Rocks, Sliggers, Smiley Smile, Smurf Dope, Smzl, Snaps, Sniff, Snow (Colorado), space Food, Spaceman, Spagack, Sparacked, Sparked, Sparkle, Speed, Speed Racer, Spin Spin Spin, Spinack, Spindarella, Spinney Boo, Spinning Spishak Spook, Spoosh, Sprack, Sprizzlefracked, Sprung (Mississippi), Spun Ducky Woo, Squawk, Stallar, Sto-pid, Stove Top, Styels, Sugar, Super Ice, Sweetness, Swerve, Syabu (Asia), Talkie, Tasmanian Devil, Tenna, Tenner, The New Prozac, The White House, Tick Tick, Tical, Tina, Tish, Tobats, Toots, Torqued, Trash, Trippin Trip, Tubbytoast, Tutu (Hawaii), Twack, Twacked Out, Tweak, Tweedle Doo, Tweek, Tweezwasabi, Twiz, Twizacked, 222 (Chicago Area) Ugly Dust, Vanilla Pheromones, Wake, Way, Wash, WE WE We, Whacked, White Bitch, White Cross (after pill form), White Crunk, White Ink, White Junk, White Lady, White Pony, White, Who-Ha, Wigg, Working Man's Cocaine, Xaing, Yaba, Yama, Yammer Bammer, Yank, Yankee, Yay, Yead Out, Yellow Barn, Yellow Powder, Zingin, Zip, Zoiks, and Zoom.

It should be noted that some of these terms are used interchangeably with amphetamine, such as "speed."

to make the drug in a manner and in quantities that do not arouse suspicion. This acquisition of supplies is called smurfing.

The meth subculture has developed other terms related to use. For example, crank, craters, crank bugs, and spider bites refer to sores on the face and body resulting from prolonged meth use. Meth mouth refers to the terrible dental conditions addicts have from long-term use.

HOW IS METH USED?

Users can inject, smoke, orally ingest, anally insert, or snort meth. The method the user selects influences how the drug is experienced. Meth is a bitter-tasting powder that easily dissolves in beverages. The powder form of the drug is often snorted, which produces a less intense but much longer-lasting high. In 1993, 42 percent of meth and amphetamine treatment admissions reported they used the drug in this manner, according to the Substance Abuse and Mental Health Services Administration (SAMHSA 2006). By 2003, only 15 percent of the treatment admissions reported they snorted or inhaled the drug. Recent Treatment Episode Data Set (TEDS) data found that in 2003, 56 percent of primary meth and amphetamine admissions reported smoking the drug, which was up from the 15 percent reported in 1993 (SAMHSA 2006). In 1993, 29 percent indicated that they injected the drug, which compares to 22 percent in 2003. Smoking or injecting the drug produces a short but more intense and pleasurable "rush." In 1993, oral ingestion represented 13 percent and "other" accounted for 1 percent of the routes of administration. By 2003, oral administration declined to 6 percent and other routes of administration remained unchanged at 1 percent (SAMHSA 2006).

Powdered meth is a hydrochloride salt form that quickly absorbs water from the air. This form of meth is smokable, as is "crystal meth" or "ice," which refers to meth grown into crystals. Although some people believe that crystal meth is a freebase form of meth, this is not true. Meth that is grown into crystals is simply easier to smoke. Meth in crystal form, rather than powder, also is more likely to be relatively pure because of the difficulty of growing crystals from impure chemicals. According to SAMHSA (2004), in 1992, 12 percent of meth and amphetamine treatment admissions reported they smoked meth. By 2002, 50 percent of the treatment admissions reported they smoked meth in its crystal form. This represents a major shift from inhaling to smoking over this 10-year span.

Another relatively new way of consuming meth is called "booty bumping." This process involves the user heating meth into liquid form and mixing it with water. The user then draws the fluid into a syringe that lacks a needle. The syringe is then inserted in the anus and meth shot into the user's body. Users rely on this technique because the drug is readily absorbed into the blood stream.

The crystal form of meth is referred to as "crystal," "ice," or "glass." If heat is introduced, the user can smoke or inject crystal meth. Smoking it is a much faster and intense way to get high than swallowing the drug. The user places a small amount of crystal in a glass pipe (often called a tooter), heats it, and inhales the resulting vapors. Crystal meth or ice melts into a liquid when heated and returns to its crystal form when cooled. Boiling crystal turns it into a semiliquid referred to as snot, which can be smoked or placed up the nose. Users view smoking meth as ideal because it can be used almost anywhere, since the vapors are odorless and undetectable.

The rush or high felt by the user is the direct result of the release of dopamine into the section of the brain that controls feelings of pleasure. The rush or high associated with its use is relatively long lasting compared to other drugs. The effects of meth use can last as long as 12 hours. If it is snorted, the user usually experiences effects within about 5 minutes. If it is orally ingested, the user will feel a rush in around 20 minutes. Oral meth use tends to lack rushing, has less euphoric effects, and tends to cause far less of a feeling of wanting to do it again than the other methods.

The fastest rushes occur when the user smokes or injects meth. The user usually experiences an immediate and powerful response. Smoking and injecting are associated with stronger, faster, and more euphoric effects. While injecting results in a faster reward, it also results in a faster crash. Users learn to manage the rapid crashes by trying to attain another rush by taking more of the drug. These effects are more associated with compulsive or addictive user patterns. The general use trend is more toward smoking meth because of this immediacy and the strength of the initial rush. It should be noted that many addicts have an aversion to using needles and never inject the drug.

Standard-shaped light bulbs are easily converted into meth pipes. Meth pipes lack a screen found with pipes used to smoke cocaine or marijuana. The user places the meth inside the bowl of the glass pipe and then heats it until it turns into a liquid and then emits a gas (vapor). Once it turns to a gas, the user inhales it through the stem of the pipe. Over time, a white milky residue builds up on the sides of the bowl. Because the glass bowl gets very hot, users will sometimes have burn marks on their fingertips from holding the hot bowls or closing off the hole at the top of the pipe to keep the gas from escaping.

After being heated, unused crystal meth returns to its crystal state when cooled by ice or a cool wet rag. Users will cool down unused liquid meth to its crystal form because it is easier to transport and use at another time.

Regardless of the method of use, meth addicts will frequently use it with other drugs such as cocaine, marijuana, and alcohol. Because of their polydrug use, it is sometimes difficult to sort out the effects of the meth from other drugs. Users rely on other drugs or alcohol to either enhance or supplement the meth high or cushion their withdrawal and depression when coming down.

Figure 1.2
Typical Design of Pipe Used to Smoke Methamphetamine

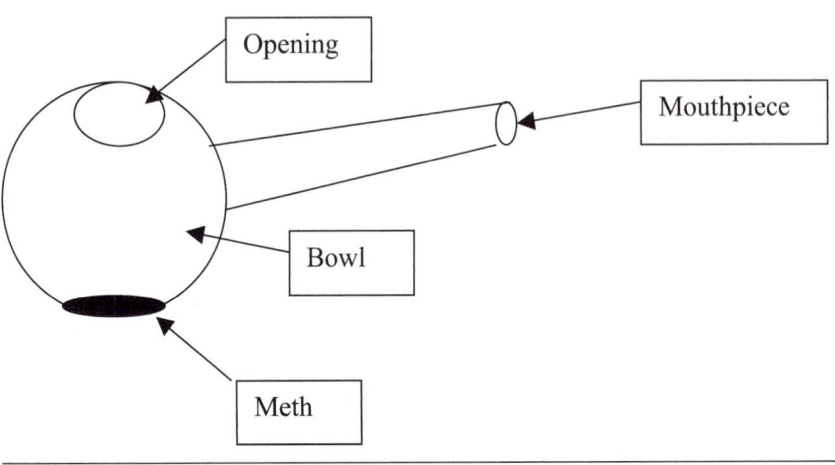

WHAT DOES METH LOOK LIKE?

Meth is usually found on the street as powder or crystal. Street meth, like many other street drugs, is often diluted or cut with other substances. Powdered meth is cut with a filler or is crushed up with amphetamine or methylphenidate (Ritalin) tablets. Sometimes street meth is not really the drug at all but some other compound. Street meth that is clear and crystal is referred to as "glass" or "crystal." Meth comes in many colors, including white, yellow, brown, orange, pink, red, or darker colors; it can also be almost transparent. The method of manufacture and chemicals used affects the color meth assumes, but most meth is white. Meth can take such forms as powder, granulated crystals (crystal meth or ice), tablets (pills sometimes called Yaba), or capsules. Crystal meth is made by adding a small molecule group (hydrochloric acid). The Yaba form is a tablet that is often comprised of meth and caffeine and is produced in Asia and Southeast Asia. The tablets are small (they can generally fit through a straw) and most often are reddish orange or green. Yaba tablets sometimes have corporate logos, such as Toyota, MTV, or Calvin Klein, that are popular in the rave scene. Examples of crystal meth, can be found in the following photo.

METH DOSES

When meth is taken in a pill or tablet form, between 0.05 and 0.1 of a gram represents a dose. When it is smoked, the amount needed is smaller—as little as 0.01 of a gram may be all that is needed. The dosage amounts differ based on the purity of the drug, tolerance of the user, frequency of use, and individual reactions that are based on body physiology, metabolism, and method

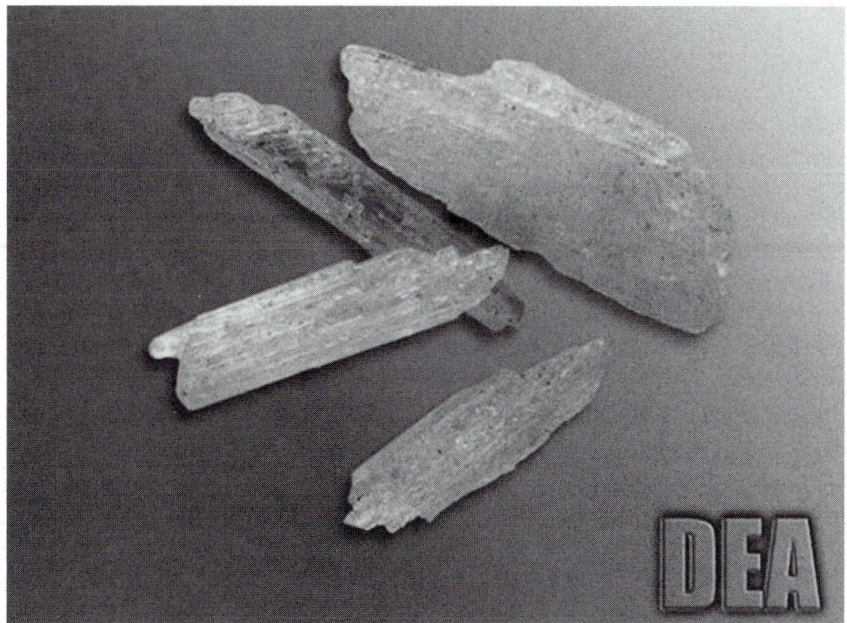

Methamphetamine in crystal ("ice") form. Photo courtesy of the Drug Enforcement Administration.

of use. The Erowid (2006) Web site provides some general guidelines for dosage amounts for an infrequent user of pure meth. Caution should be taken with any dosage amount because of the varying individual reactions to the drug. Thus, the Table 1.1 lists what some are indicating are dosage estimates and should not be considered a guide for anyone.

The important things to remember about the doses are that a number of factors influence the amount needed to get high—the doses can be very small, and with prolonged use, more of the drug is needed to get the desired results. Erowid (2006) identified vomiting, headaches, dizziness, cold sweats, shaking, and, ultimately, death as possible results from overdosing on meth.

METH USE AND DRUG TESTS

Meth is detectable using standard drug tests of urine from three to five days following use. It is detectable in hair tests for approximately 90 days and in blood samples for one to three days. A number of substances can result in false positives including ephedrine, pseudoephedrine, and other substances found in such over-the-counter medications as Sudafed, Allerest, Contact, Nyquil, Robitussin, and others. Diet aids, nasal sprays, asthma medications, and several prescription medications may suggest meth use when it has not been used.

Table 1.1
Approximate Doses by Method of Abuse

	Oral Dosages	Insufflated (Snorted)	Smoked	Injected (IV)
Threshold	5 mg	5 mg	5–10 mg	5 mg
Light Stimulation	5–15 mg	5–15 mg	10–20 mg	5–10 mg
Common	10–30 mg	10–40 mg	10–40 mg	10–40 mg
Strong (some rushing)	20–50 mg	30–60 mg	30–60 mg	30–60 mg
Very Strong (rushing)		50+ mg	50+ mg	50–100 mg (strong rushing; intense euphoria)
Onset	20–70 minutes (depending on form and stomach contents)	5–10 minutes	0–2 minutes	0–2 minutes
Duration	3–5 hours	2–4 hours	1–3 hours	1–3 hours
Coming Down	2–6 hours	2–6 hours	2–4 hours	2–4 hours
Normal Aftereffects	up to 24 hours	up to 24 hours	up to 24 hours	up to 24 hours

WHY DO PEOPLE USE METH?

People use the drug for a number of reasons (Morgan and Beck 1995). The short-term effects of meth use are desired: the sense of euphoria and pleasure; a high that lasts 8 to 12 hours or more; energy enhancement and alertness; weight loss because of decreased appetite; decreased fatigue; relief from chronic depression; a sense of social bonding with other users; and improved sexual pleasure and drive. Rawson (2005) found that more than 35 percent of the women who used the drug said they did so to lose weight, compared to 10 percent of meth-using men. Rawson also found that about 35 percent of the women used it to relieve depression, compared to about 25 percent of the men. Meth users have reported on what it feels like to use the drug. One indicated, "It made me feel confident, self-assured," then added, "Then it took on a whole new meaning to me. I became a partier" (Bonné 2004). Another said she felt "this very intense surge of energy through the body." She added, "I felt like I was superhuman because I would think more, I could accomplish more."

Meth users also experience negative short-term effects that are not desired, including increased respiration, higher pulse rate (irregular heartbeat or cardiac arrhythmia), higher blood pressure, increased body temperature (hyperthermia), convulsions, irritability, hyperexcitability, grinding of teeth, nervousness, dilated pupils resulting in an aversion to light, and death, according to the National Institute on Drug Abuse (2002), Anglin and Burke et al. (2000), Anglin and Kalechstein et al. (1997), and Leshner (2000).

LONG-TERM UNDESIRED EFFECTS OF METH USE

Several agencies, including the Drug Enforcement Administration (DEA) and other authorities (Greenwell and Brecht 2003; Leshner 2000; London et al. 2004; National Institutes of Health 2001, 2004; Volkow et al. 2001a; Volkow et al. 2001) have identified long-term effects of meth use that include severe psychological and physical dependence (addiction), violent behavior that eventually gets coupled with paranoia, making the users even more dangerous, chronic fatigue, talkativeness, overall lifestyle disruption, sleep problems such as insomnia (inability to sleep), cognitive impairments and reduced functioning, confusion, fight-or-flight responses to stimuli, visual and auditory hallucinations, uninhibited sexual functioning with prolonged use, severe depression, picking at the skin and scratching imaginary bugs, which causes open sores and infections. Morals and values are abandoned. The inability to think and act sequentially is impaired and, with heavy, prolonged use, disappears. For example, meth users find it difficult to follow directions or listen to instructions. Heavy use may also lead to homicidal or suicidal thoughts.

Physically, long-term use may result in seizures, chest pain, dry mouth, cardiac valve thickening, death, dramatic weight loss because users lose interest in food and eventually suffer from malnutrition, and brain damage (methamphetamine is neurotoxic). Prolonged use can lead to what is called "amphetamine psychosis," resulting in paranoia, auditory and visual hallucinations, self-absorption, irritability, and aggressive and erratic behavior. Amphetamine psychosis is a disorder similar to paranoid schizophrenia. Individuals with amphetamine psychosis may exhibit bizarre behavior that is sometimes violent.

PATTERNS OF METH USE — LOW INTENSITY, BINGE, AND HIGH INTENSITY

There are three basic patterns of meth use: low intensity, binge, and high intensity. Low intensity is a pattern of use where the user is not psychologically addicted to meth but relies on it for specific perceived benefits, such as a work enhancer or diet-aid drug. Typically, low-intensity users snort or swallow the drug.

Low-Intensity Users

According to Narconon (2002), low-intensity use is characterized by the snorting of powdered meth or ingestion of pills. Users at this level use meth to keep themselves awake and alert for special tasks, or to lose weight. Users at this level are able to hold down jobs, attend school, and otherwise appear to act normal and operate normal lives. Some over-the-road truckers, overtime workers, night-shift workers, stay-at-home parents needing to get several tasks done, and students use it for these purposes. Low-intensity users are unlikely to come into contact with law enforcement, social service, health, or child welfare caseworkers because of problems resulting from this pattern of use.

Professionals may encounter or be working with low-intensity users and not be aware of their use of meth. It is important to note that chronic low-intensity users often view it as a "functional drug." That is, they see it as helping them get things done, such as lose weight, focus on tasks, or get work done. They believe that they "can stop anytime" or "have it under control." Over the long run, this functionality turns out to be a myth.

Narconon (2002) notes that, while use of meth in this fashion seems to be managed, low-intensity users are a short step away from becoming binge users. Low-intensity users have experienced the rush associated with heavier use and generally only need to smoke or inject to cross over the line into binge-use patterns. When they do so, the problems with their use escalate.

Binge Users

Binge users smoke or inject to experience the euphoria that comes from a more intense use of meth. During a binge, the user will periodically use the drug to maintain the high. It is these strong euphoric experiences that move the user from a low-intensity to a psychologically addicted user. A common and unhealthy use pattern for meth is to re-dose repeatedly for several days in a row. Depending on whether the intention is to stay awake, remain high, or attempt to continue to get "rushing" effects, doses are repeated every 3 to 8 hours to stay awake, or every 30 minutes to 4 hours to remain "high." A user re-dosing often takes the same amount of meth as the first dose. As re-dosing continues beyond 48 hours, the user's dosages tend to increase.

High-Intensity Users

High-intensity users have a goal of never crashing or coming down but maintaining a state of euphoria and the perfect rush. Given the nature of meth and its effects on the body, this becomes an impossible goal. For the chronic user, following the first injection or smoke, each successive rush or high becomes more difficult to obtain, and more of the drug is needed. The user remembers the initial high but can never reach that point again no matter how much of the drug is used.

High-intensity users may start out with a pattern of needing from $20 to $40 a day to support their addiction. This increases several-fold as more and more of it is needed to maintain the high they are seeking. The high cost of heavy use drives many to criminal behavior to support their addiction. For some, crime is the only alternative.

Phases of High-Intensity Use

High-intensity users experience meth use as a series of phases. Depending on how often they use, their history of use, method of use, and dosage amounts, the length and nature of each phase differ but follow a general pattern. In order of occurrence, the general phases follow.

The Rush

The rush is the initial sense of intense euphoria that the user experiences immediately after smoking or injecting meth. Low-intensity users do not experience a rush when snorting or swallowing the drug. During the rush, the user experiences an intense feeling of pleasure and burning sensation. The initial rush can last between 5 and 30 minutes, which is longer than the rush associated with the stimulant cocaine. Some users, especially injectors, report an initial burning sensation as the meth is introduced into the body. During the rush, the user's metabolic rate increases, blood pressure elevates, and pulse soars. Users compare the experience of the rush as being the equivalent to having multiple sexual orgasms.

The reason for the rush is that meth triggers the adrenal gland to release a hormone called epinephrine (adrenaline), which puts the body in a battle mode—fight or flight. In addition, the physical sensation the rush provides results from the explosive release of dopamine in the pleasure center of the user's brain. Dopamine is released in the brain's pleasure center. Long-term users find that much of their life is devoted to maintaining a constant rush.

The High

The rush is followed by a high that can last between 4 and 16 hours. This is a longer period than that experienced by cocaine users. Some circles refer to being high as the "shoulder." While being high on meth, the user has a sense of being smarter, more focused, argumentative, and aggressive. High users frequently interrupt those around them.

The Binge

When the user continues to use while high, this is known as binging. Binging is an effort by the user to maintain a prolonged high by taking more meth. During the binge the user becomes hyperactive. Because of severe depression and other negative effects that begin when the drug starts to wear off, users try to avoid crashing or coming down. They may binge to stay high and awake for many days at a time. The law of diminishing returns operates for the user, as the desired effects of meth diminish with each dose. This may cause the user to consume even more to reach the initial rush or stay high. Eventually, there is no rush or high resulting from further consumption, and the user stops.

Tweaking

When the binge ends, a stage of the cycle known as tweaking occurs. The user has a sense of emptiness and dysphoria. Taking more meth will not alleviate the negative feelings experienced by the tweaking user. This stage is not comfortable for the user and some turn to other drugs to self-medicate their feelings. For some, alcohol or other illegal substances are used for self-medications. Tweaking is assumed by many to be the most dangerous stage to professionals, such as law enforcement officers and social workers. Tweakers have not slept for days and as a result are irritable. Think about how moody you get when you don't have enough sleep and then multiply this feeling several times over. Tweakers are unpredictable and short tempered. Tweakers sometimes are frustrated because they can't find enough of a dose to experience that initial high, and this frustration translates into a sense of unease and aggression. When coupled with the paranoia that results from long-term use, they are loose cannons on the deck able to go off at any time.

Tweakers appear to have rapid and brisk movements. They are overstimulated. Their eyes will rapidly dart around, speech will be rapid, eyes will be clear, and speech concise. A tweaker's eyes may roll back into the head. Tweakers are obsessive about things. For example, they will clean the same thing over and over but ignore other things that need cleaning. The kitchen may be spotless but the house or yard may be full of unfinished projects and filth. In addition, tweakers can become obsessed with dismantling things, such as appliances, with no idea of why they are doing it. They might dismantle a television, washing machine, or any number of objects without a clue about how to put things back together.

Because tweakers hear and see things differently, it can be difficult for law enforcement or caseworkers to predict what, if anything, will set them off. Tweakers have such an altered sense of reality that virtually anybody or anything could set them off into a rage or confrontation. Because many become paranoid, a caseworker, law enforcement officer, family member, or other person could become an unsuspecting target. Because some users fear authorities, they have many weapons around the house. This requires that caseworkers and other professionals be cautious around tweaking individuals.

There is considerable folklore on how long a user can tweak. Reports of 15 to almost 40 days without sleep have been reported to the authors of this book. While it is true that addicts do stay awake for very long periods of time, what is likely is they actually take short naps and float in and out of consciousness. They never fall into a deep and replenishing sleep until later in the cycle. While meth is not a hallucinogen or a psychedelic, it is easy to understand how prolonged sleep deprivation would result in bizarre behaviors and thoughts. Sleep deprivation can result in profoundly disturbing hallucinations. For example, many addicts will describe the "shadow people" that seem to appear and be very real to them (Holthouse and Rubin 1997).

The Crash

Eventually, because of a lack of sleep and loss of epinephrine, the body becomes exhausted and falls into a deep sleep. This is known as the crash. When high-intensity users stop taking meth they experience depression, anxiety, fatigue, paranoia, aggression, and an intense craving for the drug (London et al. 2004; National Institute on Drug Abuse 2002). Tweakers sleep like they are dead when the time comes to crash, and they sleep for days afterwards. The crash can last for days, as the body replenishes its supply of epinephrine. Users may try to cushion the crash by using tranquilizers or downer drugs, such as marijuana, heroin, or alcohol (Gibson et al. 2002). Users that are crashing usually pose no real threat to caseworkers, law enforcement officers, or other professionals. However, crashing parents or guardians cannot provide basic care to children and often are neglectful of them and may place them at risk. Protecting, feeding, and overseeing children are not possible for the crashing user, and sometimes their children go without food, sleep, care, and supervision. Some children learn to survive on their own when parents or guardians are crashing. They eat and drink whatever they can find. Crashes may last between one and three days.

Normalcy

Meth addicts eventually return to a state of normalcy for a few days. This stage can last between 2 and 14 days depending on frequency of use. The high-intensity user never really gets back to complete normalcy because of the physiological damage done to the body, specifically the brain. This is not to say the high-intensity user cannot recover and lead a normal life.

Withdrawal

Users who withdraw from meth experience symptoms of physical distress. Withdrawal from the drug is a prolonged process, and users in withdrawal experience depression and are initially unable to experience pleasure. They also may experience fatigue, paranoia, and aggression and have psychotic symptoms that may persist for months or years following use (Office of National Drug Control Policy 2005). They become lethargic and have no energy. Users, because of poor eating habits, also may experience extreme hunger. If the cravings for meth are strong, some may become suicidal. If more meth is used, their sense of pleasure increases and their depression will temporarily be alleviated. Some suggest that this is a major reason why meth addicts are some of the most difficult to treat and why recidivism rates are high.

Experts agree that meth is a highly addictive stimulant drug (National Institute of Health 2001). According to the U.S. Drug Enforcement Administration (2005), "Methamphetamine has a phenomenal rate of addiction, with some experts saying users can get hooked after just one use." Anecdotal accounts and clinical experience suggest that addiction can occur in less than a year. The Center for Substance Abuse Treatment (1999) *Tip 33: Treatment for Stimulant Use Disorders* notes in chapter 2 that addiction typically occurs after using the drug for 2 to 5 years. Prolonged or binge use of meth causes significant tolerance and psychological dependence. Some report addiction after the first use, but this is not typical for most.

THE PHYSICAL APPEARANCE OF METH USERS

It would be inaccurate to stereotype high-intensity meth users as looking a certain way. There is no set appearance for all meth users and addicts. They can assume a variety of appearances depending on a number of factors, including the amount and frequency they are using. Low-intensity meth users can look reasonably normal in appearance. However, if the individual is using meth on a regular basis, obvious physical indications develop over time. It should be noted that as dramatic as the insert photos appear, there is also physiological damage occurring on the inside of the body. Three excellent Web sites that have examples of the progression of deterioration from meth use are: 2stopmeth.org; www.co.multnomah.or.us/sheriff/faces_of_meth.htm; and www.mappsd.org. The reader can view some examples of the physical deterioration resulting from prolonged meth use in the insert section of this book.

Crank Bugs and Meth Mites

The color insert photos show the deterioration that results from prolonged meth use, but also what are termed "crank bugs" or "meth mites." The open sores on the skin shown in the photos are the result of the individual scratching imaginary "crank bugs" or "meth mites." Long-term meth users develop the sensation that insects are crawling on their skin, causing them to scratch themselves. The scratching associated with these imaginary insects (known as formication) eventually leads to lesions in the skin, topical infections, sore areas, and scabs. These open sores are aggravated by the addict continuing to scratch and thus spreading the infection. The user's lack of proper hygiene contributes to the spread of infection. Those who inject frequently develop abscesses, ulcerations, and scars around the injection sites. These injection sites may become infected and also a target of scratching. The reader can view the color insert for additional examples of crank bugs and meth mites.

"Meth Mouth"

The long-term or heavy use of meth also leads to severe dental problems, which professionals and addicts refer to as "meth mouth." The American Dental Association (2005) concluded that "the oral effects of methamphetamine can be devastating." Long-term drug addicts, especially those using meth, do not take good care of their teeth and do not visit their dentists on a regular basis. Meth addicts do not brush their teeth often, have poor diets, and avoid medical and dental professionals to hide their addiction. Meth acts on the gums and teeth as a corrosive. It softens the teeth, and they basically melt away. When a user smokes meth, the chemicals used to make it, such as sulfuric or muriatic acid, are heated and vaporize and spread around the mouth. The user's mouth is irritated and burned by the chemicals, and sores eventually develop that become infected. This infection spreads throughout the mouth and gums. When coupled with the corrosive action of chemicals on tooth enamel, eventually the teeth rot away to well below the gum line. The gums are also affected because meth use causes blood flow to decrease and thus gums to break down and become diseased. For these and other reasons, it is common for the roots to show and the loss of teeth to occur.

The decay occurring can also be attributed to the effect of meth use on saliva production, or what is medically referred to as "dry mouth" (American Dental Association 2005). Meth dries out the salivary glands and thus the production of saliva. Normally, the body uses saliva to clean the teeth and neutralize acids, and to control harmful bacteria. With less saliva, the user's mouth cannot perform these functions. Consequently, the acids in anything consumed are free to decay the teeth and gums. The sense of a "dry mouth" or "cottonmouth" (xerostomic) causes some users to drink lots of sugary sodas, which also add to tooth decay (American Dental Association 2005). Damage to the mouth is not limited to those who smoke the drug; it can also be caused by snorting meth, as caustic chemicals flow through the nasal passage to the back of the mouth.

Another fundamental process that destroys the user's teeth is the grinding that occurs during use. Meth use causes the user to feel anxious or nervous, and the unintentional teeth grinding that consequently occurs leading to cracks and breaks. Meth users often grind their teeth down hard, causing teeth to break and nerve endings to become exposed. The user may also lose fillings because the teeth grinding causes them to fall out. Just breathing through the mouth and having air pass over the teeth and gums can cause some users to feel pain. Whether from smoking or snorting, the user will eventually develop meth mouth, and many users simply use more meth to alleviate the pain.

The best way to visualize and understand meth mouth is to view some of the images of the mouths of long-term users. The color insert section contains examples of meth mouth and the corresponding tooth and gum decay resulting from prolonged meth use. The consequences of meth mouth go beyond pain and disfiguration. Some long-term recovering users with damaged teeth may be reluctant or unable to find dental help. If they do find it, they may lack the money for dental repairs. With poor teeth, they find it difficult to obtain work because potential employers are turned off by unsightly teeth (mouths), and users face social rejection.

THE COMPARATIVE LOW COST OF METH

In addition to the desired effects of meth on the user, one of the reasons for the drug's popularity is its relative low cost. It is relatively inexpensive to produce, but more importantly lasts longer than alternative stimulants, such as cocaine. Prices for the drug vary across the United States:

- It costs $20 to $60 for a quarter gram, which is slightly lower than cocaine but lasts significantly longer (Bonné 2001).
- The National Council of State Governments estimated a $100 batch of methamphetamine would sell on the street for about $1,000 (Kraman 2004).
- Meth prices range between $5 and $15 a dose (Leinwand 2003).
- The Drug Enforcement Administration in 2001 provided a price range from $3,500 to $23,000 per pound, $350 to $2,700 per ounce, and $20 to $300 per gram (Drug Policy Information Clearinghouse 2003).

The price of crystal meth runs higher because of its purity and additional manufacturing steps. The National Drug Intelligence Center (2005), using Drug Enforcement Administration data, reported the prices for powdered and crystal meth shown in Table 1.2.

Although prices seem high to the nonuser, they represent a good value to the addict. The long-term high of the drug is a good value compared to cocaine or other substances. Likewise, meth quickly becomes expensive as addicts must use increasing amounts of the drug and do so more frequently over time in pursuit of that lasting high and avoidance of the crash. The consequence is that the price of meth becomes very high for children as their needs compete with the meth for family resources.

HOW DOES METH COMPARE TO COCAINE?

Because both are powerful psycho stimulants, meth is often compared with cocaine (National Drug Intelligence Center 2002). Users who have used both drugs report similar experiences, such as a sense of euphoria. Users of both drugs report experiencing an initial rush, and a longer high and sense of euphoria with meth. If the cocaine is in crack form, the rush and high are much shorter. Users can smoke, inject, snort, or swallow either illicit drug. Both drugs may produce anxiety, increased blood pressure, increased temperature, higher pulse

Table 1.2
National Price Ranges of Methamphetamine, 2003

Quantity	Powder	Crystal
Pound	$1,600–$45,000	$6,000–$70,000
Ounce	$270–$5,000	$500–$3,100
Gram	$20–$300	$60–$700

Source: National Drug Intelligence Center 2005.

rates, and possible death. Short-term effects of both include increased activity, decreased appetite, and respiration. Prolonged use of either drug can lead to psychotic behaviors, hallucinations, mood disturbances, and or violence. When users of either drug withdraw, they report craving, paranoia, and depression (London et al. 2004).

Differences between the two drugs exist. Cocaine is derived from the refined leaves of the South American coca plant; consequently, almost all cocaine in the United States is imported. The meth found in the United States is also imported from Mexico, Southeast Asia, and other countries. However, unlike cocaine, it can be domestically manufactured in large or small operations. Large spaces, while often desirable, are not required for production. Meth can be produced in small rooms or spaces. The production of meth is relatively easy compared to importing cocaine. All of the necessary chemicals to produce meth are relatively available, thus making law enforcement control of the illicit drug difficult.

Cocaine and meth abusers have different use patterns. For example, meth users report that they use the drug on a more regular basis than that reported by cocaine users. Meth's effects require less-frequent administration than cocaine, because meth leaves the system more slowly and thus has a longer half-life than cocaine. Meth has a half-life of between 10 and 12 hours, compared with only about one hour for cocaine (Wermuth 2000). While cocaine is quickly and almost completely metabolized in the body, meth has a longer duration, and a larger percent of the drug remains unchanged in the body (Center for Substance Abuse Prevention/National Prevention Network 2006; National Institute on Drug Abuse 2002). Thus, the brain is affected for more prolonged spans of time. Cocaine is not neurotoxic to dopamine and serotonin neurons, but meth is neurotoxic. "Meth has more long-term, serious effects on the brain than cocaine" (National Institute on Drug Abuse 2002).

Another difference is cost. Meth is cheaper on the street than cocaine. Meth has a longer duration for the initial rush and high. Crack cocaine offers a high of about 15–20 minutes and meth a high of 8–24 hours. The perceived cost-benefit ratio to the user is much greater for the meth addict. Rawson and Anglin et al. (2002, p. 7) wrote, "Methamphetamine effects are long lasting and methamphetamine users typically spend about 25 percent as much money for methamphetamine as that spent by cocaine users for cocaine."

According to research by Dr. Sara Simon sponsored by the National Institute on Drug Abuse (NIDA), abuse patterns differ between meth and cocaine abusers (Zickler 2005). Meth abusers typically take the drug early in the morning and in two- to four-hour intervals, similar to being on a medication. In contrast, cocaine abusers typically take the drug in the evening and take it over a period of several hours that resembles a recreational-use pattern. They typically continue using until all of the cocaine is gone. In addition, another pattern showed that continuous use was more common among meth abusers than among those abusing cocaine. According to other NIDA- sponsored research by Dr. Simon, the effects of meth and cocaine abuse resulted in similar cognitive deficits, but meth abusers had more problems than cocaine abusers at tasks requiring attention and the ability to organize information (Zickler 2005).

In the 1980s cocaine use became epidemic, but in recent years use has declined among the middle class. Crack cocaine remains a serious blight in some inner cities. Cocaine's use, similar to other drugs, is cyclic, with periodic increases and decreases (Rawson and Anglin et al. 2002). In contrast, meth has the potential of enduring, similar to marijuana and alcohol.

Cocaine addicts typically experience profound life changes in a relatively short time frame because of higher costs of use and use patterns, which involve binging. Cocaine users typically hit bottom sooner than many meth users. Meth addicts experience the same losses and also hit bottom, but in many cases do so over a longer period. Some meth addicts use at levels that allow them to maintain jobs, homes, some money, and at least the appearance of being in control.

CHAPTER 2

Prevalence of Use and Manufacture of Methamphetamine in the United States—Is the Sky Falling or Is It Not Really a Problem?

Herbert C. Covey, Ph.D.

INTRODUCTION

Methamphetamine has been available for years; why all of the recent alarm? The answer is easy—many of the indicators of illegal substance use indicate that meth use is spreading throughout much of the United States, and authorities report that meth use has increased to "epidemic" proportions (Rawson and Anglin et al. 2002). This spread has been likened to an epidemic moving from the West and Southwest to the rest of the country.

Is this spread unique to the United States? No. The World Health Organization recently reported that amphetamine and methamphetamine are the second most abused drugs in the world. The World Health Organization estimates that over 35 million people use or abuse amphetamine or meth (Rawson and Anglin et al. 2002). This compares with 15 million for cocaine and 10 million for heroin. Meth abuse has taken over in some countries as the illegal drug of choice. For example, in Thailand methamphetamine abuse now accounts for almost 70 percent of addictions, and other Asian countries report a similar pattern of increasing abuse (Zickler 2005a).

THE SPECIAL CHALLENGES OF METH

Does meth pose special challenges for agencies and staff trying to curb its use or address its affects on children and families? Some authorities suggest that meth use and addiction are similar to other stimulants, such as cocaine, and should be addressed using the same approaches. Others conclude that meth use and addiction are unique and require special strategies. Its use does, in fact, pose special challenges.

The drug is relatively abundant compared to illegal substances that have to be imported across national boundaries. It is often locally produced in home laboratories using materials such as household batteries and cold medicines (Bonné 2001). Although authorities have made efforts to control the precursor chemicals used to produce meth, it is impossible to eliminate them altogether (Rawson and Anglin et al. 2002) because they are found in multiple household products (see chapter 3).

Meth manufacture has been targeted in rural areas, which are attractive for dealers and manufacturers because the odors and by-products of meth production are more easily concealed from authorities and thus they are less likely to be discovered. Some of the methods of production involve chemicals and substances that are associated with farming and ranching, and their possession is not viewed as extraordinary. For example, anhydrous ammonia and iodine, both chemical precursors for meth manufacture, are both commonly used on farms and ranches.

Meth can be produced on a small scale for personal use. Authorities have found labs in car trunks, mobile homes, microwave ovens, and small rooms. For example, one child welfare caseworker found a lab set-up in a suitcase she planned to use to pack a child's clothing during the child's removal from a home.

More than a decade ago illicit meth production was restricted to a few "cooks" who kept their recipes relatively secret. Today, instructions for making meth are readily available in publications and over the Internet. Any Internet search engine will generate numerous recipes for producing meth. Internet chat rooms are full of self-proclaimed chemists (cooks) who are willing to provide free advice to aspiring cooks. For example, www.totse. com has a Web site that provides amateur recipes for cooking meth and making other illegal substances. If the Internet is not used, there are books that provide easily accessible recipes on how to produce the drug. The most widely known is Uncle Fester's (2002) *Secrets of Methamphetamine Manufacture: Including Recipes for Mda, Ecstasy, and Other Psychedelic Amphetamines* (6th Edition). Other similar books are available.

Another challenge of meth is that it is intense and powerfully addictive. It affords a strong sense of euphoria from its first use onward and does so for a relatively low cost when compared to other stimulants, such as crack cocaine. Because of its effect on the brain and nervous system, heavily involved addicts have difficulty experiencing pleasure that is comparable to being high on the drug.

Users perceive other attractive benefits beyond being high on meth. Initial users and addicts view the drug as effective in reducing fatigue and allowing them to work for prolonged periods of time. For example, over-the-road truck drivers use meth and amphetamines to stay awake on long road trips. Some students view it as a study aid that allows them to study and stay focused for hours. Other individuals, especially females, view it as an effective way to lose weight.

Treatment approaches must be modified to the special needs of the meth addict. For example, treatment information must be easy to understand (simple) and repeated. This is due partially to the effect meth has on brain functioning. The reasoning portion of the brain is affected by prolonged use. Meth addicts struggle with sequential thinking and instructions. In addition, the depression associated with long-term withdrawal must be addressed.

The distribution of meth is different from other illegal substances. It is not generally a street drug but is sold or provided by family, friends, and associates. This makes law enforcement activities challenging, as the drug is less on the street than marijuana, heroin, cocaine, and other street drugs.

TRENDS IN THE UNITED STATES

Many substance abuse authorities believe that meth use and distribution has been a significant problem that is expanding in the United States (Freese et al. 2000; Gibson et al. 2002; Herrell et al. 2000; Hser et al. 2005; Huber et al. 2000). Some basic data indicate this growth:

- Meth is showing up in the workplace. Between 1999 and 2003, the percentage of positive workplace drug tests containing amphetamines doubled, from 4.5 percent to 9.3 percent (Center for Substance Abuse Research 2004).

- There are indications that it is spreading among white, low-income, rural Americans (Bonné 2001; Kraman 2004).

- The National Drug Intelligence Center (2002) reported that crystal meth's availability is expanding in several states. The center reported that 31 percent of all state and local law enforcement agencies considered meth their primary drug threat, and 58 percent considered the availability of the drug in their communities to range from medium to high (National Drug Intelligence Center 2003).

- The Office of National Drug Control Policy (2003a) reported that federal meth lab seizures increased from 327 in 1995 to 13,092 in 2001. This represents an increase of over 4,000 percent, or a 40-fold increase in the number of labs seized. This number does not reflect all of the undiscovered labs or small and undetected operations.

- The methamphetamine problem is becoming so large nationally that at the 2005 National Association of Counties (NACo) annual meeting, members viewed meth as an "epidemic" and voted to request the president to provide more funding for meth research, treatment, enforcement, education, and cleanup (Leinwand 2005; National Association of Counties 2005). In the same vein, NACo released two surveys on the impact of meth on hospital emergency rooms and the challenge of treating its abuse (National Association of Counties 2006, 2006a).

- *National Drug Threat Assessment 2003* data reveal that, nationally, 36.2 percent of state and local law enforcement agencies identified meth as their greatest drug threat, ranking second only to cocaine (37 percent). State and local law enforcement agencies in the Pacific (90.9 percent), West Central (80.2 percent), and Southwest (51.6 percent) regions were more likely to identify meth as their greatest drug threat than were agencies in the Great Lakes (29.4 percent), Southeast (28 percent), and Northeast/Mid-Atlantic regions (2.7 percent) (National Drug Intelligence Center 2004, p. 1).

MEDIA ATTENTION

In addition to some general indicators, the topic of meth has recently been the subject of television, the press, music, and film. The mass media and pop culture have embraced the topic of meth use and manufacture, which had always been present but were less visible to the general public. As a result of all this attention, increased public awareness of meth, and increased media attention, it seems that the drug is reaching epidemic proportions in many regions of the country.

The Drug Enforcement Administration (DEA) Web site at www.usdoj. gov/dea/pubs/pressrel/meth and the partnership for a Drug-Free America at www.drugfreeamerica.org contain examples of recent press releases regarding meth, as do other Web sites. There are a number of other examples of recent media titles and press clips regarding meth use:

- "Meth's Deadly Buzz—Sioux City, Iowa." In many ways, this article observes that meth is the crack cocaine of the new millennium. Much like crack, which swept across the nation in the 1980s and 90s, meth use has hit epidemic proportions in the past several years. Crack plagued inner cities and the black community; methamphetamine is thriving in cities like San Francisco, sweeping across the Midwest and headed east. It has quietly become America's first major home-grown drug epidemic (Bonné 2001, 2001a).

- "Methamphetamine's Young Victims' Homes Doubling as Drug Labs Pose Serious Dangers to Kids," *Denver Post*, October 20, 2002 (Herdy 2002).

- "The Meth Epidemic: Inside America's Drug Crisis" (*Newsweek*, August 8, 2005).

- "Potent Mexican Meth Floods in as States Curb Domestic Variety," *New York Times*, January 23, 2006 (Zernike 2006).

- "Methamphetamine Use Increasing: Public Health Officials Voice Concerns about Infants Born to Addicted Mothers," *American Medical News*, July 26, 2004 (Elliot 2004).

- "Children of Ice." A series of articles about methamphetamine addiction in Hawaii noted, "The ice epidemic has touched tens of thousands of lives in Hawaii. It has an impact on our families, our children, our schools, our crime rate, our prisons, our businesses. Our community has never faced a problem quite like this, and we are still searching for the right responses" (*Honolulu Advertiser*, September 14, 2003).

- "Counties Say Meth Is Top Drug Threat." This article noted that meth is a bigger problem than cocaine, marijuana, or heroin for most communities, according to a survey of law enforcement agencies in 500 counties in 45 states by the National Association of Counties (*USA Today*, July 4, 2005).

Documentaries and films have been produced on meth use and production. For example, a journalistic documentary titled *Crank—Made in America* (2003) shows meth use and the interpersonal relationships among users. The PBS documentary *Frontline* (2006) produced a special titled "The Meth Epidemic."

The music industry has also paid attention to meth. The industry has produced songs about the risks and experiences of meth use. The following songs all refer to use: Eminem, "These Drugs"; Third-Eye Blind, "Semi-Charmed Kind of Life"; Bush, "The People That We Love: Speed Kills"; Eminem, "Purple Pills"; and Green Day, "Brain Stew." The song "Brain Stew" provides typical lyrics that describe meth use.

With all of the attention meth has received in the media in recent years, in an open letter, Dr. David Lewis and Dr. Donald Millar (July 27, 2005) warned that caution should be exercised in drawing unproven conclusions about what meth use means to the unborn and newborns. They and others criticize recent media references to "meth babies" or "ice babies" as being unfounded and damaging. Such labels are detrimental, because as they grow up, such children face lower expectations and harmful stereotypes about their abilities. They cite recent media coverage, such as *CBS News*, "Generation of Meth Babies" (April 28, 2005) at *CBSNews.com* as an example of the misuse of the label "meth baby" in the mass media. They also contend that there is no such thing as a "meth-addicted baby," because babies do not act compulsively in spite of adverse consequences as addicts do.

Lewis and Millar and other substance abuse experts are concerned that stating that meth use by pregnant women results in severe health consequences for infants has not been established by medical research and may actually do more harm than good. As was the case for "crack babies" in the 1980s and 1990s, they argue that there has not been enough scientific research to warrant any medical or addictive conclusions about meth use and infants. With at least two decades of research on the effects of the use of the stimulant cocaine on fetuses and newborns, they observe that the feared epidemic of "crack babies" never materialized and the same may be true for meth. Although they do not specifically refer to there being a panic, they do stress that the media has consistently overexaggerated meth at a social cost to infants and new mothers.

WHO USES METH? IS THERE A PROFILE OF METH USERS?

What populations are more likely to use meth? Summarizing the literature, Wermuth (2000, p. 423) wrote, "Low-income and unemployed young white men continue to be the group most likely to use methamphetamine, but by the mid-1990s the drug had increased in popularity in more diverse populations and regions." Numerous studies have found that meth use is predominantly a white phenomenon (Anglin et al. 2000; Yacoubian and Peters 2004). According to the SAMHSA's (2005b) *DASIS Report*, January 7, 2005, treatment admissions for methamphetamine or amphetamine abuse in 1992 were 55 percent male, and that percentage remained stable through 2002. The mean age for treatment admissions increased to 29 years in 2002. In 1992, 62 percent of treatment admissions were white. Whites increased to 66 percent of the admissions in 2002. Of those being admitted for treatment, 25 percent indicated that they had part-time or full-time jobs. A SAMHSA Report (2005a) estimated a prevalence of about 0.7 percent for whites.

However, meth users come from a wide variety of socioeconomic profiles. For example, one Sacramento, California, study found that users came from all walks of life, and some users started in their teens (Gibson et al. 2002). The penetration of meth into other demographic circles is occurring. Anglin et al. (1997) reported that other groups such as Latinos, gay-bisexual males, older adult arrestees, and adolescents are increasingly involved. Joe (1996) found and reported on meth abuse among Asian-Pacific women in Honolulu, San Francisco, and San Diego. There are numerous anecdotal reports on the broad spectrum of users, such as those describing high-achieving students who use the drug to perform better in school and college, and others, such as athletes, cheerleaders, beauty pageant participants, and models who use it to improve performance (Rawson and Anglin et al. 2002).

While many are at risk of meth addiction, some populations identified in the literature are of special concern:

- Women who have emotional relationships with males who are addicted to meth. The males encourage and often demand that the females in their lives also use meth to "bond" with them. If the male is using, it is likely that the female is also using. Anecdotally, a common pattern is for an older male to introduce the drug and encourage its use of meth by a younger female. Another group to use it is stay-at-home adults, usually females, who begin using meth for its short-term benefits such as its energy boost, to treat depression, or for its related weight loss (Rawson 2005).

- Workaholics or low-income adults who use it to stay awake and perform in multiple jobs. Working low-income individuals find meth attractive because they must work several jobs or long hours to support themselves or their families. They find that higher energy and alertness (ability to stay awake for prolonged periods) helps them cope with the demands of multiple jobs. Probably the best example of this are over-the-road truckers, some of whom use meth (or amphetamine), allowing them to keep driving long distances.

- Gay men who use meth to enhance their sexual experiences and stimulate sexual behavior. According to Freese et al. (2000), urban gay males living along the West Coast of California represent a large segment of the meth-using population. The user's sense of euphoria from using the drug reduces normal inhibitions about sex and multiple partners. Meth use can increase the libido, but long-term use may result in sexual dysfunction. There are reports of gay men using meth to prolong and enhance sexual encounters with several partners without appropriate protection, thus increasing the potential for transmission of HIV among this population. Some suggest that associating the use of meth among this population is important to addressing the spread of HIV (Rawson and Anglin et al. 2002; Specter 2005). Aware of the association between meth use and the spread of HIV, some activists have made posters that proclaim, "Buy Crystal. Get HIV for Free," or "Crystal Free and Sexy" (Join Together 2005). Because of this tie to sexual activity, the gay community poses unique challenges for meth treatment. The problem has grown to such a level in New York City that the gay community has developed Meth Anonymous support groups (New York State Office of Alcoholism and Substance Abuse Services 2004). Some authorities are also concerned about the spreading of HIV through the sharing of needles, which is common among injectors (Gibson et al. 2002).

- Rural residents who are interested in manufacturing meth for profit and personal use. Meth is particularly attractive in rural areas where farming and the economy are in decline (Wermuth 2000). North Carolina profiled the typical user as, "young, white, small-town residents with limited education and a blue-collar career" (North Carolina Division of Social Services and the Family and Children's Resource Program 2005). One study comparing rural with urban illegal substance use in Nebraska found that while meth use was present in urban Omaha, in rural areas meth use was more common (Herz 2000). One report found that rural and small town youth were more likely than their urban counterparts to become substance abusers (National Center on Addiction and Substance Abuse at Columbia University 2000). The same report found that rural eighth graders were 104 percent more likely than urban eighth graders to use amphetamines. This same group was 59 percent more likely to use methamphetamine than urban eighth graders.

- Heterosexuals drawn to sexual experimentation and sexual experiences who use the drug to alter their sexual pleasure (Wermuth 2000). Meth is known to lower sexual inhibitions, making it attractive to those interested in sexual activity and seduction.

- Youths and young adults involved with the rave subculture who mix meth with other substances for entertainment and excitement.

- Native Americans, including those living on reservations. Native American meth use is spreading across the reservations. In a special *Newsweek* report, journalist Andrew Murr (2004) found that it was becoming a "scourge" affecting Native Americans living on reservations. The SAMHSA (2005a) estimates the prevalence of meth use among American Indian and Alaska Native at about 1.7 percent. Freese et al. (2000) summarize the literature by noting that new approaches need to be designed to address the meth problem in Native American communities. They noted that Native American communities in Wyoming and Montana are moving forward in addressing the problem at the community level.

Evidence indicates that meth use has the potential to spread to other populations. Rawson and Anglin et al. wrote:

Meth use is expanding from a purely Caucasian, English-speaking clientele to Hispanic and Asian populations. Although the use of methamphetamine appears to be minimal among African Americans, increases among Hispanics and Asians suggest expansion of the methamphetamine problem to new markets. (Rawson and Anglin et al. 2002, p. 8)

Whether meth spreads to new ethnic and cultural groups remains to be seen. Some research has found that strong ethnic identification and segregation may offset some drug risks (Zickler 2005b). For example, meth use has not made serious inroads into the African American population. The Drug Abuse Warning Network (DAWN) is a public health surveillance system that monitors drug-related visits to hospital emergency departments (EDs) and drug-related deaths investigated by medical examiners and coroners. DAWN data reflect less popularity of meth use among African Americans than among whites and Hispanics (Wermuth 2000). This pattern may or may not hold steady over time.

What is apparent is that users come from a wide variety of backgrounds. As they continue to use and move on to heavy use, their outward appearances, lifestyle disruptions, thought patterns, and behaviors become more similar. They begin the race at different points and end at the same place, becoming more similar with each dose.

GENDER DIFFERENCES AND METH USE

Research has been conducted on gender and patterns of meth acquisition, initiation, use, motivation, problems, treatment, and manufacture. Before the 1980s, female use of any substance was viewed as dependent upon relationships with men. Females were either viewed as "good" citizens with addiction problems, or "bad" ones whose drug use mirrored their roles as deviants (Morgan and Joe 1996). Since the 1980s, increasing amounts of research has found that women have reasons for drug use outside of their relationships with men.

Today, researchers are exploring gender differences among male and female meth users. For example, Brecht et al. (2004) studied 350 people engaged in substance abuse treatment. They found gender differences in selected aspects of meth involvement. Some of the differences found were:

- Females were more likely than males to be introduced to meth and gain access through spouses or boyfriends than were males from girlfriends or spouses. Males were more likely to be introduced and gain access through friends and co-workers.
- Males were more likely to be injectors than were females.
- Males more likely to sell it than were females.
- Females were more likely to report skin and high-blood-pressure problems than were males.
- Females had longer first-time treatment episodes than males did.
- Male polydrug use included a wider variety of drugs than females reported.

Hser et al. (2005) also studied gender differences in meth users in a sample of treatment programs in California. In summary, Hser et al. (2005, p. 84) concluded, "Women in our sample, most of whom were of childbearing age or had children, demonstrated more severe problems than did men." They added, "Many were unemployed, relied on public assistance, and suffered from severe psychiatric problems." Hser et al. (2005) specifically found:

- Women reported meth use at an average earlier age (19.2 years) than males (20.6 years).
- Both genders used meth regularly for about the same number of years (8.7–8.8 years).
- Women reported significantly more numbers of prior treatments for drug use.
- The majority of women in the study had children under 18, but most did not live with their children within the last 30 days. Women were significantly more likely to be living with their children than were men. Though the findings were not statistically significant, more women than men had someone else taking care of their children through court order and had their parental rights terminated.

Research findings support gender differences regarding treatment needs. Hser et al. (2005) summarized the literature and concluded that females in treatment tend to have more psychological symptoms, lower self-esteem, heightened anxiety and depression, and higher rates of childhood sexual abuse than males. Women also had greater issues regarding employment, children, job skills, and incomes than males. Women have additional concerns if they are pregnant because of preliminary research suggesting negative effects of meth use on the fetus. Females are more concerned with child-rearing responsibilities, work, and the other seemingly overwhelming demands on their lives than males. This can affect their willingness to stop using a drug that they believe helps them get it all done. In contrast, males were more likely to be involved in criminal activities and be under criminal system supervision.

MEASURES OF THE EXTENT OF METH USE IN THE UNITED STATES

It is possible to get a sense of the extent of meth use and manufacture in the United States by looking at a number of national statistical indicators. While no measure captures everything, when a number of measures are viewed together, a sense for its use in the United States is possible. The following are some national indicators that give a sense of the extent of meth use, manufacture, and treatment.

A number of national efforts are made to track the extent of drug use, treatment, production, arrests, and other data. These data are useful in identifying trends. One of the most widely known is the Monitoring the Future Survey (MTF). This study is an annual national survey that assesses the beliefs, attitudes, and behaviors of high-school students in grades 8, 10, and 12 as well as young adults. The study does not include school dropouts, which could represent a high-risk group for meth use. The MTF study surveys about 50,000 subjects. Since 1999, meth has been included in the survey. Table 2.1 shows that meth use is not common among high-school-aged youths. The numbers are low, which is encouraging. However, before becoming too optimistic, one must realize that the usage reported is at least three years old and does not capture recent regional expansion of the drug. In addition, note that the percent of 12th graders indicated a decline in lifetime use from 1999 to 2005 from 8.2 percent to 4.5 percent, respectively.

Emergency Department Drug Mentions—Drug Abuse Warning Network (DAWN)

Drug-related emergency department (ED) mentions are provided by the SAMHSA through its Drug Abuse Warning Network (DAWN), which provides national information on morbidity and mortalities related to substance abuse, including meth, collected from short-stay medical and medical examiner offices across the United States. The DAWN study is an annual

Table 2.1
Percentage of Methamphetamine Use by Secondary School Students by Grade, 1999–2005

				Lifetime				
Grade	1999	2000	2001	2002	2003	2004	2005
8th	4.5%	4.2%	4.4%	3.5%	3.9%	2.5%	3.1%
10th	7.3	6.9	6.4	6.1	5.2	5.3	4.1
12th	8.2	7.9	6.9	6.7	6.2	6.2	4.5
				Annual				
Grade	1999	2000	2001	2002	2003	2004	2005
8th	3.2%	2.5%	2.8%	2.2%	2.5%	1.5%	1.8%
10th	4.6	4.0	3.7	6.1	3.3	3.0	2.9
12th	4.7	4.3	3.9	6.7	3.2	3.4	2.5
				Past 30 Days				
Grade	1999	2000	2001	2002	2003	2004	2005
8th	1.1%	0.8%	1.3%	1.1%	1.2%	0.6%	0.7%
10th	1.8	2.0	1.5	1.8	1.4	1.3	1.1
12th	1.7	1.9	1.5	1.7	1.7	1.4	0.9

Source: National Institute on Drug Abuse 2005.

Table 2.2
Number of Emergency Department Visits for Methamphetamine Mentions (Drug Abuse Warning Network), 1995–2003

				Year				
1995	1996	1997	1998	1999	2000	2001	2002	2003
15,933	11,002	17,154	11,486	10,447	13,505	14,923	17,696	25,039

Source: Substance Abuse and Mental Health Services Administration 2004.

survey of emergency department episodes from metropolitan areas. The DAWN data are useful in understanding meth and other substance abuse patterns. The DAWN data show that meth-related deaths and emergency department episodes have increased in many urban areas over recent years. For example, in 2003, according to the DAWN data, meth was involved in 25,039 emergency room visits (SAMHSA 2004). Table 2.2 shows DAWN data from 1995 to 2003. The data show that emergency department meth mentions have increased from 1995 to 2003 by 57.1 percent.

Treatment Episode Data Set (TEDS)

The Treatment Episode Data Set (TEDS), once labeled the Client Data System, collect data on clients admitted to substance abuse treatment programs. TEDS is an annual compilation of data on the demographic characteristics and substance abuse problems of those admitted for substance abuse treatment. In 1992–1993, with 42 states and the District of Columbia reporting, admissions due to meth abuse increased in 23 out of 29 reporting states for a net increase of 43 percent (Wermuth 2000). Meth was the primary substances of abuse in over 116,595 substance abuse treatment admissions in 2003 reported to TEDS (SAMHSA 2005). In comparison, the same TEDS data show that the number of meth admissions for 1993 was 20,776, which indicates that admissions increased by 461 percent over this 10-year span. The SAMHSA (2005) reported that from 1992 to 2002 the amphetamine and meth treatment admission rate in the United States increased from 10 to 52 per 100,000. In California, a state at the forefront of meth use and manufacture, publicly funded meth treatment increased 226 percent from 1992 to 1998 (Brecht 2001). The state of Washington treatment admissions increased more than 1,000 percent from 1992 to the first half of 1998 (Mills 1999). Nationally, this trend continued as reported admissions to publicly funded treatment for meth abuse grew from 12,122 in 1992 to 55,582 in 2002, representing more than a four-fold increase (Hser et al. 2005). This may be reflective of increased interest by meth addicts in getting treatment and/or of more court-ordered treatment.

SAMHSA's March 15, 2006, *DASIS Report* summarized that meth and amphetamine were identified in more than 136,000 cases as the primary substance of abuse in treatment admissions. This represented about 7 percent of all treatment admissions. The same report noted that between 1993 and 2003, the meth and/or amphetamine admission rate increased from 13 to 56 admissions per 100,000 population aged 12 or older. This represents a 330 percent increase over the period. The report also noted that 18 states had meth and/or amphetamine treatment rates that were higher than the national average of 56 per 100,000 population 12 or older. In addition, the report found that, "The proportion of primary methamphetamine/amphetamine admissions referred to treatment by the criminal justice system increased from 36 percent in 1993 to 51 percent in 2003." This later conclusion indicates that methamphetamine and amphetamine users are being ordered into treatment by the courts more frequently.

Reported Lifetime Use

Another way to measure substance use is to survey a sample of households. The National Household Survey on Drug Abuse (NHSDA) is an annual national survey of drug use by household. During the year 2000, the DEA found that 4 percent of the U.S. population reported trying meth at some time over their lifetime (SAMHSA 2001a). According to its 2004 survey, about 12 million people aged 12 and older reported they had used meth at least once in their lifetime. These people represent about 5.3 percent of the total population. The percents of reported use from the 2004 household survey broken down by age are shown in Table 2.3.

Quest Diagnostics Data

Quest Diagnostics, a private substance use testing firm, develops an index of use every six months as part of its substance testing operations. Quest conducted 7.1 million drug tests in 2003 and has been indexing the results of drug tests since 1988. Quest Diagnostics makes its index of positive results available on its Web site, www.questdiagnostics.com. The company reported major increases in the positive test results for amphetamines and meth. It recently reported:

Drug tests suggest that greater use of Meth among a large group of general U.S. workforce employees during 2003 may have caused the increase in amphetamines use overall. For this group of workers, the incidence of positive drug tests attributed to methamphetamine increased by more than 68% in 2003 from 2002, reaching 0.32% of all drug tests. During 2002, methamphetamine was 0.19%. (Quest Diagnostics 2004, p. 1)

For the period between January and June 2005, Quest Diagnostics data indicate that of the over 3 million general workforce members that took drug tests between January and June of 2005, .50 percent tested positive for amphetamine use, which includes meth (Quest Diagnostics 2005). This percent was slightly down from the 2004 tests.

Meth Arrests and Seizures

The Drug Enforcement Administration (DEA) tracks the number of drug seizures made each year by reporting law enforcement agencies. The number of seizures only reflects the general amount of drug trafficking known to law enforcement authorities. Law enforcement agencies vary in their effectiveness

Table 2.3
Percentage of Lifetime Methamphetamine Use among U.S. Population by Age Group, 2004

Age Group	Lifetime	Past Year	Past Month
12 and over	4.9%	0.6%	0.2%
12–17	1.2	0.6	0.2
18–25	5.2	1.6	0.6
26 and older	5.3	0.4	0.2

Source: Substance Abuse and Mental Health Services Administration 2005a.

and efficiency in seizing illegal drugs. Thus, these data tend to undercount the amount of true activity. Table 2.4 shows the DEA drug seizures for the United States from 1990 to September 2005. For this time span, the number of meth kilograms seized increased by 500 percent. In comparison, seizures for the illegal stimulant cocaine increased by 48.9 percent.

Arrestee Drug Abuse Monitoring Program (ADAM)

The Arrestee Drug Abuse Monitoring Program (ADAM), established in 1987 but no longer in existence, collected urine samples from arrestees in 42 jurisdictions across the United States. It was one of the few national efforts to collect verifiable data on actual drug use by urine specimens. ADAM data for adults are available from 1987 to 2003.

ADAM data from 1991 to 2001 indicate that western states had the highest concentration of positive tests for meth among adult arrestees (Yacoubian and Peters 2004). ADAM 2002 data reveal that the median percentage of adult male

Table 2.4
Drug Enforcement Administration Drug Seizures, 1990–September 2005

Calendar Year	Cocaine kgs.	Heroin kgs.	Marijuana kgs.	Methamphetamine kgs.	Hallucinogens Dosage Units
Sept. 2005	84,959	479	222,943	1,817.7	8,425,499
2004	117,622	672	264,714	1,647.5	2,483,663
2003	73,720	789	254,188	1,676.9	2,879,528
2002	61,594	705	195,644	1352.8	11,661,811
2001	59,426	752	271,785	1634.1	13,756,939
2000	58,627	546	331,964	1771.4	29,306,453
1999	36,167	351	337,832	1,488.8	1,716,954
1998	34,448	371	262,176	1,202.7	1,075,257
1997	28,630	399	215,348	1,143.2	1,100,912
1996	44,765	320	190,453	751.0	1,719,096
1995	45,326	876	219,830	875.1	2,768,165
1994	75,051	491	157,182	767.6	1,366,817
1993	55,158	616	143,030	559.8	2,710,063
1992	69,323	722	201,507	352.7	1,305,177
1991	67,016	1,170	98,601	289.6	1,295,874
1990	57,031	532	127,694	274.5	2,826,966

Source: Drug Enforcement Administration 2006.

arrestees that tested positive for meth use in 2002 was 5.3 percent. The highest proportions of arrestees testing positive for meth were in the West Coast, Southwest, and West Central regions. Honolulu led all ADAM reporting cities for the percentage of male arrestees (44.8 percent) in 2002 who tested positive for methamphetamine. Hawaii has a long history of crystal meth abuse.

Regionalization of Meth

Meth use and manufacture is not evenly distributed across the United States. For years meth use and production was concentrated in Hawaii, California, and the western United States. Across the border, Mexico is a country noted for meth production, with targeted sales in the United States. Motorcycle gangs often operated clandestine labs in California and western states and for years held advantage in production. Meth use in other regions, while occurring, remained relatively rare. This regionalization of meth is rapidly changing as the drug is creeping across the United States. For example, midwestern states, such as Missouri, are now major areas of meth production.

In recent years, production has been spreading to other regions of the country. Some states have passed laws that have slowed this progression down but not halted it entirely. There are several reasons why this is occurring. The popularity of the drug, tightening of the borders due to the war on drugs, and the Internet are among the possibilities. The Internet has probably played a critical role in the spread of the manufacture of the drug because of the easily accessible Web site recipes for its manufacture. Virtually anyone who has access to common household chemicals can find a recipe for cooking meth within a few minutes of searching the Internet. The ability to produce small batches of the drug at home has made users throughout the country less dependent on western or Mexican sources of the drug. The trend continues that most users buy the drug rather than manufacture it for personal use.

Map 2.1 displays three maps that show the percentage of agencies in each state for the years 2003–2005 reporting meth as their greatest threat, broken down by year. States with 0–24.9 percent of agencies reporting meth as the greatest threat are shown in black; 25–49.9 percent in middle gray; 50–74.9 percent in light gray; and 75–100 percent in dark gray. According to the Drug Enforcement Administration (2006), in 2003, black states were Connecticut, Delaware, Florida, Illinois, Louisiana, Maine, Maryland, Massachusetts, Michigan, New Hampshire, New Jersey, New York, North and South Carolina, Ohio, Pennsylvania, Rhode Island, Vermont, Virginia, West Virginia, and Wisconsin. Middle gray states were Alabama, Alaska, Georgia, Indiana, Kentucky, Mississippi, and Texas. Light gray states were Arkansas, Colorado, Missouri, New Mexico, and Tennessee. The dark gray states of Arizona, California, Hawaii, Idaho, Iowa, Kansas, Minnesota, Montana, Nebraska, Nevada, North and South Dakota, Oklahoma, Oregon, Utah, Washington, and Wyoming reported meth as their greatest threat. In 2004, West Virginia changed from black to middle gray; Georgia changed from middle gray to light gray; and Arkansas changed from light gray to dark gray. In 2005, Tennessee changed from light gray to middle gray; Louisiana changed from black to middle gray; Alabama, Alaska, and Indiana changed from middle gray to light gray; and New Mexico and Colorado changed from light gray to dark gray. The maps show that meth is marching from the West to the East and South. It has not made serious inroads in the Northeast.

Clandestine Labs Identification

Karen P. Tandy, administrator for the Drug Enforcement Administration, testified before a congressional hearing that meth was "most frequently produced clandestinely in the United States" (Tandy 2004). These labs can be anywhere. Missouri often shows up as a state with numerous meth labs. It is ideal because of its central location and rural landscape that helps cooks hide their labs from officials. Leinwand (2003) reported, "In fiscal 2002, local police and U.S. agents shut down 1,039 labs in Missouri, 321 in Illinois, 89 in Florida, and 85 in Georgia." She added for comparison, "Seven years earlier, officials had reported finding 29 labs in Missouri and two each in Illinois, Florida, and Georgia." Other states have reported similar experiences:

- California reported 1,262 meth lab busts from Sept. 30, 2002, to Sept. 30, 2003, more than double the number from seven years earlier (Leinwand 2003).
- The number of DEA meth lab seizures rose from 8,000 in 1999 to 10,000 in 2003
- The DEA reported breaking up more than 16,203 clandestine labs in 2002 and 2003 (Ray 2004).
- The Hazardous Substances Emergency Events Surveillance (HSEES) system reported that meth-related health events increased from 184 in June 2000 to 320

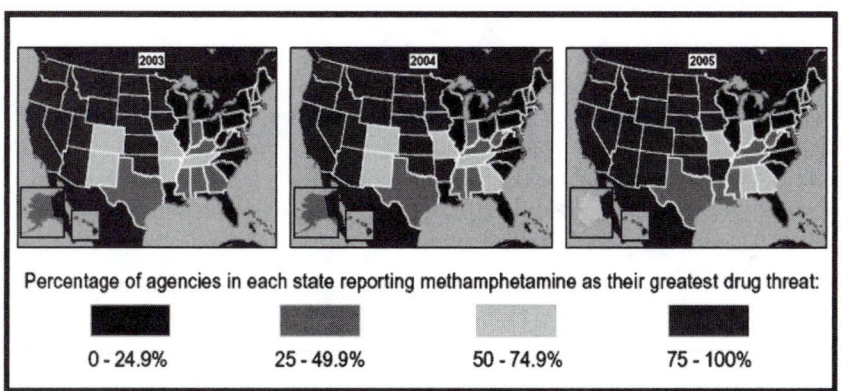

Map Showing Methamphetamine Threat Progression, 2003–2005
Courtesy Drug Enforcement Administration, 2006.

in June 2004. The system reported a total of 1,791 events in 16 states that use the reporting system in 2004. These events resulted in 960 injuries (E. Edwards 2005).

The number of lab seizures may undercount the true extent of the lab problem. As states have passed restrictions on the purchase of precursors, illegal meth labs have become "fractured." Fractured means the production process and acquisition of precursors is spread out over larger geographical areas to avoid detection by authorities. For example, with fracturing, cooks buy precursors from different stores in different towns to avoid detection from law enforcement.

PREVENTION EFFORTS TO CONTROL THE SPREAD OF METH

Prevention is an important component of any community response to meth use and manufacture. Many of the Web sites, such as www.methresources.gov, www.mappsd.org, stopmeth.org, www.preventionpathways.samhsa.gov, and www.modelprograms.samhsa.gov, and documents referenced throughout this volume provide prevention brochures, ads, video clips, fact sheets, literature, strategies, links, and materials. Some Web sites, such as www.justthinktwice.com and www.montanameth.org, provide prevention materials geared toward youth. The Montana Meth Project (www.montanameth.org) has films, posters, radio clips, and other excellent prevention resources. SAMHSA can provide prevention documents and materials to any community wanting to prevent meth use. States such as California, Hawaii, Illinois, Indiana, Iowa, Kansas, Michigan, Missouri, Montana, New York, Oregon, South Dakota, Tennessee, and others have launched meth prevention efforts. These are summarized in Chapter VII of the SAMHSA-funded (Center for Substance Abuse Prevention/National Prevention Network, 2006) *Methamphetamine: A Resource Kit.*

In addition, the Methamphetamine Interagency Task Force (2000, 2000a) made specific prevention recommendations that are worth noting:

- Address meth issues through broad-based drug prevention and education efforts that target all forms of drug use and that are based on research and established prevention principles.
- Develop science-based prevention program planning and intervention guidelines in communities where meth is already a problem.
- Involve the entire community in prevention efforts, including educators, youths, parents, vendors of materials used in meth manufacture, law enforcement officials, business leaders, members of the faith community, social services providers, and representatives of government agencies and organizations.
- Identify the changing population characteristics of users, their motivations, risk factors, and demographics.

- Involve parents and other adults in prevention and education programs for youths, particularly in the areas on monitoring for "latchkey" children, enhancing parent-child communication skills, and providing consistent family/home rules for youth behavior and leisure time activities.

- Ensure that media campaigns proceed with caution, focusing on raising awareness of meth and using messages designed to minimize unintended effects, such as arousing curiosity about meth.

- Develop or augment programs aimed at educating those communities in which meth is an emerging or chronic problem.

In an effort to prevent manufacturing of meth, lawmakers in several states and Congress have been active in taking precursors and drugs such as pseudoephedrine off of store shelves and restricting access to them. Law enforcement agencies in some jurisdictions have worked with local merchants to monitor suspicious or high-quantity sales of over-the-counter medicines (those containing pseudoephedrine) and chemicals (including fertilizer) that might be used for the purpose of manufacturing meth.

The Comprehensive Methamphetamine Control Act of 1996 identified selected chemicals, such as iodine, as List II chemicals. Using iodine as an example, the Drug Enforcement Administration (DEA) requires that detailed records be maintained for sales of iodine crystals that exceed the threshold of 0.4 kilogram (about 14 ounces) of iodine crystals to anyone or any entity. The Act also requires that distributors and retailers report any suspicious activities to the DEA. Section 21 U.S.C. 841 § (c) (1)-(3) prohibits any person from knowingly possessing or distributing a listed chemical with the intent, knowledge, or belief that the chemical will be used to manufacture a controlled substance, such as meth. Section 21 U.S.C. 843 § (a)-(7) prohibits the individual from knowingly or intentionally manufacturing, distributing, exporting, or importing any equipment, chemical, or material that may be used to manufacture a controlled substance or listed chemical. Penalties for conviction for each violation are 10 years of imprisonment, a $250,000 fine, or both, and they double with a second or subsequent convictions. States have passed laws to stiffen the penalties. For example, in North Carolina, individuals possessing ingredients in quantities sufficient to make the drug can be punished with up to five years in prison if prosecutors can prove intent to manufacture meth (Eisley 2004).

Some states have passed laws that hold store owners accountable for large quantity sales of precursors (ingredients) used to make meth. States that have passed legislation that restricts the sales of precursors are Arkansas, Georgia, Iowa, Illinois, Kentucky, Mississippi, Oklahoma, Oregon, South Dakota, Tennessee, West Virginia, and Wyoming. There are a number of states that have passed laws that restrict the sale of precursors used to manufacture meth:

- Iowa passed legislation that restricts access to over-the-counter cold medicines that can be used to cook meth.

- California, a state with some of the earliest laws restricting the sale of precursors needed to produce meth, believes that it has had positive effects in controlling the spread of meth. After it enacted laws limiting the sale of key chemicals, such as ephedrine and pseudoephedrine, lab busts were cut in half, from 2,090 in 1999 to 1,130 in 2002 (Lacour and Gregory 2004). California also has strict regulations regarding the sale of iodine crystals. California Code (11107.1) requires all sales to be recorded, limits the quantity, and has other limits.
- Oklahoma passed legislation that requires that pseudoephedrine be kept behind the counter.
- In April 2004, the Food and Drug Administration (FDA) banned drugs containing the stimulant ephedrine. In 2005, a Utah Federal Court limited the scope of a Food and Drug Administration rule banning the sale of all ephedrine-alkaloid dietary supplements. The judge ordered the FDA to develop rules for the legal distribution of the drug.

Short of passing restrictions, other efforts have been made to control the distribution of precursors. For example, Illinois issues bulletins to farmers and fertilizer sellers encouraging them to protect their supplies of anhydrous ammonia. In addition, as part of this anti-meth campaign, some farmers and supplies have secured their anhydrous ammonia storage tanks (known in some meth circles as "white buffalos") with fences, motion detectors, and locks.

CLOSING OBSERVATIONS

Meth accounts for a small percent of the total number of people affected by drug and alcohol problems. However, almost all of the data in this chapter reveal that meth use, manufacturing, and distribution are increasing throughout much of the nation. Some have likened the spread of meth to an epidemic in some regions of the country (Anglin and Kalechstein et al. 1997). It is clear that meth has impacted the West, Southwest, and Midwest and is beginning to expand into the Northeast. How extensive this expansion will be is unknown. The other question is whether meth use will grow in prevalence in minority populations. To date Latino, Hispanic, and African American populations have not embraced meth to the extent that Anglos have. If this changes, its negative effects could be substantial. Whether the upward spiral of meth use and manufacture continues remains to be seen. How communities, service agencies, law enforcement, families, elected officials, treatment providers, the courts, and businesses respond to the challenge will influence how, and even whether, this trend can be reversed.

PART II

The Human Side of Clandestine Methamphetamine Labs and Health Risks of Exposure

The chapters in part II address the human side of methamphetamine labs and those impacted by them. Meth, unlike many other drugs, can easily be manufactured by using mixtures of household products. Many of the products and by-products of cooking meth are toxic, explosive, corrosive, and pose serious health hazards to those exposed. Often children and others are exposed to these harmful substances.

Lynn Riemer's chapter 3 presents information on meth lab identification and the signs that meth is being cooked. The chapter guides the reader through the manufacturing processes. Makeshift labs have been found inside automobiles, trucks, homes, motel rooms, barns, trailers, and roadside rest areas. Some of these labs are highly mobile; some can fit easily into a suitcase or duffle bag. This chapter identifies signs that indicate the cooking of meth. This is important information for anyone whose work requires that they visit homes, are first responders, or otherwise have contact with individuals possibly involved with manufacturing the drug.

This chapter also covers the chemical dangers of such production to all who come into contact with the lab environment. Meth labs, as this chapter reveals, need to be taken seriously as a highly dangerous situation posing life-endangering risks to children, staff, and families. This includes child protection workers, law enforcement officers, public health officers, neighbors, family members, and children.

Experts agree that exposure to meth labs and use of meth are unhealthy for children, newborns, and adults. Dr. Wells' chapter 4 focuses on what we know about the short- and long-term medical effects of exposure to or use of meth.

How does meth affect the body and its functioning? This chapter highlights some of the health hazards of meth use for the user and those around them. It focuses on the research on the effects of meth use on children and fetuses. Because meth addicts use other drugs that are known to contribute to birth defects, such as alcohol and cigarettes, and practice poor nutritional habits, researchers have found it difficult to determine the effects of meth on fetuses. However, according to the Director of NIDA, Dr. Nora Volkow (2005), in her testimony to Congress, the few studies that exist suggest that meth use during pregnancy results in premature delivery, early separation of the placenta from the wall of the uterus, stunted fetal growth, and brain and heart abnormalities.

The illegal manufacture of meth is hazardous and environmentally destructive. The manufacture of meth creates considerable amounts of toxic waste, such as acid vapors, heavy metals, solvents, and other harmful materials that can be absorbed by the body. The Drug Enforcement Administration's (2004a) *FACT Sheet* estimated that one pound of meth generated six pounds of waste. In addition, some of the ingredients are highly explosive and pose a serious fire hazard. Manufacturers of the drug call the bags containing the waste from the processes "death bags" for a good reason: They can kill or disable anyone breathing sufficient fumes from them.

Meth labs are very expensive to clean up. In 2002, the Drug Enforcement Administration estimated that the average cleanup cost was about $3,300 and by 2005 had dropped to $2,000 (Rannazzisi 2005). Large-scale labs cost considerably more to clean up. Toxic chemicals used to produce meth often are dumped in rivers, fields, lakes, and forests, causing environmental damage that results in high cleanup costs. For example, DEA's annual cost for the clean up of clandestine laboratories (almost entirely meth laboratories) in the United States has increased steadily from fiscal year 1995 ($2 million), to fiscal year 1999 ($12.2 million), to fiscal year 2002 ($23.8 million). Moreover, the Los Angeles County Regional Criminal Information Clearinghouse, a component of the Los Angeles High-Intensity Drug Trafficking Area (HIDTA), reports that in 2002 lab cleanup costs in the combined Central Valley and Los Angeles HIDTA areas alone reached $3,909,809. Statewide, California spent $4,974,517 to remediate meth laboratories and dump sites in 2002 (National Drug Intelligence Center 2004, p. 1). California's experiences are mirrored in other states. For example North Carolina's estimated typical cleanup costs for a meth lab are between $4,000 and $10,000 (North Carolina Department of Justice 2004).

Meth labs also pose a serious threat to the general public and the community. When they are done, it is common for cooks to dump the dangerous by-products in drains, streams, public facilities, roadsides, and other convenient locations, placing others at risk of serious harm. Because clothing and other articles are so easily contaminated by meth production, toxins can quickly spread from one place to another, requiring involved cleanup. Meth cooks often discard dangerous chemicals in public and in appropriate locations. Meth cooks will dispose of dangerous lab waste by dumping it in public trash containers, burning it, dumping it in streams, fields, and down toilets, or simply leaving it behind in hotels, on roadsides, and in other public areas. One Colorado highway worker was seriously injured and hospitalized after he opened a seemingly innocent trash bag at a roadside rest area. He accidentally inhaled phosgene gas from a disposed "death bag" and is lucky to have survived.

It is also true that meth labs are typically messy for reasons other than production. Meth cooks do not maintain or care about having clean homes or living quarters. Clutter, trash, and filth, are all common to lab sites. This is because addicts and cooks are focused primarily on production of the drug, not cleanliness. This has important implications for caseworkers and the children they are trying to protect, as well as the families under investigation. There are a number of health hazards, such as disposed needles that can carry hepatitis or other biohazards, that might be present in the household. Caseworkers and other first responders need to exercise caution because of risk of injury and serious health problems. For example, the Hazardous Substance Emergency Events Surveillance (HSEES) system reported that meth-related events increased from 184 in June 2000 to 320 in June 2004. In 2004, 1,791 events occurred in 16 states that use the HSEES system, resulting in 960 personal injuries. First responders, such as police and fire department staff, were the most often injured, according to the Centers for Disease Control (Centers for Disease Control 2000, 2005). Caseworkers and social workers have also been harmed and need to be aware of the risks they encounter and how they may accidentally expose others, such as family members and coworkers, to these risks.

Once a lab has been identified and ceases to operate, agencies and property owners need to be involved in the cleanup of the location. Meth cooks use ingredients such as lithium, ammonia, fertilizer, toluene, solvents, muriatic acid, and meth that can have devastating affects on ground water, soil, dwellings, and the environment. Cleaning up a lab in a home can result in noninvolved residents, such as grandparents and children, needing to vacate the property. Cleanup can take weeks to months, resulting in homelessness.

Chapter 5 describes the Colorado meth lab cleanup procedures and standards. The state of Colorado passed legislation that required standards for lab cleanup to be established by the state health department and implemented by local health departments. The chapter provides an example of how one state has addressed the issue of lab cleanup. Without adequate cleanup, people may unknowingly come into contact with highly toxic environments long after the lab has operated.

Some political jurisdictions have passed laws or ordinances that require sellers of property (homes) to disclose whether or not the property was ever a site used to cook meth. Some states require that home sellers provide written disclosers of all known structural problems to the purchaser. This would include the previous presence of a lab. Indiana passed a law to control environmental pollution that made it a felony to dump waste from the manufacture of controlled substances, including meth.

CHAPTER 3

Methamphetamine Production—Lab Identification and the Dangers of Making Methamphetamine to Families, Children, and Professionals

Lynn Riemer, BS

Methamphetamine is more than just a drug; it is hazardous chemicals, toxic gases, deadly vapors, paranoid behavior, and violence. Meth labs are dangerous to human health and well-being. Recognizing that you may be in this type of environment may save your life. This chapter will address awareness and recognition of chemical hazards associated with manufacturing methamphetamine, the dangers associated with those who come in contact with this toxic environment, and what to do if you find yourself in a lab.

Being aware and looking for the signs that indicate you may be in a meth lab are much easier than most think. It is important to think outside the box when dealing with labs. Everything is not what it seems, and it's not so much what you find as where you find it. It's well known that you don't keep HEET (gas line cleaner for your car) or starting fluid (also for your car) in the baby's room or in the bathroom; Coleman fuel and acids are not kept in the refrigerator. When you put starting fluid in your carburetor, you don't open the can from the bottom. If you notice holes in the bottom of starting fluid cans, that's not normal. The ether may be being used in starting fluid to make meth. Pay attention to things that look out of place or unusual.

THINGS TO LOOK FOR—RECOGNITION AND PROCESS

Common household chemicals are used to manufacture meth, some of which are displayed in the following photo. Not one ingredient needed to manufacture meth is illegal. Ingredients can be bought at local grocery stores, hardware stores, farm feed stores, and on eBay. One of the major obstacles law enforcement faces in combating this problem is the Internet. You can find everything you need to know about manufacturing meth online; eBay sells all the essential ingredients for manufacturing meth including the nice "chemistry glassware," complete with instructions on how to set it up. Try typing "manufacturing methamphetamine" into a search engine and you will get over 125,000 hits. These sites contain thousands of recipes on how to "cook" (manufacture) meth. There is even a recipe on "How to Cook Meth with Bert and Ernie." It's not exactly right, but some would lead you to believe that Sesame Street is getting into the act.

There is also a recipe on how to reextract meth from one's urine (CSAlert 2005). It's very easy to do and produces a purer form of meth because your body has filtered out some of the by-products but also introduced biological hazards to the urine. It also requires gallons of urine from one or several people. According to CSAlert (2005, p. 1), "In general, 40% of the methamphetamine ingested is excreted unchanged." We often find yellow liquids in labs and now send samples for analysis to see if it's clean urine to pass a Urine Analysis (UA) test, or "dirty urine" they may be getting ready to extract.

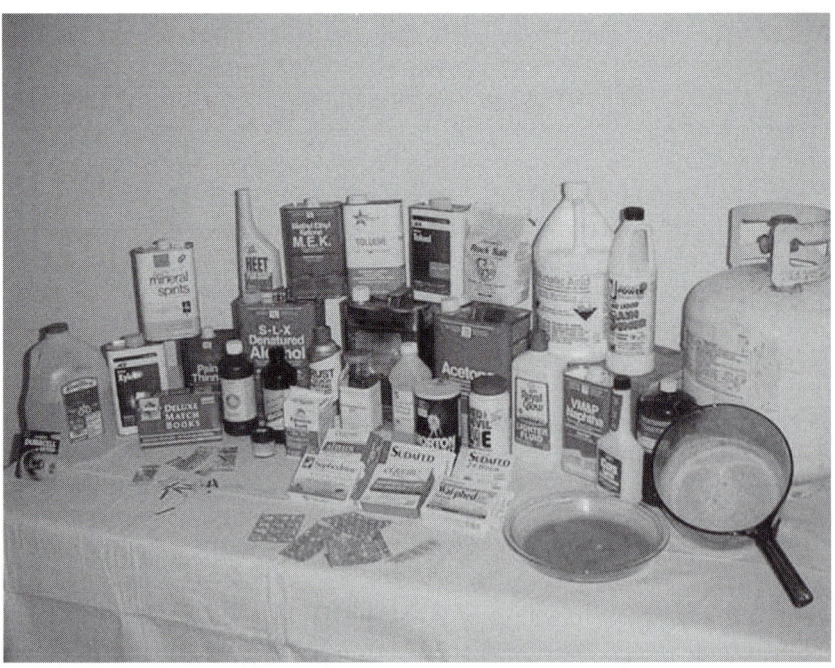

Common household items that could be used to produce methamphetamine. Photo courtesy of North Metro Task Force.

In some Web sites there is a "chat room" where meth cooks (manufacturers) share recipes and troubleshoot problems. You can set up as a first-time cooking process in the bathroom, or the kitchen or baby's room, get into a chat room, and type your question: "I just added this, this, and this and it turned green. What do I do?" A meth cook will respond almost immediately, telling you to add this, and when it turns yellow, to get back to them. Basically you can have a cook (meth manufacturer) and personal advisor at your fingertips to help you throughout the whole process. Beware: Not all cooks know what they are doing.

LAB EQUIPMENT TO LOOK FOR

The glassware used to manufacture meth ranges from the nice, expensive scientific glassware to mason jars or pickle buckets. (See the following photo for examples of glassware used to produce methamphetamine.) Anything that holds heat and pressure will work. Coffee pots and Visions brand name cookware are very popular among meth cooks because they can handle heat and pressure. One recipe on the Internet suggests, "Just use a coke bottle or champagne bottle and put some tubing in it." For separating liquids a separatory funnel is ideal (a separatory funnel is used to separate liquids of different densities); however, they are costly, so tea jars with spigots, turkey basters, and sport drink bottles are used instead. The cooks use these containers with spigots to drain off what they do and don't want. A large variety of jars and drink bottle are also found.

Tubing coming out of anything should be a strong indicator something isn't right—tubing coming out of red gasoline containers, plastic bottles, or kitty litter is not normal. Coffee grinders with red, blue, yellow, or orange powders should get your attention—coffee is brown. Discolored coffee filters are also important when it comes to recognizing meth labs. We all know what coffee filters should look like—they are not blue, pink, yellow with red powder, or green. The color of the coffee filter is indicative of the color of the cold tablet they are extracting. Multicolored and layered liquids are another indicator that you may be in a lab. Cooks will hide all chemicals and glassware but leave multicolored and layered liquids on counters, tables, in the baby's room, in the bathroom, and in the bedroom. If you notice two-layered liquids that are blue on top and clear or reddish on the bottom, that is not Italian salad dressing, but possibly liquids being made into meth. The following photo shows examples of multicolored and layered liquids being used to make meth.

WAYS TO COOK METH

Only three ingredients are needed to manufacture meth; all the other chemicals are used to convert it into a usable form (Colorado Regional Community Policing Institute and Rocky Mountain High-Intensity Drug Trafficking

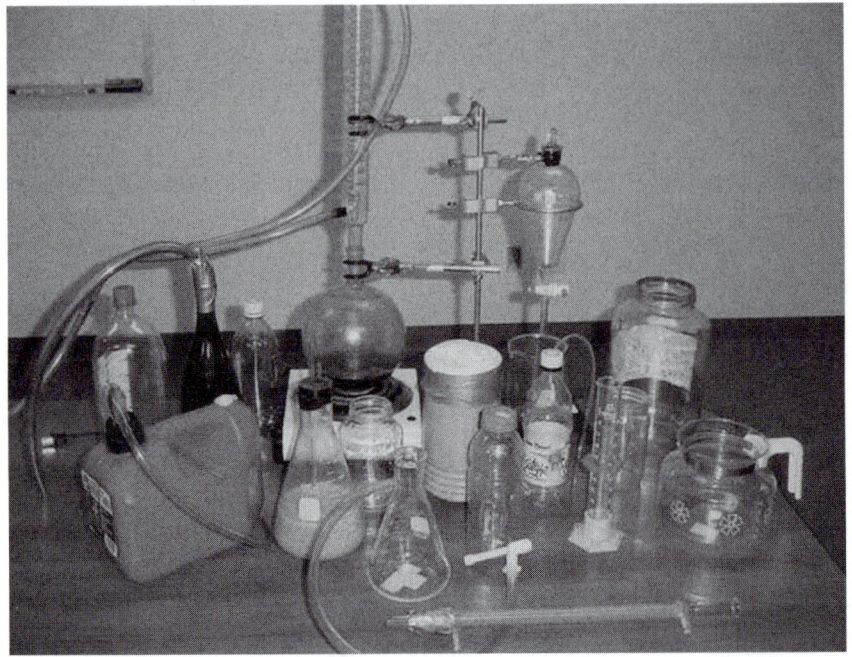

Examples of glassware used to produce methamphetamine. Photo courtesy of North Metro Task Force.

Area 2003; Department of Justice 2003). Most of us have a number of these chemicals in our homes. It is very easy to make meth; if you can make oatmeal cookies or macaroni and cheese, you can make meth. It requires solvents (i.e., Coleman fuel, toluene, lighter fluid, paint thinner, mineral spirits, starting fluid), acids, drain cleaners, ammonia, camera batteries, cold tablets, matches, salt, hydrogen peroxide, and iodine. These chemicals are safe when used as directed; however, meth cooks are not using them for their intended purpose. For example, if you are in a house with clogged toilets, yet you notice a case of Red Devil lye (drain opener) or other drain-opening chemicals, you may be in a lab. Let's take a closer look at the chemicals and process involved.

Most of the labs we find are for personal use and small-quantity distribution only. They are not "super labs" producing large quantities for distribution. The most common method used today is known as the ephedrine or pseudo-ephedrine reduction method, meaning the removal of one oxygen molecule off of the ephedrine or pseudoephedrine molecule. This process is much faster and produces a higher quality of meth than the phenyl-2-propanone or the P2P method. The number one ingredient necessary for manufacturing meth is ephedrine or pseudoephedrine. For the basis of this subject, without going into great depth of chemistry and isomers, ephedrine and pseudoephedrine

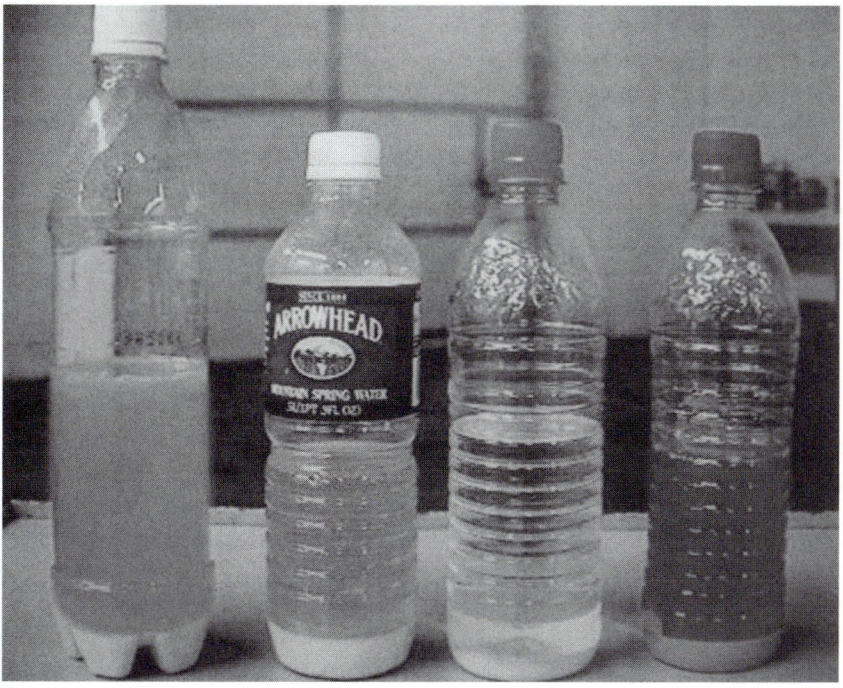

Examples of layered liquids. Photo courtesy of North Metro Task Force.

are considered identical. Pseudoephedrine is the precursor, defined as a raw material that becomes part of the finished product through a chemical reaction. Without it, meth cannot be manufactured.

The first step is the "pill pull," separating the pseudoephedrine from the binders, cellulose, and other substances in the cold tablets. This is done by crushing the cold tablets and soaking them in a water-soluble solvent. HEET gas-line cleaner is most common; however, alcohols, acetone, and water can be used. The pseudoephedrine dissolves in the liquid, leaving the binders and other material from the tablet on the bottom (note: a two-layered liquid). The liquid is filtered off, the binders, cellulose, and other materials are tossed, the liquid is evaporated, and the remaining powder is the pseudoephedrine. The pseudoephedrine is scraped out and put into scientific glassware, a coffee pot, or anything that will hold heat and pressure. Adding iodine, red phosphorus, and a little water to the pseudoephedrine, known as the Red P method, creates a violent reaction that removes the oxygen molecule from pseudoephedrine. Thus, we have meth in its acidic form; we then need to take three additional steps to convert it into a usable form.

The other method of ephedrine reduction is known as the ammonia method, "Nazi" method, or Birch method. This process requires the addition of anhydrous ammonia and lithium or sodium metal to the pseudoephedrine. Hitler did not invent this method; it is known as the "Nazi" method because the first lab found using this process had swastikas on the walls and Nazi paraphernalia throughout the lab. You need just three ingredients to manufacture meth by either method, then multiple chemicals to convert it into a usable form.

CHEMICAL HAZARDS

The chemicals found in labs are safe when used as directed; however, meth cooks are not using them for their intended purpose. Iodine is the world's oldest antiseptic, but the liquid used to disinfect cuts and wounds is a tincture and not pure iodine crystals. Iodine crystals are one of the three essential ingredients used in the manufacturing process. The problem with iodine crystals is that they will sublime, meaning they will go from a solid state into a vapor in no time. A yellow cloud of iodine can do severe damage. Iodine is immediately dangerous to life and health (IDLH) at 2 parts per million (ppm), which converts into .0002 percent in air. Approximately one square inch on a football field can kill you. Just to give you an idea about iodine's toxicity, sarin gas (nerve gas) has an IDLH of 3.5 to 5 parts per million. In vapor form iodine is more toxic than sarin gas, and we find pounds of iodine crystals in labs all the time (Keep in mind that iodine is an essential nutrient in our diet).

If you don't have the iodine crystals needed, you can make them. Take tincture of iodine, hydrogen peroxide, and a small amount of any acid and the crystals will fall out of the tincture of iodine and can be filtered out. The problem with this process is the "waste" solution generated from the mixture. Tincture of iodine has alcohol in it. If you mix alcohol with a peroxide and acid, you get peroxide salts, which are explosive. If the "waste" solution evaporates and thickens to the consistency of honey and you agitate it, it will explode. Cooks are generating explosive hazardous waste just to obtain the drug they crave. Iodine crystals do have legitimate uses; they are used for water treatment and to kill "foot rot" disease in cattle. However, veterinarians tell us that newer, more effective medicines are available to deal with this disease.

The only good thing about iodine is that it leaves a yellow stain, a footprint that it has been around. Yellow-stained walls, floors, paper, counters, coffee filters, and gloves can all be signs that iodine is present. Indication of iodine staining can be tested with spray starch. When sprayed, if the stain turns purple, we know it is iodine.

Red phosphorus is most often obtained from the striker plates on matchbooks, although you can also buy chemical grade red phosphorus on eBay or from a chemical supply company. The striker plate on the matchbook can be dipped in an alcohol or acetone, loosening the glue, and the phosphorus scraped off. This takes quite a while to accomplish, and a very large number of striker plates are needed to obtain enough phosphorus to manufacture meth.

This is also very dangerous in that you are dipping the phosphorus in a flammable solvent and then scraping it. If the scraping of phosphorus creates a spark, the matchbook soaked in a flammable solvent can easily catch fire. The alternative is to cut off the striker plates, soak them in a jar of alcohol until the red phosphorus falls to the bottom, take out the striker paper, filter off the liquid, and keep the red powder to process the meth. Either method of removing the phosphorus off the striker plate is hazardous. If you don't want to deal with striker plates, you can use hypophosphorous acid (known on the streets as Hypo or water) as your source of phosphorus. Hypophosphorous acid is a colorless, oily liquid with a sour smell and is on the Drug Enforcement Administration (DEA) chemical watch list. Because it is regulated it is not as easy to obtain as cases of matches. Hypophosphorous acid is a strong acid and a powerful reducing agent used in chemical synthesis. Lately meth cooks have been putting their "HYPO" in baby bottles in the refrigerator and taping the tops. The tops are taped to keep dangerous fluids and gases from escaping from the tops of the bottles.

The biggest problem with either source of phosphorus is the generation of phosphine gas, which is colorless, odorless, and deadly. Phosphine gas is a severe pulmonary irritant, which means that it harms the lungs and respiratory system. Any time you heat phosphorus, whether it is red phosphorus or hypophosphorous acid, you generate phosphine gas. This occurs during a number of stages of the cooking process. Phosphine gas is immediately dangerous to life and health (IDLH) at 50 parts per million (ppm). Cyanide gas is also toxic at 50 parts per million; therefore, phosphine is as toxic as cyanide. The only difference between the two is that cyanide has an almond odor and phosphine is odorless. During the cooking process, gases are vented off in the initial reaction (mixing of the three essential ingredients) into a container of kitty litter, also known as a "death bag." This is used to collect the phosphine gas and hydriodic gas. Phosphine is a very small particulate and remains inert in the kitty litter as long as it in not agitated. Once you shake up the kitty litter, phosphine can become airborne. This is why those doing an initial assessment of a meth lab wear self-contained breathing apparatuses (SCBA); no filters are made that can block out phosphine gas. Another problem with heating red phosphorus is that when overcooked, it can turn into yellow and then white phosphorus. White phosphorus is pyrophoric, meaning it can explode with the introduction of air. This creates a whole new problem when it comes time to deal with an actively cooking lab.

A large number of acids and bases are found in these labs: Sulfuric acid (drain opener), muriatic acid (cement or brick cleaner), and hypophosphorous acid (metal etcher) are most common. Phosphoric acid, hydriodic acid, and chemical grade hydrochloric acid are found as well. The most common base found in these labs is Red Devil lye (drain cleaner), also known as sodium hydroxide. The problem with acids is they can cause burns to the mucous membranes (eyes, nose, and throat) as well as to the skin. If you spill acid on your skin you know it immediately, because your skin starts to burn and you can wash it off and get the burn treated. The toxic vapors off the acids can cause severe burning to the respiratory tract and lungs, possibly even death through respiratory failure at high levels of exposure.

In contrast, if you get a base (caustic) burn, it is a deeper tissue burn attacking the fat in your tissue and thus making your skin feel soapy or slimy (saponification). It is much harder to wash off and causes a much deeper burn. The most dangerous acid found in these labs is hydrofluoric acid, a glass etcher. If you spill this acid on your skin it will attack the calcium in your bones; it is not easily washed off, and unless immediately treated with an antidote, the only way to stop it is amputation. It comes in a plastic bottle with a teal colored top and can be bought at hobby stores. It has been seen a number of times in labs the Denver Narcotics team has processed, however is not commonly seen.

Generating hydrogen chloride gas is an essential part of manufacturing meth. Meth to be absorbed by our bodies needs to be in its salt form, its hydrochloride form—methamphetamine hydrochloride. Our bodies are made mostly of water, and salts dissolve in water; therefore meth needs to be in its salt form for our bodies to process it. The easiest way to do this is mix salt and sulfuric acid together in what is known as a gas generator. A gas generator is a red gasoline can with tubing coming out of it, or just a water or soda bottle with tubing coming out of it. Pouring in the salt and some sulfuric acid immediately causes hydrogen chloride gas to be generated. Hydrogen chloride gas in water is hydrochloric acid (muriatic acid).

There are a number of problems with this. One, there is no recipe for generating the gas—it's not one teaspoon of salt to one cup of acid. Cooks just pour in salt and then pour in acid. Gas generation doesn't stop until all of the salt and acid react. The meth can fall out of the solution, yet the hydrogen chloride gas will continue to generate. Sometimes meth cooks they will put the gas generator in the refrigerator or freezer thinking if they cool it down it will stop, but it doesn't—it just contaminates any food that may be in there. Another problem is that acid gases react with metals. The air-monitoring equipment taken into labs to get air readings to help determine how to deal with the environment can become damaged or ruined in a high acid vapor environment.

The biggest problem with a high acid vapor environment is the fact that these vapors have to go somewhere; the furniture, carpet, clothes, or drywall absorbs them. For example, in one case a deputy went into a house on a domestic violence call, then realized he was in a lab and got the people outside. On the way out one law enforcement officer brushing up against the couch within fifteen minutes had a large chemical blister oozing on his arm. In another example, task force detectives patted suspects down and handcuffed them only to have the skin on the palms of their hands start peeling off within a few minutes.

If you go into a lab with a high acid gas vapor dressed, dressed in normal clothes, those vapors can get on your skin. If you go outside and get a wet wipe or wet washrag and start wiping down your hands or face, you can convert the vapors on your skin into hydrochloric acid and you can get severely burned. Large amounts of water are needed when dealing with a high acid vapor environment; this is one of the reasons everyone that is found living in a lab must be decontaminated. Child protection workers and other professionals face the same hazards and must be careful if they accidentally are exposed to a meth lab. They will need to decontaminate themselves or run the risk of spreading dangerous acids and bases (chemicals), iodine, solvents, and meth contamination to their families, friends, coworkers, and others.

Solvents such as Coleman fuel, toluene, lighter fluid, HEET, acetone, methanol, ethyl ether, and alcohols are needed during various stages of manufacturing meth. All solvents are neurologic toxins. The first solvent extraction, the "pill pull," is a very dangerous process, because heat is applied to evaporate off a flammable liquid, thus causing the potential for fires and explosions. The same is true for the extraction of red phosphorus off the matchbook strikers.

A well-publicized meth lab fire that killed two women happened because they spilled some Coleman fuel on the floor in the basement and dry-mopped it. They created a larger surface area of the spill by using a dry mop. Most solvent vapors are heavier than air so they travel low, close to the floor. The pilot light on the basement water heater did not have a cover, and vapors found the flame of the pilot light. A wall of fire prevented the women from getting out. Two males were downstairs with them at the time and ran through the wall of fire to escape. The women retreated to a cubbyhole to wait for help and died of smoke inhalation.

A source of heat or flame is not necessary to cause a fire or explosion. Two days before the lab fire that killed the two women, there was another house fire in Denver. A meth lab was set up in a bathroom. No death bag was attached to the reaction, so phosphine gas, which is explosive, was filling the room. There were also some open containers of solvents off-gassing in the bathroom. The meth cooks closed the bathroom door and left. When they came back, they opened the bathroom door to check on their batch of meth. Oxygen was introduced into the bathroom, and the room, a high vapor content environment, exploded and caught fire. They received severe burns, and significant damage to the building occurred.

The use of lithium or sodium metal in the production of meth has created a whole new problem for firefighters. Sodium and lithium metal are water reactive, meaning they create fire when mixed with water. On a very humid day the lithium or sodium metal can react with the moisture in the air, creating a very intense fire. When firefighters respond to a fire they used to think arson or accident; now they need to consider the possibility of a meth lab. If they respond to a meth lab using anhydrous ammonia and lithium metal that has caught fire, and put water on it, they could blow up the neighborhood, depending on how much exposed metal is present. Blocks of sodium metal can be purchased on eBay; however, we find lithium metal from lithium batteries, in particular AA or camera batteries, is most commonly used.

Anhydrous ammonia is a farm fertilizer being put into propane tanks, fire extinguishers, and coolers and stolen from co-ops and farms to make meth. Anhydrous ammonia reacts with the brass fittings on propane tanks, turning them a deep bluish purple and degrading the valve. If you come across one at a propane exchange, do not take it home and attempt to hook it up to your barbecue grill. These need to be treated as bombs; call the fire department or police immediately.

To be a liquid, anhydrous ammonia needs to be very cold, like liquid nitrogen. It is so toxic that it requires a hazardous material placard to be transported on the highways. Anhydrous means without water, so it's a very strong, concentrated form of ammonia. It will seek out moisture in your skin if you spill it on you, plus it's very cold so it will freeze-dry your skin. It can also do severe damage to your lungs if inhaled. Because our lungs have a very large surface area and are very moist, even the smallest amount can take your breath away. Anhydrous ammonia can cause severe irritation to your eyes, respiratory tract, and skin and is so potent that the tychem suits worn to process labs won't last more than 30 minutes in an anhydrous vapor.

Because anhydrous ammonia is so cold, when meth is made with it, a heavy thick frost, almost like snow, occurs on the outside of the container. This thick condensation on jars, buckets, or containers in a home, with or without an ammonia odor, may indicate the presence of a meth lab. Farmers are being hit hard by the theft of anhydrous ammonia. Some universities in the Midwest are looking at ways to reduce the use of this fertilizer in the manufacturing of meth. One has created a pink-colored dye, called GloTell, to help prevent the theft and use in meth production. GloTell will stain everything it comes in contact with—containers, hands, and clothes will be bright pink for about 48 hours.

RECOGNIZING THE SIGNS AND YOUR SAFETY

Recognizing the signs and chemicals used to manufacture illicit drugs is vital to your safety (Goin 2002). All of the aforementioned chemicals have legitimate uses; however, when it comes to manufacturing meth they become toxic hazardous waste, contaminating the lab surroundings and environment. Look for yellow staining on walls, floors, sinks, and any drains. Move pictures to see if the color is consistent. Check the smoke detectors in hotels. Pay attention to unusual odors, especially if your eyes, nose, and throat start burning or become irritated. Today's labs do not have a distinct odor like the P2P labs did; they do not smell like cat urine or have a fishy odor. Today's labs have a solvent or acrid smell from all the solvents used, very similar to the smell of a garage. They may contain plastic bags with items from such stores as Wal-Mart. There may be unusual glassware or chemicals, two-layered liquids, and tubing coming out of containers. The environment is probably filthy, with an unidentifiable odor.

When you are in an unknown home with some of these characteristics for any reason, it is recommended that you do not sit on furniture or the floor.

Needles are everywhere in drug homes, and often under sofa cushions. It is recommended that if you do make home visits you make up a personal decontamination bag and keep it in your car. It should include towels, an extra pair of shoes and clothes, bottles of water, wet wipes, and trash bags of all sizes. These items can be very handy in a variety of situations.

If you find yourself in a lab, calmly get out. Act as if your boss has paged you or is calling on the phone and excuse yourself. Walk down the street and call the police. Stay in the area until the police arrive to obtain your information. Do not get in your car and speed away; you may need to be decontaminated. Do not get into a confrontation with meth users; they can be very unpredictable and dangerous. If a child is present, leave the child. The police have ways of dealing with the situation under exigency. It is always better to be safe than sorry.

SUMMARY OF THINGS TO LOOK FOR

Medium- and large-scale meth labs are difficult to conceal from the public. Typically, the labs use pungent chemicals. In addition to the previously mentioned signs of the presence of a lab, there are other things that suggest a lab, including the following:

- Strong chemical odors
- Covered windows, sometimes with aluminum foil, to block people from looking inside and to keep sunlight out
- Persons coming and going at all hours of the day and night
- Excessive traffic, often for a short stay
- Tubing coming out of containers or bottles
- Exhaust fans in constant use, such as open windows in the winter or fans blowing odors outside
- Filthy living conditions, inside and outside of the house
- Numerous propane tanks that are the size used for barbecue grills (look for the blue discolored valve)
- Coffee grinders or blenders with colored powder residue and coffee filters with reddish-yellow or non-coffee-colored stains
- Heavy fortification and security measures, such as numerous surveillance cameras, bars on windows, and big dogs
- Large quantities of blister packs and boxes of cold tablets (such as Sudafed)
- Thermos or plastic liter pop bottles that have suspicious liquids in them or have their tops taped closed
- Chemical containers discarded in the trash
- Large quantities of matches, match book covers with the striker plates missing, acetone cans, lithium batteries, and other methamphetamine-making ingredients
- People coming outside buildings to smoke
- Drug paraphernalia such as pipes

NEW TRENDS

One way to combat the meth epidemic is to control or restrict the availability of the precursor pseudoephedrine. Target and Wal-Mart stores have stepped up to do their part, keeping the boxes behind the pharmacy counter and limited the quantity. Oklahoma, similar to other states, passed a law making certain pseudoephedrine-containing products Schedule V–controlled substances, and many states are looking at specific regulations to reduce the availability of cold tablets containing pseudoephedrine. Liquid cold medications can also be used to manufacture meth if they contain the precursor pseudoephedrine. It is very easy to extract pseudoephedrine out of the liquid, and since most people are just thinking of the tablets, lots of liquid cold medication boxes might indicate the presence of a lab. In January Pfizer Inc. made Sudafed PE available. This cold tablet contains phenylephrine instead of pseudoephedrine. The big question is whether meth can be made with this new product. We know cooks will use Sudafed PE by mistake, but we will have to wait to see what research chemists determine. Early reports indicate that phenylephrine does not behave in the same way as pseudoephedrine and thus requires some different techniques at various stages of the cooking process. Time will tell what develops.

Urine-extraction labs are popping up across the country. Unbelievable as it may seem, as states put more and more restrictions on chemicals and cold tablets, the country will see variations on ways to obtain meth. Recipes using urine can be found on the Internet, and it is a very easy extraction. It is believed that about 40 percent of ingested meth will be excreted unchanged; therefore, drug manufacture requires very large quantities of urine—gallons and gallons. Large quantities of yellow liquids along with some solvents, Red Devil lye, acids, and containers with tubing may indicate a different type of lab.

As all of the ingredients used to make meth become harder and harder to obtain, cooks will come up with other ways to manufacture the drug. With farmers using a dye in anhydrous ammonia and some farm feed stores refusing to sell it anymore, cooks learned how to make their own anhydrous ammonia, using ammonium nitrate (the farm fertilizer that was used to blow up the federal building in Oklahoma City), Red Devil lye, dry ice, acetone, some containers, and tubing. From this process of generating and condensing the ammonia vapor comes the newest process being seen nationwide, the "One-Pot" Method (CSAlert 2004). The forensic scientists at Washington State Patrol Marysville Crime Laboratory obtained an Internet recipe and put it to the test. It involved combining the following in a two-liter bottle and letting it sit about three hours: crushed pseudoephedrine tablets, ammonium nitrate, starter fluid, lithium metal strips, Red Devil lye, and a very small amount of water. This reaction has its own set of hazards, but is "easy," self-contained, has less odor than the ammonia method, and is a fast and efficient way to manufacture methamphetamine in small quantities.

CHAPTER 4

The Short- and Long-Term Medical Effects of Methamphetamine on Children and Adults

Kathryn M. Wells, MD

HISTORY OF MEDICAL USE

Methamphetamine is a drug that has been around and known to the medical community for many years. Chemically, it is a synthetic drug that belongs to the amphetamine class of drugs. Medically, its stimulant effects act on both the central and peripheral nervous systems. Throughout history it has had various medical uses, but it has increasingly been used illicitly.

Meth was first synthesized in 1887 by a German chemist. It was not used therapeutically until the 1930s when it began to be promoted by American pharmaceutical companies for various ailments and was thought to be without risk of addiction. At about the same time, Japan began to produce large quantities of meth in the pill form for domestic consumption. After the war, Japanese pharmaceutical companies launched a large campaign to increase the use of over-the-counter meth pills that were in abundance in former military warehouses. This consequently led to the first large-scale epidemic of meth use and abuse (Kato 1990). In the United States, a prescription was still needed to legally obtain amphetamines, but by the 1950s, the nonmedical use of amphetamines had spread to the civilian population, most commonly being used by individuals who needed to stay awake for long periods of time or to perform well at monotonous tasks. Additionally, meth was being prescribed for the treatment of hyperactivity, obesity, narcolepsy (a disorder causing spontaneous sleep), and depression (Beebe and Walley 1995).

The "second wave" of the meth epidemic in the United States occurred in the 1960s when intravenous use of the drug became more popular. These users were the first individuals to take the drug solely for its euphoric effects (Wolkoff 1997). During this period, users had created a way to manufacture meth on the street called the P2P (phenyl-2-propanone) method. This wave was controlled by law enforcement and public efforts to educate potential abusers and treat users. This method of manufacturing meth used lead acetate as a chemical reagent and, because there were often large quantities of lead in the final product, placing the user at risk for lead poisoning, there was the risk of hepatitis, nephritis, and encephalopathy (Allcott et al. 1987).

The "third wave" of meth use in the United States occurred in the 1980s as a result of the advent of another, faster and easier method for meth manufacturing called the pseudoephedrine reduction method. This method, further discussed elsewhere in this text, contributed to the rapidly rising accessibility and popularity of the drug on the street in the 1990s and 2000s. It produced a more potent and psychoactive form of the drug with a higher percentage of the dextro-isomer of the drug compared to the P2P method, which produced equal proportions of the dextro- and levo-isomers (Burton 1991; Cho 1990; Center for Substance Abuse Treatment 1997). This is important because dextro-methamphetamine is three to four times more potent to the central nervous system than levo-methamphetamine (Sowder and Beschner 1993). The extent of the potential consequences of the impurities of this manufactured form of meth is unclear (unintended by-products and reagent residuals as well as processing errors), but this is of great concern, as many of these laboratories are operated by uneducated "chemists" who get their recipes from unpublished sources or through the Internet and who are frequently using the drug while processing it.

Additionally, on the street a potent, smokable form of meth, known as "crystal," "glass," or "ice," began to gain popularity, and its use grew rapidly because of the more potent and longer "high." For these reasons, many cocaine users began to be attracted to the use of meth (Wolkoff 1997). By the 1990s, the use of prescription meth was almost completely discontinued due to the understanding of its potential for addiction. Meth is currently classified as a Schedule II stimulant, meaning that it is known to have a high potential for abuse and is available only by prescription. The only accepted medical indications for use of meth are for the treatment of narcolepsy and attention-deficit/hyperactivity disorder, and the dosages prescribed are much smaller than what is used by the abusers.

HOW IS METH USED?

Meth may be snorted, smoked, orally ingested, injected, or absorbed through any mucous membranes such as sublingually, rectally, or vaginally. It is readily absorbed from the gut, nasopharynx (back of the nose and throat), muscle (when injected), mucosa, and placenta. It alters the mood differently depending on the route of ingestion. When the drug is snorted or taken orally, the user describes a feeling of euphoria or a feeling of extreme well-being called a "high." Smoking or injecting the drug results additionally in a more immediate, brief, intense sensation called a "flash" or a "rush." Users describe this as extremely pleasurable, and it has been characterized by some individuals as being equivalent to multiple orgasms. This is then followed by the euphoria. The "high" and the "rush" are both a result of the release of very high levels of the neurotransmitter dopamine into areas of the brain that regulate feelings of pleasure. Further description of the effect of this drug on the brain will be discussed in a later section.

Different methods of use produce different response within the user's body. The length of time until onset of symptoms is dependent upon the method of use. If the drug is snorted, effects occur within 3–5 minutes due to the rapid uptake of the drug through highly vascular nasal passages. If, however, the drug is ingested orally, it must be taken up through the lining of the digestive system, with effects not occurring for 15–20 minutes. Smoking meth usually allows the drug to reach the brain even more rapidly than injecting it (MacKenzie and Heischober 1997). This is felt to be related to the small particle size of the drug, allowing it to penetrate deep into the lung tissue, where it rapidly crosses into the pulmonary circulation. In fact, meth is available to the body and brain very rapidly after use as it, unlike cocaine, does not have to be converted to a "free base" in order to be smoked effectively (MacKenzie and Heischober 1997). The stimulant effects of meth have been reported to last up to 24 hours, most commonly 8–12 hours, compared to cocaine's high of only 20–30 minutes (National Institute on Drug Abuse 1998). Additionally, the route of administration plays a role in the potential for dangerous and unintended consequences or side effects. Intravenous use is frequently associated with additional illnesses related to the administration of the drug (i.e., sharing of needles) such as hepatitis, HIV infection, tuberculosis, pneumonia, cellulitis (tissue infection), bacterial or viral endocarditis (infection of the lining of the heart), wound abscesses, sepsis (blood infection), thrombosis (blood clot in the blood vessels), thrombophlebitis (infection of lining of the blood vessel), and kidney injury (Šlamberová et al. 2005; Sowder and Beschner 1993). Snorting the drug may be associated with sinusitis (infection of the sinuses), loss of the sense of smell, congestion, atrophy (thinning) of the nasal mucosa, nosebleeds, perforation or damage to the nasal septum, hoarseness, and difficulty with swallowing (Sowder and Beschner 1993; Gold 1997).

Meth is commonly used in a "binge and crash" pattern—this means that the user will continue to use the drug ("binge") until they completely "crash." Many users go on a "run," during which time they may forgo food and sleep while binging. This period of use can last for several days. After the heavy binge cycle and before the "crash," the user may experience extreme paranoia, hallucinations, aggression, and agitation. This period of use is called "tweaking" and is felt to be the most physiologically dangerous time for the user as he or she may have a tremendous amount of drug in their body. It is also the time period when the user is potentially the most dangerous, due at least in part to their propensity for violence and feelings of paranoia. The "crash" is believed to occur because the chemical messenger (neurotransmitter) dopamine is depleted from the nerve terminals. It will slowly reaccumulate (at least to some level) while the user is crashing, but during this time the user may sleep for days, not even awakening to take care of regular bodily needs such as eating. Unfortunately, this often leads to increased use of the drug following the crash and eventually to difficulty in feeling any pleasure at all as the nerve terminals become injured. This is further discussed below in the section on central nervous system effects.

Tolerance to meth occurs within minutes, and the pleasurable effects disappear even before the blood concentrations fall. This partially explains the lack of direct correlation between blood level and clinical effects seen with meth. Tolerance means that users often need to take repeatedly higher doses and dose more frequently to get the desired effect. In addition, users often change their method of intake to a method that provides the additional "rush" or "flash" but is also more addictive (injection or smoking). However, there is no tolerance for the negative effects on the user's judgment, impulsivity, aggression, and susceptibility to paranoia, delusions, and hallucinations. In fact, it frequently takes an increasingly smaller amount of the drug to produce these symptoms.

When users discontinue their meth use, they will experience at least some symptoms of withdrawal. The more problematic and prominent withdrawal is the psychological withdrawal, which consists of depression, anxiety and agitation, fatigue, paranoia, aggression, and an intense craving for the drug. Physical withdrawal may also occur and is characterized by excessive hunger (polyphagia) and excessive sleepiness (hypersomnolence). Seizures may occur when the user is withdrawing from this drug. Studies have shown that there are brain abnormalities similar to those seen in people with mood disorders such as anxiety and depression (London et al. 2004) in individuals who have recently discontinued their meth use. This poses additional challenges for individuals in treatment for this addiction, as discussed in chapter 7 on treatment.

CLINICAL EFFECTS OF METH USE

There are many factors that may contribute to how a person's body responds to meth use and abuse. The clinical effects from the use of meth are related to the form of the drug used, the dose, the frequency of use, the route of administration, and the length and amount of use. Additionally, the user may have underlying mental health problems for which he or she is trying to self-medicate with the use of the meth. The user may also be using other drugs in conjunction with meth, which may compound and complicate the effects of the drug. Finally, the methods of manufacturing this drug vary greatly, as does the purity of the final product. Therefore, the chemicals used in the manufacturing process as well as unwanted by-products may remain in the final product. This makes if very difficult to differentiate the effects of the drug alone from the effects of the other chemicals and by-products present. These variables also make it very difficult to predict, with any great certainty, the effects of the drug on each individual user.

Short-Term Effects

Pharmacologically, meth is a strong stimulant and is therefore in a class of drugs that includes cocaine, caffeine, and amphetamines. It is structurally similar to amphetamine as well as some of the body's natural neurotransmitters (chemical messengers) such as dopamine, serotonin, epinephrine (adrenaline), and norepinephrine. Meth has a much greater effect on the central nervous system than other amphetamines. Additionally, it seems to exert fewer peripheral nervous system effects (Beebe and Walley 1995).

Many users report that they began taking meth to try to increase their alertness and to stay awake for longer periods of time, while others begin taking the drug use to lose weight. Still other users begin using to increase their sexual appetite, using it socially to go dancing or "clubbing."

A large portion of the acute physiological symptoms displayed after the use of meth are related to its peripheral effects on the autonomic nervous system and include dilated pupils, dry mouth, suppressed appetite (and consequent weight loss), elevated blood pressure (hypertension), tachycardia (high heart rate), rapid respiratory rate (tachyon), bruxism (involuntary teeth grinding), insomnia (inability to sleep or decreased need for sleep), tremors, and blurry vision. Additionally, meth is a vasoconstrictor of peripheral blood vessels, which causes decreased oxygen delivery to the extremities, resulting in poor circulation. This may contribute to the multiple skin lesions that users often have, which are further worsened by the frequent picking behavior that the user demonstrates while perseverating on the lesions. Users also often perseverate on other tasks such as taking electronic items apart but then are unable to focus adequately in order to reassemble them (Center for Substance Abuse Treatment 1999).

The central nervous system effects of meth ingestion are the result of the structural similarity of meth and the neurotransmitters active in the brain (dopamine, serotonin, epinephrine or adrenaline, and norepinephrine). Meth use can initially create feelings of euphoria (well-being), elevated energy, increased sensory perception, improved attention, excitation, intensification of emotions, perception of elevated self-esteem, increased alertness, agitation, aggression, restlessness, irritability, repetitive stereotyped behaviors, and increased physical activity (Jaffe 1995). Conversely, it can decrease physical appetite with subsequent often marked and rapid weight loss. Users may have pressured speech and flight of ideas with rapid shifts in thinking, poor concentration, exaggerated self-esteem, hypervigilance, enhanced sensory awareness, fearlessness, suspiciousness, impaired judgment, poor impulse control, aggression, and emotional lability (Center for Substance Abuse Treatment 1999).

Users have described markedly increased feelings of sexual desire, but despite this increased libido (sex drive) they usually begin to have difficulty in sexual performance. It is believed that the result of meth-stimulated serotonin release in the brain gives an initial antidepressant effect and elevates feelings of empathy. However, it is also responsible for bizarre mood changes, psychotic behavior, aggressiveness, and bruxism (involuntary grinding of the teeth). Some users may also experience feelings of nausea and dizziness.

The central nervous system effects of acute ingestion may include psychotic behaviors such as hallucinations and paranoia, which can lead to bizarre, irrational, and even violent behavior. These effects may persist for days or weeks after the drug was discontinued (Beebe and Walley 1995). These individuals may therefore have a great potential for violence, are at risk for homicidal and suicidal behavior (Szuster 1990), and can be very dangerous to approach in any setting. A condition called methamphetamine psychosis has been described in the literature (Murray 1998). This illness consists of several features including extreme paranoia, well-formed delusions, hypersensitivity to environmental stimuli including light and sound, stereotyped "tweaking" behavior, panic, extreme fearfulness, and a high potential for violence. In fact, there is a described "hyperviolence syndrome" where the victim is frequently a part of the perpetrator's delusional belief system. A weapon such as a knife or gun is commonly used in committing a crime and frequently there are multiple wounds inflicted, sometimes even days after the victim's death (MacKenzie and Heischober 1997). Additionally, agitated delirium has been described in cases of meth-psychotic states and has also been linked to sudden cardiac death in meth users.

Overdose of the drug may be lethal and can even occur in a first-time user who ingests a single large dose (Jaffe 1990). Acute symptoms of toxic ingestion may include dizziness, tremor, irritability, confusion, hostility, hallucinations, panic, headache, skin flushing, chest pain, palpitations, increased core body temperature (hyperthermia), irregular heart rhythms (arrhythmias), vomiting, cramps, excessive sweating, and severe high blood pressure (hypertension). This can result in brain hemorrhage or stroke, heart attack (myocardial infarction), and acute pulmonary edema (abnormal accumulation of fluid in the lungs) (Nestor et al. 1989, 1989a; Furst et al. 1990). Additionally, the hyperthermia may be exacerbated by increased muscular activity due to agitation and can result in massive muscle breakdown (rhabdomyolysis) and potentially kidney failure (Beebe and Walley 1995). The development of a very high fever, rapid heart rate, severe hypertension, convulsions, toxic delirium, and cardiovascular collapse may signal a life-threatening situation (Ellinwood and Sudilovsky et al. 1973; Rowbotham 1993; Wetli 1993).

Medical treatment for overdose of meth consists primarily of supportive care. Other potential causes of presentation must be excluded. There are no specific medications or antidotes for the treatment of meth intoxication.

Sedation and rapid cooling may be used to manage the hyperthermia and agitated movements (Ellinwood and Sudilovsky et al. 1973; Gold 1997). Ventilation and oxygenation may need to be provided and medications may need to be used to manage hypertension and seizures. Evaluation for cardiac arrhythmias and injury may need to be undertaken as well.

Long-Term Effects

The long-term effects of meth use can be particularly challenging when dealing with a chronic meth abuser. The use and abuse of this drug commonly leads to progressive social and occupational deterioration. Many who work with meth addicts report that the changes caused by the drug lead to a complete rearrangement of the user's priorities. For this reason, meth causes the heavy user to withdraw from anything and everything that is important to them. The reality is that studies now show that these effects are related to brain changes, many of which may be permanent. Individuals who have used meth for long periods of time demonstrate many features of dependence. It is clear that meth is highly addictive and may lead to a chronic, relapsing disease. Addiction to meth is characterized by compulsive drug-seeking behavior, which is the result of functional and molecular changes in the brain. There is a stronger potential for addiction when utilizing the more rapid-acting routes of administration such as injection or smoking the drug, since there is stronger positive reinforcement for the use with the extremely pleasurable feelings that immediately follow (National Institute on Drug Abuse 1998).

Chronic users often exhibit concerning behavioral changes, which consist of paranoia, auditory and visual hallucinations, mood disturbances, and delusions. This may result in homicidal or suicidal thoughts. Chronic users may also demonstrate excessive anxiety, confusion, insomnia, weight loss, and extremely violent behavior. It is important to be aware of this when dealing with someone addicted to the drug as they may exhibit very dangerous, unprovoked rages. Additionally, long-term users may display unusual motor movements that appear very similar to a Parkinsonian tremor. When the drug is discontinued, the user may experience depression, anxiety, fatigue, paranoia, aggression, and an intense craving for the drug. Studies have shown that the behavioral changes may persist for months or years after use of the drug is discontinued (National Institute on Drug Abuse 1998). Chronic meth abuse may lead to the "kindling" phenomenon or "reverse tolerance" where the user can be pushed into frank psychosis by even very small amounts of any stimulant (methamphetamine, amphetamine, caffeine, or nicotine). This is felt to involve alterations that occur in the brain (Jaffe 1990). Recent studies have suggested that meth psychosis may also spontaneously be brought on by mild stressors (Yui et al. 2000). Finally, there is another condition called chronic psychosis or "withdrawal" or "abstinence" psychosis, but it is unclear if this may be related to latent schizophrenia that was uncovered by the meth use (Streltzer and Leigh 1977; Tomiyama 1990).

Another feature of long-term meth use and abuse relates to the heightened sexuality linked to the use of this drug. After meth use for any length of time, users frequently describe changes in their sexual behaviors. They report that frequently activities that would previously give them sexual gratification no longer do, which leads many users to turn to increasingly bizarre sexual behaviors to meet their sexual needs. This can lead to predatory sexual behavior, increased promiscuity, and the extensive use of pornography. Frequent, often unprotected, sexual activity results in many unplanned pregnancies as well as the transmission of sexually transmitted and blood-borne infections including HIV/AIDS and multiple forms of viral hepatitis (particularly Hepatitis B and C). These risks are increased further when the users are injecting the drug and sharing the injection equipment. In fact, the use of methamphetamine is so closely linked to sexual behavior that some studies have shown that sexual photos presented to meth users can trigger desire to use, even after long-term abstinence.

Dental decay has become a hallmark of chronic meth use and abuse. This complication has been termed by many as "meth mouth" and is likely multi-factorial. First, meth use markedly reduces the production of saliva, causing a very dry mouth (xerostomia). Since saliva normally serves to bathe the teeth and reduce decay-causing bacteria, its reduction may lead to dental decay. Additionally users often have a high intake of sugary soft drinks, which, coupled with a lack of oral hygiene as well as poor nutrition, may contribute to dental decay (Shaner 2002). Finally, the significant vasoconstriction caused by meth use may also decrease blood flow to the teeth through the dental pulp, causing further damage. Another hallmark of chronic meth abuse is skin lesions. This is discussed in detail below in the section on the dermatologic system.

MEDICAL COMPLICATIONS OF METH USE

Meth use can affect any major organ system in the body. It has the most profound effect on the brain and central nervous system, but can also affect other organs.

Central Nervous System

The greatest systemic medical concern about meth use is the serious effect that the drug has on the brain of the user. The effects of meth on the central nervous system are numerous. First, this drug affects the brain at the very cellular level, causing nerve damage and loss.

In order to understand the complex effect that meth has on brain cells, it is important to understand the way that brain cells normally work. Nerve cells pass messages from one cell to another through the assistance of chemicals called neurotransmitters. These chemicals are necessary, because the nerve cells do not actually touch and therefore must pass their messages by the release and uptake of a neurotransmitter. These chemical messengers, such as dopamine, epinephrine, norepinephrine, and serotonin, are stored in structures called vesicles that float around in a fluid called cytoplasm within the presynaptic (sending) nerve cell. They remain there until the cell is given the signal to release the chemical. At that time the vesicle moves to the edge of the presynaptic cell, binds to the cell wall, and releases the neurotransmitter into the synapse (the space between the two nerve cells). The message is then picked up by the postsynaptic (receiving) cell when the neurotransmitter attaches to a receptor on the cell wall. If there is more neurotransmitter in the synapse than is needed, it will either be destroyed or taken back up into the presynaptic cell for storage until it is needed again. This is done through a mechanism in the cell wall of the presynaptic cell called a transporter.

Dopamine is the neurotransmitter most affected by meth, because the two chemicals are very similar in structure. Dopamine is normally released when something pleasurable occurs, since it acts in the regions of the brain that regulate feelings of pleasure. It also elicits effects in the areas of the brain that regulate movement, emotion, judgment, and motivation. Once meth enters the body, regardless of the manner, it makes its way to the brain cells, among other places, where it causes the cells to release dopamine into the nerve synapse. This is what creates the stimulant effects of the drug that the user desires. Early studies showed that meth decreased the transporter function in dopamine neurons (Brown and Hanson et al. 2000). However, newer studies have shown that the meth actually enters the presynaptic cell and causes massive release of dopamine from the storage vesicles into the cell cytoplasm as well as an additional massive release of dopamine from the presynaptic cell. This causes flooding of the synapse with the dopamine. There are only a limited number of receptors on the postsynaptic cell, and once they are full of the dopamine, they can no longer take up more of the chemical. Therefore, there is an excess of dopamine left in the synapse. Researchers believe that the excess dopamine is broken down by chemicals in the synapse and is ultimately turned into breakdown products that are toxic to the nerve cells. Additionally, the excess dopamine released into the presynaptic cell's cytoplasm is believed to be damaging to the cell.

Studies using a noninvasive brain imaging technique called magnetic resonance spectroscopy (MRS) have shown that the damage done to nerve cells is long-term and is similar to that caused by strokes or Alzheimer's disease (Ernst et al. 2000). Another study by Dr. Volkow used positron emission tomography (PET) scans to show that dopamine transporter levels in the striatum of the brain were 24 percent lower in meth users than in control subjects. Additionally, the meth users performed more poorly than nonusers on tests that evaluated brain function associated with the striatum including fine motor skills, gross motor skills, and memory. The reduction in performance was proportional to the deficits in dopamine transporters. She concluded that compared with the normal 6–7 percent reduction in dopamine transporters found in aging, users saw losses roughly equivalent to 40 years of aging (Volkow et al. 2001a).

Damage caused by meth to the dopamine system has been compared to that seen in patients with Parkinson's disease, a brain disease characterized by the progressive loss of dopamine neurons in the regions of the brain involved in movement. Although damage to the brains of Parkinson's patients is more severe than that in meth users, researchers now believe that long-term meth use may lead to symptoms very similar to Parkinson's disease (Volkow et al. 2001a). It is unknown if sustained abstinence from meth use will result in recovery of brain changes. Early studies suggested that abstinence was accompanied by dopamine transporter recovery, but a parallel recovery in cognitive function has been more difficult to identify. It is clear that recovery is related to the individual's baseline prior to use, the length of use, and the length of the abstinence (Volkow et al. 2001a). A recent study using proton magnetic resonance spectroscopy suggested that following cessation of meth use, adaptive changes occur in the brain, which was felt to potentially contribute to some improvement in function (Nordahl et al. 2005). However, another recent publication suggests that meth use causes persistent hypometabolism in the frontal white matter of the brain with impairment in frontal executive function (Kim et al. 2005). Many studies are ongoing in this important area.

The release of serotonin is also stimulated by meth ingestion. This neurotransmitter has been implicated in states of consciousness, mood, depression, and anxiety. It is believed that meth has a little bit less serotonin effect than dopamine effect. However, damage to cells responsive to this chemical may explain the problems with depression that recovering addicts face.

As the nerve terminals are injured, the user eventually is unable to feel the pleasure that they began to use the drug for. This can contribute to the cycle of addiction and many of the chronic effects that are seen in long-term users.

Meth use can cause seizure activity, strokes, and spontaneous brain bleeds. It can also lead to chronic psychosis as well as movement disorders.

Cardiovascular System

Because meth is a stimulant, it has multiple effects on the cardiovascular system. These effects appear to be manifest at all dose levels and routes of administration even in otherwise healthy young adults. Virtually any kind of heart disease has been linked to meth use and abuse. First, use of this drug causes an increase in heart rate (tachycardia) as well as elevation of blood pressure (hypertension), both of which can be marked and very dangerous. Additionally, meth use can cause sudden cardiac death as well as the sudden rupture of an aneurysm. Meth is a blood vessel constrictor (vasoconstrictor), and that abnormal constriction of blood vessels of the heart can cause heart damage or a heart attack. This may be worsened or exacerbated by the fact that meth use causes increased platelet aggregation, which may clog cardiac vessels. Primarily because of the catecholamine (epinephrine and other neurotransmitted) excess, meth abuse may result in cardiotoxicity. This may be manifest as inflammation of the heart muscle (myocarditis) or the heart lining (endocarditis) and abnormalities in the heart muscle itself (cardiomyopathy) (Hong and Matsuyama et al. 1991; Gold 1997). Finally, chronic meth abuse can cause damage to any vessels throughout the body, further damaging the tissues those vessels supply.

Respiratory System

Respiratory system complications from meth abuse include shortness of breath (dyspnea) and severe chest pain. Coughing spasms following inhalation of the drug may result in pulmonary barotrauma and consequent leakiness of air into the pleural cavity, chest cavity (mediastinum), and soft (subcutaneous) tissues of the chest. Pulmonary edema (excess fluid in the lungs) has been noted in meth fatalities and is felt to be the result of deep inhalation of the drug and subsequent aggravation of preexisting conditions (Nestor et al. 1989, 1989a). Granulomas may form as a result of chronic irritation from adulterants added to the drugs, and constriction of the blood vessels in the lungs may ultimately affect oxygen exchange, potentially leading to chronic lung disease (Center for Substance Abuse Treatment 1997).

Dermatologic System

The skin of the chronic user is often in poor condition and may be covered in sores. Poor circulation to the skin, poor nutrition, and tactile hallucinations all contribute to this quickly identifiable problem. Users often report that they believe that there are bugs crawling on their skin (a phenomenon called "formication") and will perseverate on trying to pick at the bugs, often with instruments such as knives. These lesions frequently have difficulty healing well and become readily apparent in chronic users. Some parents will even believe that their children have bugs on their skin and cover the children in insect spray or pick at the child's skin. These lesions may be confused with another skin disorder if the drug use is not identified.

There may be evidence of healed burns if the user participated in manufacturing and was burned—often these individuals do not get medical care for the burns when they occur and attempt to treat the injury themselves. Recent data in the literature suggests that if such a burn patient seeks medical care, they need to be managed differently than routine burn patients, requiring two to three times the usual amount of fluid resuscitation (Warner et al. 2003).

Immunologic System

Drug abuse has been linked to increased risk of HIV and Hepatitis B, C, and D infection due to high-risk behaviors of users such as unprotected sexual activity and the sharing of injection paraphernalia. Preliminary animal studies have suggested that meth may also affect HIV disease progression by a more rapid and increased brain HIV viral load. Another study suggested that HIV-positive meth users may be at a greater risk of developing acquired immune deficiency syndrome (AIDS) than non-meth-using HIV positive patients. Finally, additional studies have suggested that interactions between meth and the HIV virus itself may lead to greater neuronal damage and neuropsychological impairment (Volkow 2005).

Other Organs

Other organs can be affected by meth use as well. Muscle damage can occur as a result of severely elevated body temperature (rhabdomyolysis). This can lead to major organ system damage including the kidney, liver, and brain. Giant gastrointestinal ulcers can occur as a result of vasoconstriction decreasing blood supply to the intestines. There have also been reports of acute liver failure following intravenous meth (Kamijo et al. 2002). One recent study showed significantly decreased calcification in the bone of chronic meth users, suggesting possible chronic effects on bone metabolism (Katsuragawa 1999).

EFFECTS OF METH USE IN PREGNANCY

Meth use during pregnancy is believed to place the unborn fetus at risk, as does the use of other illicit drugs and alcohol. However, the full extent of maternal use of meth on the fetus and newborn infant is not completely known, and the fact that a mother uses a drug while pregnant does not, in and of itself, ensure that the unborn fetus will be affected. In fact, it is very difficult to differentiate the effects of meth exposure from a multitude of other factors such as maternal nutritional status and health, genetics, socioeconomic status, lack of prenatal care, and concomitant exposure to other drugs, including nicotine and alcohol. Additionally, the effect of any prenatal exposure on the fetus is also related to the gestational period during which the drug was used as well as the amount and form of use (Plessinger 1998). Exposures in the first and second trimester of pregnancy are more likely to result in systemic abnormalities, while exposures later in pregnancy are linked with growth abnormalities. There is currently a multicenter study underway to further describe this issue but, preliminarily, the investigators report that the effects appear to be similar to those of cocaine-exposed infants. However, although meth and cocaine are both sympathomimetic agents, it is known that meth has a much longer duration of action, potentially complicating its effects further.

There are several components of the potential risk to the fetus in a pregnancy complicated by maternal meth use. First, the effects of the use of the drug on the mother and father, including fertility, must be considered. Studies have shown that chronic, high-dose stimulant use affects reproductive and sexual functioning in both males and females. Male users report loss of sexual interest, impotence, and difficulty in maintaining an ejaculation, while female users may have abnormalities in their menstrual cycles leading to amenorrhea and infertility, as well as difficulty in achieving an orgasm (Gold 1997). In the pregnant woman, meth may cause hypertension (high blood pressure), tachycardia, and vasoconstriction. Additionally, the mother's poor nutritional habits, high-risk behaviors, and commonly poor prenatal care may contribute to potential risk to the fetus.

Next, the risks to the placenta and the fetus must be considered. Based on its sympathomimetic function, meth is thought to have direct cardiovascular effects on both the fetus and the placenta, potentially causing fetal hypertension (high blood pressure), tachycardia (high heart rate), and vasoconstriction. These effects may result in premature delivery, intrauterine growth retardation, placental hemorrhage, fetal distress, or spontaneous abortion. Additionally, because the placenta provides the source of nutrition for the fetus, constriction of these blood vessels, as caused by meth, may result in reduced blood flow to the fetus and ultimately reduced oxygen and nutrient supply. These findings are consistent with the pharmacologic properties of meth, as it is known that elevated levels of norepinephrine can cause placental vasoconstriction and increased uterine contractility (Sherman and Gautieri 1972; Lederman et al. 1978). One sheep study released in 1993 showed that methamphetamine readily crosses the placenta and produces significant and long-lasting maternal and fetal cardiovascular effects (Stek and Fisher et al. 1993). It is also known that meth passes through the placenta to the fetus and can cause elevated fetal blood pressure, potentially leading to prenatal strokes and heart or other major organ damage. The drug can cause an increased or extremely variable heart rate in the fetus and slowing or alteration of fetal growth. Additionally, simultaneous with an increase in maternal blood pressure following meth abuse, there is a decreased blood supply as well as oxygen supply to the placenta and fetus. This impaired oxygen supply can retard fetal development (Stewart and Meeker 1997). Another study in sheep, released in 1994, showed that maternal administration of meth was found to be associated with a short-term increase in circulating fetal catecholamines, which was followed by hyperglycemia, lacticacidemia, and hyperinsulinism. This began to suggest an alteration of fetal sympathoadrenal activity, which may contribute to the perinatal complications seen with meth use (Dickinson and Andres et al. 1994). Additionally, it has been shown that the norepinephrine transporter and, to a lesser extent, the serotonin transporter are cellular targets in the human placenta for both amphetamine and meth (Ramamoorthy et al. 1995).

Another aspect of prenatal meth exposure that must be considered is any possible direct effect on the fetus. Fetal development abnormalities have been described sporadically in the medical literature, but no true syndrome specifically linked with maternal use of meth in the prenatal period has been described. There are limited numbers of studies in this area, particularly studies focusing on human infants. Additionally, most of the research in this area combines all amphetamines (often including cocaine), and only few studies isolate meth exposures. It is known that because of its low molecular weight and lipid solubility, there is considerable transfer of meth from maternal to fetal blood. This, in addition to the immaturity of fetal metabolic activities, may account for the reason that the drug remains in fetal circulation much longer than it does in maternal blood (Stek et al. 1993; Inaba and Cohen 1993). Multiple studies looking at human exposures to amphetamines have indicated an association between meth or amphetamine use during pregnancy and cleft lip (Little et al. 1988; Nelson and Forfar 1971; Saxen 1975; Thomas 1995), cardiac defects (Little et al. 1988; Nelson and Forfar 1971; Nora et al. 1967; Nora et al. 1970), low birth weight (Little et al. 1988; Oro and Dixon 1987), growth reduction and reduced head circumference (Eriksson et al. 1981; Little et al. 1988; Oro and Dixon 1987), biliary atresia (Golbus 1980; Levin 1971), prematurity and stillbirth (Ericksson et al. 1978), hyperbilirubinemia requiring transfusion (Ericksson et al. 1978), cerebral hemorrhage (Dixon and Bejar 1989), low body fat, and undescended testes (Little et al. 1988). Although these things have been noted to be associated with meth or amphetamine use prenatally, there is little data to suggest any kind of causative relationship, and the direct link between fetal abnormalities and maternal methamphetamine use is not clearly discernable. One study by Oro and Dixon showed that in utero exposure to cocaine or methamphetamine was adversely, negatively associated with gestational age, birth weight, length, and occipitofrontal circumference. They also showed that "the increased rate of prematurity, intrauterine growth retardation, and perinatal complications associated with prenatal exposure to cocaine or methamphetamine was greater than that predicted by coexisting risk factors and was consistent with the pharmacologic properties of these drugs" (Oro and Dixon 1987). Another study by Smith et al. showed an association between decreased growth in infants exposed to meth throughout pregnancy relative to those infants only exposed in the first and second trimesters (Smith and Yonekura et al. 2003). Therefore, it is felt that birth outcomes may improve if the mother stops using the drug in the last one to three months of pregnancy. In addition this study revealed significantly more small-for-gestational-age infants in the methamphetamine-exposed group than those in the nonexposed group (Smith et al. 2003). There also appeared to be a significant decrease in growth in the meth-exposed infants who were born to mothers who additionally smoked cigarettes compared to those who did not smoke (Smith et al. 2003). Finally, these infants may be at increased risk of blood-borne diseases such as HIV, Hepatitis B, and Hepatitis C because of the frequent high-risk behaviors of the mother.

Early studies of amphetamine-exposed infants indicated that many of these infants had difficulties with poor feeding and extreme drowsiness throughout the first several weeks to as long as a year of life (Ericksson et al. 1978; Eriksson et al. 1981; Ramer 1974). Some of these infants (like infants with exposures to narcotics) may display an array of behavioral disturbances after birth characterized by tremors, irritability, abnormal sleep patterns, and poor feeding, which may represent direct drug effects rather than withdrawal, as the metabolites were found in the infants' urine for up to seven days after birth (Oro and Dixon 1987). One study that analyzed 294 mother-infant pairs (134 exposed and 160 unexposed) found that 49 percent of exposed infants displayed evidence of withdrawal symptoms and documented the need for pharmacologic intervention for the treatment of withdrawal symptoms in 4 percent of these infants (Smith et al. 2003). Following this initial hyperirritable phase (usually only displayed in the first several days of life), some meth-exposed infants were so extremely drowsy that they required tube feedings, approximating the prolonged sleep, lethargy, and depression ("crash") seen in adult users (Oro and Dixon 1987). This period of time through the first four weeks of life is felt to be related to the dopamine depletion syndrome and may be characterized by lethargy in the infant with excessive periods of sleep, poor suck and swallow coordination, sleep apnea, and poor habituation (Shah 2006). Exposed infants may have irregular sleep patterns, poor feeding, tremors, and increased muscle tone. Their poor ability to habituate or self-regulate, especially under stressful situations, will be further intensified if their environment is noisy and chaotic. They will not tolerate this well, which will likely lead to increased irritability and potential for abuse. In the next four months of life, the infant may display symptoms of CNS immaturity, including effects on motor development, sensory integration problems including tactile, defensive, and texture issues, and neurobehavioral symptoms affecting their interaction and social development. This period is frequently followed by a symptom-free period or the honeymoon phase from 6 to 18 months. However, from 18 months to 5 years, the children may again begin to exhibit difficulties with sensory integration, poorly focused attention, easy distractibility, poor anger management, and aggressive outbursts (Shah 2006).

Because of the multitude of confounding variables such as other potential drug exposures, genetic predisposition, and environmental factors, it is difficult to identify postnatal features that are directly related to in utero meth exposure. However, scientists have begun to study infants exposed to meth in utero to attempt to identify potential outcomes. One study by Hansen et al. of infants exposed to meth in utero has identified visual cognitive effects (poorer visual recognition memory—a measure correlated with subsequent IQ) and changes in behavior that appear to be permanent in these infants (Hansen et al. 1993). Several additional studies in rats have demonstrated similar concerns for spatial learning in adult animals exposed to meth in utero (Williams et al. 2002; Crawford et al. 2003; Williams et al. 2003).

Several studies have shown that prenatally meth-exposed infants may go on to exhibit further difficulties in childhood. Children exposed to meth in utero may face difficulties with what is called executive-level functioning. This functioning is related to the brain's ability to absorb information, interpret the information, and make decisions based on it. Difficulties in this level of functioning may help explain the problems that many of these children face with impulsivity, judgment, and connecting behavior with consequence. Although there are mounting studies on the effects of meth on adult brains, studies on the brains of infants exposed to meth in utero are limited but beginning to emerge. One study by Smith et al. attempted to study the possible neurotoxic effects of prenatal meth exposure on the developing brain using brain proton magnetic resonance spectroscopy (Smith et al. 2003). In this study, the researchers found the suggestion of an abnormality in the energy metabolism in the brains of children exposed to meth in utero, but acknowledged the need for more studies and the interpretation of this study with caution due to their small sample size and limited behavioral assessments (Smith et al. 2003). The study, however, may have important clinical implications, since the area found to be affected is the frontal-striatal pathway, which is involved in executive-level functioning.

Studies done in Sweden following the short-term legalization of drugs of abuse in the 1960s looked at populations of children exposed to amphetamines prenatally who were then monitored for their progress and performance (Plessinger 1998). Several reports indicated difficulties with altered growth and behavior in the exposed children (Plessinger 1998). Looking at matched groups of exposed and unexposed children at 8 year and then 14 years of age, a larger number of amphetamine-exposed children did more poorly than unexposed controls in mathematics, language, and physical training (Ericksson et al. 1978; Eriksson 1981; Cernerud et al. 1996). These studies also showed that once these exposed children were past puberty, the boys were taller and heavier and the girls were shorter and lighter than the Swedish standards used for comparison (Cernerud et al. 1996). These findings may suggest an effect of in utero exposure of methamphetamines on normal neural development and maturation of the adenohypophysis, which raises concern that the use of amphetamines during pregnancy may cause a wide variety of effects (Plessinger 1998).

Additional work is being done in an effort to better define any association there may be between prenatal drug exposures and later drug use and medical complications in young adults and adults. One recent study at the University of Chicago indicated that males who were exposed to meth in utero and then went on to take the drug themselves as teens or adults may have hastened onset of brain disorders such as Parkinson's Disease (Heller et al. 2001).

Finally, there have been reports of deaths in fetuses and infants felt to be related to maternal meth use. Although the actual number of these cases reported in the literature is low, there is concern about the risk of death in infant's exposure to this drug either prenatally or in the postnatal period. One study reviewed the deaths of eight fetuses/infants aged from 20 weeks estimated gestational age to a 1-month-old infant (Stewart and Meeker 1997). In these cases, it was believed that the maternal use of meth played a role in the deaths of the fetuses/infants, and the authors cited the increased vulnerability of the developing nervous system and potential compromise due to fetal acidosis, hypoxernia, decreased uterine blood flow, changes in fetal blood gases, and an increase in fetal glucose levels (Stewart and Meeker 1997). There have also been some studies suggesting a possible link between cocaine exposure in utero and sudden infant death syndrome (SIDS), but the nature of this connection is unclear. However, because of this potential link as well as the possibility that the infant may have ingested the drug, California law now requires that all SIDS deaths be tested for certain drugs including meth.

PARENTING ISSUES IN METH USE

A very important factor that must be considered regarding children that are exposed to meth is the environment in which the child is raised. There are additional and potentially very dangerous consequences that may occur if a child grows up in an environment where there is active use of methamphetamine. These risks include the actual environment, which may include many hazards including the exposure to the drug itself as well as the actual quality of parenting that the child receives.

The environment of a meth abuser is one that may contain many risks for growing children. These risks include exposure to the actual drug itself (see the next section), weapons, an unkempt and dirty home, inadequate food, inappropriate sleeping conditions, multiple unsavory visitors, and exposure to violence and sexual content and activity. The child may be neglected while the parents sleep for long periods of time during a "crash." They frequently do not receive adequate medical, dental, emotional, and educational care. Additionally, children living in these homes are at an increased risk of sexual abuse, either from witnessing sexually explicit activity or material or from becoming the actual targets of bizarre sexual activity in the home. They may also be physically abused or even killed when the parent becomes easily frustrated or the child becomes the target of the parent's homicidal ideations.

There are few studies in this area, but one study in which meth was administered to premating, gestational, and lactational rat pups demonstrated that the drug had a negative effect on maternal behavior toward the pups (Šlamberová et al. 2005).

EFFECTS ON CHILDREN

When meth is used in a home where children reside, there are several routes of potential exposure and subsequent danger to the children. First, when there is active use in the home, the drug itself is frequently readily accessible to children, often lying on surfaces within easy reach of a curious child. Children display frequent hand-to-mouth behavior, placing them at risk for picking up the drug itself and ingesting it, resulting in a continuum of possible effects ranging from minor physiologic response to significant intoxication, seizures, and death. Although this is not an uncommon event, there are only a few such cases reported in the literature. In 1998 Kolecki reported 18 cases in which children less than 13 years of age were confirmed to be victims of oral methamphetamine poisoning. In these cases, the drugs had been left out with easy access for the children. The children displayed agitation (9), inconsolability (6), increased heart rate (18), abdominal pain, vomiting (6), seizures, muscle breakdown, fever (1), and ataxia (1). Prior to identification of the cause for the children's illness, multiple tests and treatments were undertaken such as head CTs (5), spinal taps (3), and administration of spider (*Centruroides sculpturatus*) antivenom (3), since the presentation closely resembled spider envenomation. In fact, one child developed an anaphylactic reaction to the antivenom (Kolecki 1998). Another case reported in 1995 by Gospe profiled the case of an 11-month-old boy who presented to medical care with irritability and transient cortical blindness and involuntary turning of the head and tested positive for meth. Symptoms resolved after 12 hours of supportive care. Mother reported that she had found the infant chewing on a small plastic bag (Gospe 1995). An additional case was reported by Narogka, who described a 13-month-old girl whose symptoms of restlessness and roving eye movements were initially felt to be from scorpion evenomation, but when she did not respond to antivenom, a urine drug screen was obtained and found to be positive for meth (Nagorka and Bergeson 1998).

Effects of exposures to meth through breastfeeding must also be considered. Meth, like most drugs, is transferred to the breast milk when a lactating mother uses the drug. Therefore, the American Academy of Pediatrics does not recommend breastfeeding when the mother is using meth, as it is believed that the infant will receive the drug through breast milk, and this has been reported to cause irritability and poor sleeping patterns (American Academy of Pediatrics, Committee on Drugs 2001).

At this time, there is not enough scientific data in the literature to fully understand the amount of exposure that a child may receive when living in an environment where meth is actively being smoked or used. There is no information on the potential for intake of the drug through transdermal absorption or passive inhalation. Research in this area is clearly needed.

CONCLUSION

Meth use and abuse in this country has far-reaching ramifications for not only the user but for society. While we currently understand a great deal about the medical effects of this drug on both adults and children, there is far more that needs to be studied. Additionally, the nature and extent of the effects on the user of the by-products and other chemicals that may remain in the meth following the manufacturing process are unknown at this time. The studies that are currently available have only addressed the effect of the actual drug. The National Institute of Drug Abuse (NIDA) is aggressively supporting a comprehensive research program to better understand meth's mechanism of action, physical and behavioral effects, risk and protective factors, treatments, and potential predictors of treatment success (Volkow 2005). Continued collaborative efforts are critical to advancements in understanding the medical effects of meth on the users and children who are exposed.

CHAPTER 5

The Environmental Cleanup of Methamphetamine Labs

Colleen Brisnehan, BS

INTRODUCTION

Methamphetamine labs are a growing problem throughout the United States. Dealing with properties contaminated by meth production has become a primary concern for many state and local regulatory agencies. The cleanup procedures discussed in this chapter are generally accepted practices for meth lab cleanup. However, the reader should be aware that state or local requirements may exist that differ from these procedures.

Typically, after a meth lab is discovered by law enforcement, meth lab–related chemicals and containers are removed. However, contamination is often left on surfaces and in absorbent materials, posing health concerns to persons exposed to them.

METH LAB CLEANUP STANDARDS

Several states and local agencies have established standards for meth lab cleanup (for example, Missouri Department of Health 2000; Washington Department of Health 1996). Authorities base most of these standards on an allowable concentration of meth detected in a surface wipe sample. These cleanup standards are not health-based, but are based on what is believed to be conservative and protective, detectable by laboratories, and achievable by cleanup contractors. While there are other chemicals of concern related to meth labs, using a meth-based cleanup standard is the most straightforward approach to determine the effectiveness of cleanup. Since common household products are often used in the drug-manufacturing process, distinguishing between meth lab–derived and legally used products can be very difficult. The rationale used to support the use of meth concentration as an indication of cleanup effectiveness is based on the assumption that if a cleanup is thorough enough to reduce the concentrations of meth, it should also be adequate to reduce the concentrations of other meth lab–related chemicals to protective levels.

Although numerous states have adopted cleanup standards for meth, until recently, none had tried to correlate these cleanup standards to concentrations with known health effects. The Colorado Department of Public Health and Environment recently performed such an evaluation in order to support the selection of a cleanup standard for meth (Colorado Department of Public Health and Environment, 2003, 2005). This evaluation focused on reconciling what is known about meth health effects with those levels currently being used as cleanup standards in other states. Three technology-based standards currently being used as meth cleanup standards were evaluated, 0.5 ug/100 cm^2, 0.1 ug/100 cm^2, and 0.05 ug/100 cm^2. Exposure estimates were made for three categories of individuals: infant (age 1), child (age 6), and adult female (childbearing age). The exposure calculations were used to estimate a high-end or reasonable maximum exposure to the individuals of concern. The exposure calculations resulted in the infant being predicted to receive the highest daily dose of meth on a body-weight basis.

Exposure estimates were then compared to what is known about the health effects of meth. This included an evaluation of the therapeutic use of Desoxyn (methamphetamine hydrochloride tablets, USP) and illicit use. Laboratory studies assessing neurotoxicity, developmental toxicity, and reproductive toxicity were also evaluated. This information was used to derive reference dose (RfD) values, or health-based intakes, that are protective of neurological, reproductive, and developmental effects for sensitive individuals in a population. The RfDs were then compared to the intakes (doses) that an infant would be expected to receive following cleanup to each of the three technology-based standards evaluated.

The comparison showed that each of the technology-based cleanup standards would be protective of residents of former drug laboratories. The estimated level of protectiveness ranges from 10- to 100-fold at cleanup concentrations of 0.5 ug/100 cm^2 and 0.05 ug/100 cm^2, respectively. It is important to recognize that the exposure calculations are based on a number of assumptions, and that these assumptions introduce uncertainty into the dose estimates. In many cases, these assumptions are intentionally conservative, meaning that they are more likely to lead to an overestimate of exposure than to an underestimate. However, some assumptions can result in an underestimation of exposure, and in other cases, it is not possible to judge whether an assumption is more likely to overestimate or underestimate exposure. Decisions regarding how a cleanup standard should be applied may allow for an extra measure of protectiveness and can help account for some of the uncertainties that are inherent in the process. For instance, by applying a cleanup standard as a "not to exceed" standard, the average concentration of meth that may be present after cleanup would be anticipated to be lower than the cleanup standard itself. Therefore, estimated doses based on exposure at concentrations equivalent to the cleanup standard will tend to be conservative.

METH LAB CLEANUP

A number of state and local agencies require cleanup of properties contaminated by meth lab activities. In addition, many states are in the process of developing requirements for cleanup. However, there are still many areas across the country where no requirements exist. The specific requirements of meth lab cleanup programs vary from state to state, with some being implemented by a state regulatory agency, and some on a local level.

Some local agencies require cleanup actions using the statutory authority to address nuisances, which either empower local boards of health to abate public health nuisances or deal with abatement of a public nuisance. Some local health departments coordinate with building departments to initiate and require the cleanup of the property and to not allow reoccupancy until cleanup standards are met as determined by the health officer. Whether this approach is possible in an area depends on what has been adopted into local ordinances. The general phases for a meth lab cleanup are outlined in the following sections.

Phase 1: Preliminary Assessment of Meth Lab Properties

Prior to beginning the cleanup of a former meth lab, a preliminary assessment should be conducted to determine what chemicals are involved, the manufacturing method used, and whether the property is fit or unfit for use. There are many meth "recipes" and manufacturing methods. Identifying the chemicals used will help to determine what kind of chemical sampling may be necessary.

Potential areas of meth lab contamination can be divided into primary and secondary areas. Typical primary areas of contamination include "cooking" areas, chemical disposal areas, and chemical storage areas. Contamination in "cooking" areas is primarily caused by chemical fumes and gases created during the heating and distilling portions of the "cooking" process, but may also be caused by spills, boil-overs, or explosions. All surfaces and materials in the vicinity of "cooking" areas are affected, including floors, walls, ceilings, working surfaces, furniture, carpeting, draperies and other textile products, and heating and air-conditioning vents. Indoor disposal areas include sinks, toilets, bathtubs, plumbing traps, and floor drains. Contamination in chemical storage areas may be caused by leaks, spills, or open containers. Outdoor cooking areas could involve picnic tables, camping stoves, or other outdoor areas where cooking could occur. Outdoor disposal areas may include soil, surface water, groundwater, dumpsters, sewer or storm systems, septic systems, and cesspools.

Secondary areas of contamination may include locations where contamination has migrated, such as hallways or high-traffic areas, common areas in multiple-dwelling structures and adjacent apartments or rooms, and common ventilation or plumbing systems in hotels and multiple dwellings. It is important that these secondary areas of contamination be evaluated during the preliminary assessment, and if necessary, cleaned in the same manner as primary areas of contamination.

Phase 2: Cleanup Procedures for Contaminated Structures

During the meth cooking process, vapors and particulates are given off that deposit on nearby surfaces and can be absorbed by porous materials. Chemical spills and careless handling of meth lab supplies and equipment can also cause contamination. Because of the potential for adverse exposures to meth lab–related chemicals, the cleanup of former meth labs should be conducted by properly trained and equipped individuals in accordance with any state and/or local requirements.

Prior to beginning cleanup of a structure, the indoor air should be field screened for volatile organic compounds (VOCs) to determine the concentration of total VOCs in the structure, which is important for monitoring exposures for worker protection. Field screening may also provide information regarding the severity of contamination and the areas to focus cleanup efforts.

Contaminated nonporous and semiporous surfaces should be thoroughly cleaned using a detergent water solution. Methanol and isopropyl alcohol may also be used, but should only be used in a well-ventilated area, and with appropriate protective equipment. Used wash-water should be properly disposed of, or it may be possible to discharge the wash-water into the sanitary sewer with approval from the local publicly owned treatment works (POTW). If a surface has visible contamination or staining, complete removal and replacement of that surface is recommended.

Some contaminated porous materials can be safely washed, or cleaned by other methods, if they exhibit little to no odor or staining. Stained materials or those with odors should be disposed of. If contaminated materials are not disposed of, the effectiveness of cleaning should be verified through sampling to ensure that concentrations of chemicals have been reduced to acceptable cleanup levels. In general, cleaning and sampling costs for these items may exceed replacement costs. If meth lab–contaminated materials are to be disposed of, the landfill should be notified of the meth lab contamination so that proper measures can be taken to ensure that it is handled appropriately.

In cases of severe contamination, or when the cost of cleanup exceeds the cost of the structure, effective cleanup may be accomplished by demolition of the contaminated structure. Debris from the demolition can be disposed of at a solid waste landfill. Prior to disposal, the landfill should be notified that the waste stream is from a former meth lab so that proper measures can be taken to handle it appropriately.

Encapsulation or Sealing

Nonporous and semiporous surfaces, such as walls, flooring, and ceilings, can be painted with an oil-based paint, epoxy, or other material suitable to create a physical barrier capable of preventing contact with or volatilization of contaminants. This procedure is often referred to as encapsulation. Some states allow encapsulation of contaminants in lieu of reducing contaminant concentrations to cleanup levels. In most cases, the surface to be encapsulated is first cleaned to reduce the concentrations of contaminants that will be left behind. There is currently no data to support the long-term effectiveness of encapsulation, and in most cases long-term monitoring and maintenance of encapsulated surfaces is not required. In addition, there are some theories and anecdotal information circulating that suggest encapsulants, such as paint, may actually act as a "wick" that draws contaminants to the surface over time. Therefore, because of the uncertainties regarding the long-term protectiveness of encapsulating contamination, some states use a more conservative approach in which cleanup levels must be achieved prior to encapsulation. In this scenario, encapsulation may add an additional measure of protectiveness, yet does not require long-term maintenance to remain protective.

Ventilation Systems

Ventilation systems tend to collect fumes and dust and redistribute them throughout a structure. The vents, ductwork, filters, and even the walls and ceilings near ventilation ducts can become contaminated. All air filters in the system should be replaced, vents should be removed and cleaned, the system's ductwork should be cleaned, and surfaces near inlets and outlets should be cleaned. In motels, apartments, or multiple-family dwellings, a ventilation system may serve more than one unit or structure. These connections must be considered when evaluating cleanup and testing procedures. One strategy is to take samples from adjacent or connected areas or units, working outward from the lab site until samples show low levels or no contamination.

Plumbing and Septic Systems

Waste products generated during meth manufacturing are often dumped down sinks, drains, and toilets. These waste products can collect in drains, traps, and septic tanks, and can give off fumes. If staining is noted around sinks, toilets, or tubs, or if a strong chemical odor is coming from household plumbing, the plumbing system should be flushed with generous amounts of water to reduce the concentration of residual chemicals.

If contamination of a septic tank or leach field is suspected, the local health department or environmental health service agency should be contacted to determine if the local regulations address such an issue. If meth lab chemicals are present, the contents of the tank should be tested and disposed of as either a solid or hazardous waste, based on the results of chemical analysis. Analysis of the septic tank contents should be based on chemicals determined to be part of the lab site chemical inventory during the preliminary assessment.

Personal Belongings

If residents of the structure need to remove personal items, they should do so only after the items have been properly decontaminated. As with household items, personal items that are visibly stained are hard to clean and may need to be disposed of. Items such as clothing that are not visibly stained can be laundered one or more times to remove any residual chemicals. Nonporous and semiporous items should be decontaminated using a detergent water wash or similar cleaning method. The effectiveness of cleaning should be verified through sampling to ensure that concentrations of chemicals have been reduced to acceptable cleanup levels.

There may be instances where the owner of the real property is not the owner of the personal property that has been contaminated by meth lab chemicals. Examples include rental properties, apartments, and hotels. In these cases, the owner of the real property will most likely not want to pay to have the personal property decontaminated. However, it may be necessary for the real property owner to go through an eviction process to legally dispose of a tenant's personal property. In addition, it may not be possible for the landlord to prevent the tenant from removing their personal property without prior decontamination. This issue of contaminated personal property may be addressed differently in different states or local jurisdictions; therefore, it is best to check with the regulatory agency overseeing cleanup to determine local requirements.

POST-CLEANUP ASSESSMENT FOR STRUCTURES

After cleanup has been conducted, small amounts of residual chemicals may remain. Post-cleanup sampling should be conducted to ensure that cleanup levels have been met. This assessment should include sampling for meth residues on surfaces using a wipe sample. Sampling of former meth labs should be conducted under the supervision of a properly qualified individual and in accordance with any state and/or local requirement.

Decisions regarding the number and location of samples to be collected can be made based on the preliminary assessment information, chemicals used and duration of lab operation, the apparent extent and severity of contamination, and professional judgment. In areas where the preliminary assessment indicates low contaminant levels or no contamination, sampling alone may be used to demonstrate that contamination does not exceed cleanup levels. In areas with low levels of contamination, cleanup may be done with limited post-cleanup sampling, based on adjacent sampling results and best professional judgment. In areas of moderate to heavy contamination, cleanup may be carried out without previous sampling if post-cleanup sampling will be conducted. On surfaces that are going to be encapsulated, sampling should be conducted either before the encapsulant is applied, or after it has cured. The decision regarding whether to sample before or after encapsulation should be determined based on state and/or local requirements and best professional judgment.

Wipe samples of nonporous and semiporous surfaces will indicate levels of contamination remaining on those surfaces. Pre-cleaning samples from these surfaces may also provide an indication of the contamination in/on adjacent porous materials. However, post-cleanup sampling of nonporous and semiporous surfaces should *not* be used to as an indication of contaminant concentrations remaining in/on adjacent porous materials. If these porous materials are not disposed of, they should be sampled to determine if contaminant concentrations have been reduced to acceptable levels.

If the phenyl-2-propanone (P2P) method of meth manufacturing was used, testing should also include airborne mercury and lead, and surface sampling for lead. If these compounds are tested for, keep in mind that the possibility of obtaining false positives for lead and mercury exists because these materials were once commonly added to paints. Homes built before 1978 may test positive for lead, and homes built before 1990 may test positive for mercury.

Written documentation showing that the cleanup has been completed should be submitted to the state or local agency overseeing the cleanup. The final report should summarize information obtained during the preliminary assessment, cleanup activities performed, and present data collected during the post-cleanup assessment. The oversight agency may review the report and determine whether the property is suitable for reoccupancy.

CLEANUP PROCEDURES FOR SOIL, GROUNDWATER, AND SURFACE WATER

If areas of potential outdoor contamination are identified or suspected, investigation of outdoor contamination may be necessary. Typically, the state or local agency that has authority over hazardous waste cleanups will be involved in the investigation and/or cleanup of outdoor contamination from meth labs.

It is important to tie the assessment of outdoor contamination to information regarding meth production, chemical storage, and waste disposal, to ensure that assessment efforts look for potential contaminants in the places they are likely to be. This type of information can be gathered from observations made by law enforcement or emergency response personnel, or by conducting a site tour to note the property's condition, looking for evidence of contamination such as stained soil or stressed (dead or dying) vegetation. Sampling and analytical procedures should be based on chemicals determined to be part of the lab site chemical inventory during the preliminary assessment.

Both natural features and man-made structures should be evaluated, including drainage systems, local topography, utilities, surface water bodies, easements, and locations of buildings, because these features can influence the migration of contaminants and restrict access to portions of the site during cleanup efforts. This information is used in conjunction with information regarding the subsurface characteristics at the site to evaluate contaminant migration pathways.

Small areas of outdoor contamination may be dealt with by removal or treatment of contaminated soils or water (such as small areas of ponded water). Contaminated soil or water removed from the site must be characterized to determine if it contains a characteristic or listed hazardous waste and must be disposed of at an appropriately licensed solid or hazardous waste disposal facility. Analysis should be based on the lab site chemical inventory and the manufacturing method used. If large areas of soil, surface water, or groundwater contamination are present, characterization and cleanup of these areas should be conducted by a professional environmental contractor, in consultation with the state or local agency with authority to oversee such cleanups. State or local authorities should also be consulted to determine appropriate cleanup levels for soil, groundwater, and surface water.

PART III

Case Management and Treatment for Methamphetamine Use— Does Anything Work?

Methamphetamine users pose unique issues for communities and responding agencies. Given the power of the drug, public agencies sometimes have to remove children from the home. In addition, before children can safely return home, the parents or guardians must have favorably addressed their addiction and abuse issues. The chapters in this part will provide guidance on how to understand and address meth use. How professionals manage these cases and answer difficult questions, such as when it is safe to return a child home or when an abuser has been "cured" will be addressed in this section.

A second topic addressed is the assessment and treatment of meth abuse and addiction. Professionals need to know the extent to which a meth abuser is using and the degree of addiction. This section covers assessment, patterns of use, and treatment approaches to abuse. Insights into what approaches work best are included as well as how to integrate the ex-user back into the community and family.

These chapters describe case management strategies for meth-involved families, treatment approaches, child welfare considerations, and statements from people who have used or had family members use meth.

Karen Mooney's chapter 6 on case planning for meth-involved families and users offers information on case management from the time children are removed from the homes of meth users, those making it, or both. Currently case managers and child protection intake and ongoing workers have little guidance on how to handle meth-involved families and children. This chapter covers what processes are unique and similar to general best-practice case management. It also covers realistic time frames for case managers regarding case progress.

This chapter also provides information on the observable patterns of use and the symptoms of use to help guide professionals, such as caseworkers, court representatives, and therapists. The purpose is to give the reader information on the signs of the degree of use and continued use of meth. What should a child protection caseworker, addictions specialist, court officer, or other professional look at to determine if use is occurring and to what degree?

Dr. Nicolas Taylor has had several years of experience working with meth-involved patients and their families. In chapter 7 on the assessment of needs and treatment of meth users, he describes how to assess the degree of meth abuse and the treatment needs of users. In addition, the chapter describes the various ways to address meth addiction. What intervention strategies work and why? What strategies are likely not to work and why not? With approximately 117,000 treatment admissions of persons with a primary meth use problem in 2003, these questions are critical (SAMHSA 2005a).

For years, Dr. Richard Rawson and his colleagues have been at the forefront of research on meth and stimulant treatment. Chapter 8 presents findings from a multisite study on treatment for meth addiction. It is one of the earliest comparison studies of meth treatment efficacy. Rawson's and other research indicates that treatment can be effective for most meth addicts. Rawson and his colleagues have pioneered research and practice in the area of meth use and treatment. This chapter represents a classic contribution to treatment and research.

Chapter 9 addresses child welfare issues and practices related to meth-involved families and children. The chapter describes important child welfare considerations at the referral, investigation, assessment, and ongoing case-work stages. The chapter also touches on some of the legal issues and important legal questions that may arise. Chapter 9 describes what law enforcement, social services, child protection, and other first responders can expect when initially coming into contact with labs and meth-involved parents or caregivers. What does exposure to the chemicals used in making meth do to children and others? The focus of this chapter is on how to treat and respond to children and older relatives who may be living in the same location as the meth lab. For example, how do you handle the removal of children from the home? How does one explain the decontamination process to small children, with the accompanying sense of loss of personal items and relatives?

Chapter 10 provides a personal account of one ex-user's experiences with being addicted to meth. Tonya's chapter demonstrates the power of this drug over the user's life. She shares her experiences with disruption, chaos, manipulation, and the other crazy aspects of chronic meth use. It also describes how she changed, what worked, and how professionals should help the addicted user.

Samantha's story in chapter 11 is a chilling first-person account of a teenager's involvement with meth at an early age and the people with whom she associated. In vivid detail, she describes the serious risks she took while using. Her story illustrates how meth use and the criminal behavior that is associated with use overcame her life and almost destroyed her. In recovery now, Samantha is moving on with her life in several positive directions.

Chapter 12 presents a mother's point of view regarding her daughter's (Samantha in chapter 11) use of meth. Samantha credits her life to her mother's dedication to helping her and never giving up. The combination of having both a daughter's and mother's point of view on the same issue provides a wonderful opportunity to understand how disruptive this drug can be to families. As destructive as it was for this family, the result for daughter and mother ends on a high note.

What we gather from these chapters is that treatment, when combined with sound case management and the desire of the user to change, can work. Treatment for meth dependency can be as effective as treatment for any other drug dependency (Luchansky 2003; Stark 2004). The view that once an addiction develops, meth addicts can never recover is a myth.

CHAPTER 6

Case Management with Parents Affected by Methamphetamine Addiction

Karen Mooney, LCSW

INTRODUCTION

This chapter provides an overview of issues related to the provision of case management services to parents of children found living in methamphetamine lab environments. Issues related to child safety and risk, although critically important, are dealt with at the appropriate level of detail in many child welfare textbooks, Web sites, and trainings (for many useful resources, refer to the Web site of the Administration for Children and Families of the United States Department of Health and Human Services at www.acf.hhs.gov, as well as to the National Center on Substance Abuse and Child Welfare at www.ncsacw.samhsa.gov/). The following provides a framework to help shape a case management perspective with parents affected by meth addiction. The chapter includes a checklist to assist the practitioner to remember a few key points.

Families affected by meth addiction have a large number of needs to be addressed if they are to function again (or for the first time) as families. The devastation wrought by many forms of addiction in families stands out in bold relief in the cases we see in the media. The media frequently highlights parents that have abandoned their children to their addictions to meth, sometimes exposing them to life-threatening situations in homes with the toxic chemicals and unsavory activities. At other times the media stresses parents and guardians who leave children to fend for themselves emotionally, physically, and mentally without money, clothes, food, education, and medical care. The chemical nature of meth, with its long half-life and easy access, renders some of these deficits particularly dramatic. At the same time, we must remember that addiction to other substances can be equally devastating for the children of addicted parents. It is not only the drug itself that produces high-risk living situations for children, but also the family's other resources, or lack thereof, that may serve to remediate or exacerbate some of the damage.

Case management services are critically important in helping families with multiple needs. It is assumed here that the reader sees and appreciates the value in helping these families. Children can be removed from homes in which meth manufacture and addiction are present; however, it may not be a foregone conclusion that the best solution for their situations is adoption into new families. Addicted parents can attain recovery, even when their primary drug is meth. Child welfare professionals frequently recognize the desires of their child clients to be with their own parents and understand that the best way to help these children is to help their parents. A commitment to, and provision of, good case management services can help to accomplish this goal. When good case management services have been provided but family reunification fails to occur, at least the professional team involved (including the family) can say that they did the best they could.

DEFINITION OF CASE MANAGEMENT

Perhaps the most helpful place to start this description of case management services with families affected by meth addiction is to define what we mean by case management. For the purpose of this chapter, we will assume that the case manager is a child welfare worker. Child welfare caseworkers play a significant case management role in the lives of their clients, brokering and advocating for services to remedy the conditions that bring the families they serve into the system.

The term case management has different meanings in different settings; within a health-care context, case management refers to coordination of services and funding sources and is often carried out by someone with a nursing background. Look up "case management" on Google, and one of the first Web sites you will find is one operated by the Society of Case Management, which is devoted to medical case management. Other sources of information on the practice of case management can be found in schools of social work. Foundation-year curricula frequently devote some attention to different social work roles, which apply to the practice of case management, such as broker, advocate, conferee, and mediator (see Woodside and McClam 2002, for further discussions of these and other roles). The Center for Substance Abuse Treatment (1998) devoted an entire publication, *Treatment Improvement Protocol Series 27* to the practice of case management for substance abuse treatment. This publication serves as an excellent introduction to this topic area for substance abuse counselors and others working with clients with addiction issues.

More recently, the National Trauma Consortium, through its participation in the SAMHSA's five-year *Women and Violence* study, moved away from the term "case management" because of its implication that a person with multiple service needs is labeled as a "case," and toward the term "resource coordination and advocacy," which more specifically describes the activity without the implied derogatory label (Moses et al. 2003).

One additional clarification before we move forward into a specific discussion of which resources need coordinating and what sort of advocacy is required with families affected by meth addiction is to make the distinction as to who is considered to be the client in this situation. In families in which the adult caretakers within the family have been involved in manufacturing meth and have endangered their children through this activity, the client at first is the child who is to be removed from the dangerous situation and who is the recipient of medical, emotional, and physical care to assure health and healing from the traumatic and dangerous environment in which she or he has been living. Following the initial removal or rescue, however, it is necessary to assess whether or not it is feasible to seek reunification between parent and child. In cases in which reunification can be explored, services must be provided to the parent in order to ascertain whether or not the family can be reunified. In this case, the terms "child-centered and family-focused," which describe the theoretical orientation currently being used by child welfare agencies, come into play. These terms also give a voice to the value embraced by most child welfare agencies that children are best cared for within their own families whenever possible.

The idea that families can be reunified when one or both parents have been active in meth use or manufacture activities is one that many professionals outside the addiction field now doubt. The notion that treatment for meth addiction is not effective is widespread among the lay population and has spread to policymakers and decision maker in many states, despite literature from within the addiction field that documents the effectiveness of treatment for addiction to this drug (Hser et al. 2005; Rawson et al. 2004). Meth addiction has become particularly stigmatized due to the portrayals in the media of the level of squalor and violence associated with the manufacture of the drug, as well as the socioeconomic status most commonly ascribed to its users. As is common when the media's attention is attracted, it is commonly described as "the most addictive drug," "the most destructive drug," or "the worst drug," and we forget that at different points in time, crack cocaine, alcohol, and even marijuana were described in those same terms. Tobacco, a substance that is blamed for approximately 438,000 deaths per year in the United States, is rarely mentioned in this vein (Centers for Disease Control 2005a).

To advocate effectively for appropriate services and resources to be provided to a family, a case manager must be able to put the different messages about meth into the appropriate context and must be able to impart hope to the family that things can get better and that the drug they have used does not render their situation hopeless. Recovery from addiction to meth is hard work and requires significant amounts of social support and encouragement over long periods of time. Change is incremental, and the process of coming to terms with one's past behavior can be very painful. But recovery is possible, and many people achieve it, even when during the active phase of the addiction it seems impossible to reach. A case manager must carry this message to the clients and can act as cheerleader and coach at times, even though other professionals may falter in their support of the family's efforts.

CASE MANAGEMENT ACTIVITIES

TIP 27: Comprehensive Case Management for Substance Abuse Treatment or *TIP 27*, details at great length the various skills and knowledge needed to carry out effective case management activities with and on behalf of clients involved in addiction treatment (Center for Substance Abuse Treatment 1998). Case management can occur on any of three different levels: within a single agency, across several agencies on an informal basis, or as a part of work among a formal consortium of agencies. Child welfare caseworkers may provide case management services at all three of these levels.

Case management within a single agency takes place when the caseworker brokers services from different parts of the same agency. This could take place within the context of a social service agency in a rural area, in which the social services agency is the only service provider with whom the client may interact, whether due to a paucity of community resources or due to lack of needed services that are accessible to the client. An example of this would be a family in which children are placed in kinship care across town from where the parents live while the family home is being cleaned of toxic meth manufacturing by-products. The social service agency might have access to housing resources as well as medical assistance for the children and may have children's mental health services co-located on site at the social service office. These different programs are all available under one roof and may all answer to the same executive director. In this situation, case management consists of coordinating resources across these programs.

Case management across several agencies on an informal basis might occur in instances in which a child welfare caseworker has several agencies with which to work, but no formal arrangements exist that would determine who has the ultimate responsibility for providing or carrying out service activities. In this case, numerous assumptions drive the delivery of services, based upon each agency's view of its own role in the lives of its clients. An example of this situation might be one in which there are a few service providers available—perhaps a mental health center that provides both addiction and mental health treatment, as well as mental health treatment for the child in the form of play therapy, and a community domestic violence treatment provider. A common dynamic here would be one in which the mental health center staff view the addiction to meth as a symptom of an underlying mental health problem (post-traumatic stress disorder due to a history of domestic violence) for the mother. The mental health center might not choose to provide the opportunity for the clients to provide urine samples to verify abstinence from substance use, viewing this as a correctional rather than a therapeutic function, thus requiring the caseworker to make other arrangements for abstinence monitoring. The caseworker would need to arrange for urinalysis testing and counseling for domestic violence with other community providers. Case management within the context of a consortium requires that roles and responsibilities of each agency and service provider are spelled out. As stated in *TIP 27*, this third scenario requires significant attention be paid to communication among the agencies involved, and sometimes this allows for less time to be spent on the needs of the clients (Center for Substance Abuse Treatment 1998). Here, the child welfare caseworker would be seen as having responsibility for coordination of services, but each provider would also be included in the decision-making process (such as decisions about risk of abuse or neglect, appropriateness of the services delivered, or whether to increase or decrease visitation), because of the information and perspective allowed by each discipline. This third arrangement takes advantage of the knowledge base of each service provider and allows, when functioning correctly, for decisions based upon multiple sources and types of information.

SKILLS REQUIRED FOR EFFECTIVE CASE MANAGEMENT

Perhaps the most important skill for a case manager is the ability to form effective cooperative relationships with families to engage and retain them in the change process. The ability to listen, ask clarifying questions, and elicit from clients their own goal statements as these relate to their parenting allows the goals being worked on to represent the wishes and desires of the clients. Skills required for this component of case management include motivational interviewing (Miller and Rollnick 1991), as well as contracting and planning for services.

Also critical for effective case management is an understanding of the different funding sources to pay for services, as well as of the mandates that come with these different sources. Sometimes these mandates can serve as barriers to effective collaboration. It is much easier to have an effective working relationship across disciplines when each partner understands the mandates under which the others operate. This prevents perceptions that those who cannot do particular things under their system's regulations are not simply being stubborn or unresponsive. One common barrier encountered by professionals working with substance abuse treatment agencies is the Federal Confidentiality Statute (42 CFR Part 2). This statute restricts and defines how and what substance abuse information can be disclosed to whom and under what circumstances. Helpful protocols when working with substance abuse treatment agencies include ways in which to obtain from clients properly executed signed releases of information. One example of this would be a social services agency that has blank release of information forms from each community substance abuse treatment agency available for clients to sign, to facilitate necessary exchanges of information.

In addition, critical to the success of a case manager is the ability to foster relationships with individuals in different systems. Knowing whom to call to get information or make treatment referrals is critical—sometimes informal relationships can allow a case manager to negotiate big systems better than going through proper channels. It is important to know when to use informal relationships and when to use formal channels, however. One way to foster these relationships is to use the traditional sales technique of never telling the customer no. The case managers should always respond to requests for information with information, if not the requested information then a suggestion as to where this might be available. This will keep communication channels open and assure that other requests and exchanges of information will happen.

KNOWLEDGE BASE FOR EFFECTIVE CASE MANAGEMENT

To work effectively with people with meth addiction issues, it is critical to understand how treatment and recovery work. A basic understanding of the different theory bases upon which addiction treatment is predicated will do a lot to help the case manager understand what her clients are saying about their experiences in treatment and can help to reinforce key concepts as they come up. As case managers also see clients in a variety of settings—in their homes and in the community—ample opportunities for the discussion of relapse and relapse prevention present themselves along the way. Participation in recreational and social activities that do not revolve around substance use are also a key component of treatment; this can be reinforced by case management plans to include and foster these activities.

In addition to a thorough familiarity with treatment principles, case managers must understand family dynamics and recovery, which are critical to the success of the client in early recovery. Children react in a variety of ways to their parents' progress in recovery, and it is helpful when the case manager understands this and can normalize it for the client. Children commonly experience considerable fear, anger, and sadness during the time they are living with their addicted parents and generally have no outlet for expression of these feelings. When parents enter recovery, the children's feelings remain powerful and can be difficult for newly sober parents to deal with.

Case managers' knowledge about available community resources is also critical to the provision of successful case management services. The skills required to establish and foster relationships with community nonprofit, charitable, and faith-based organizations are the same professional relationship skills required for other case management activities. Knowledge of funding mandates and participation requirements for different forms of social service programming can assist the case manager to broker appropriate resources for the family and can help to make the best match between a service agency and the client. Many case managers have resource binders they have put together with information about various services available in their communities. For a very helpful, in-depth treatment of case management within a child welfare practice setting, the reader is referred to *Helping in Child Protective Services*, 2nd Ed. (Brittain and Hunt 2004).

ATTITUDES REQUIRED FOR EFFECTIVE CASE MANAGEMENT

As stated in the introduction to this chapter, the most helpful attitude for a case manager to take with clients affected by meth addiction is one of support and caring. Values inherent to the practice of motivational interviewing, which call for a client-centered, counselor-directed interaction, provide for an attitude of mutual respect and carefully earned trust, which in turn elicits motivation for change from the client. This stance toward provision of services may seem to run counter to the practice of most social service agencies, which can foster caseworker and court-driven agendas with which the client must either comply or have parental rights terminated. Such approaches may appear effective, especially in the short term; however, much damage can be done to families and children through such activities. Recognition of this damage led to the development of the Homebuilders Model of family preservation services in the mid-1990s; however, alarm regarding the dangers of meth addiction and manufacture has now led many social services agencies away from this philosophy.

In keeping with the philosophy of family preservation, families must be seen as the best experts regarding their circumstances. It may be tempting to adopt a correctional approach to meth-addicted families (after all, use and manufacture of meth are illegal activities), which then drives a punishment-based approach to dealing with their problems. Unfortunately, though it has long been recognized in the field of addiction treatment that punishment is an ineffective way to stop substance abuse (otherwise the jails and prisons now full of people with substance-related problems would be turning out clean and sober model citizens), many professionals outside of the addiction treatment field do not have the experience to recognize the futility of this approach.

CASE MANAGEMENT ROLES

As mentioned above, case managers can play a variety of roles in working with families. Perhaps the most common of these, particularly within the context of child welfare practice, is that of broker—linking clients to needed services. With parents addicted to meth, substance abuse treatment is critical. In making referrals to substance abuse treatment providers, case managers can facilitate engagement and retention in treatment if they are prepared to align with the treatment program to which they are referring their clients. Providing as much information as possible about the client and the situation that brings them into contact with the child welfare agency assists the substance abuse counselor to formulate a more accurate assessment of the client's strengths and challenges and to tailor treatment to meet the client's needs. Too often, clients are referred to treatment with no collateral information being provided, which leaves the counselors to try to figure out on their own information that the caseworker had all along. This can lead to fragmented delivery of services, which slows the treatment process dramatically and discourages both clients and professionals.

Linkage to other resources is also very important. Treatment is much less likely to be effective if families have no place to live, if they have no access to transportation or medical care, and if there are few opportunities for them to engage in activities without the use of drugs or alcohol. Often, people who have been addicted to meth have been living in a subculture from which they need to disengage in order to enter recovery. In these situations, groups such as Crystal Meth Anonymous can be very helpful, because they provide both a sober social outlet and role models in others who have made it into recovery.

Sometimes the case manager serves as an advocate. The stigma that addiction to meth carries with it can be very difficult to face, especially for someone newly in recovery. Employers may be reluctant to hire people in recovery, particularly when their primary drug has been meth, and there are criminal records to consider. In larger communities, there are employers and treatment providers who have worked together to arrange enough structure in the workplace to support those who are trying to pull their lives together despite these histories. Many county Temporary Aid to Needy Families (TANF) offices have experience in working with clients in these situations and can offer guidance and assistance.

Similarly, school personnel, guardians ad litem, landlords, and others may express negative views of people who have used meth. Some clients, especially at first, may need and appreciate support when interacting with people in these roles to help them to form relationships that will last long past the case manager's involvement in their lives. People in recovery from meth addiction may find that some people question their ability to remain abstinent from drug use because they have heard and give credence to the notion that it is impossible to quit using meth. In this case, a case manager can advocate by providing accurate, science-based information about meth addiction and treatment to counteract this misinformation.

Sometimes conversations between case managers and clients about the family's progress toward sobriety and reunification with children become impromptu counseling sessions. It is at these times that the case manager's listening and reflection skills become very important in moving the progress of the case along. If a mutual trust is established early in the case management relationship, the case manager's knowledge base and skills can be frequently called into play. A mother who is beginning her substance abuse treatment may have doubts about whether or not she can be successful; a case manager who knows that these misgivings are

Figure 6.1
Case Management Checklist

Case Management Checklist:

___ Client's current living situation.

___Contact information of someone who will know client's whereabouts in case

above contact information becomes invalid? (Remember to get a signed release of

information for this person!)

___ Needs documented:

    ___Immediate safety needs (is client in physical or emotional danger?)

    ___Housing

    ___Food

    ___Medical needs

    ___Dental needs

    ___Children

        Names, ages?

        Location?

        Available, allowed to visit?

        Protective orders?

        Next court hearing date/type?

___ All collateral case information shared with substance abuse counselor with

referral

---

common and that depression almost always accompanies early abstinence from meth use can help to reassure her client that these feelings are normal and that they do not mean that she will not be successful. These messages must be readily available from all of the professionals in this mother's life, and not just from her substance abuse counselor.

HARD SERVICES AND LINKAGES TO OTHER SYSTEMS

Now that we've discussed activities, attitudes, knowledge, roles, and skills necessary to work with parents affected by meth addiction, let us turn our attention to their particular needs. The term "hard services" refers to concrete, tangible needs that people have and must have met in order to live. Referrals to food banks, soup kitchens, and the like can meet short-term needs for food. Linkage to the local food stamp office can provide a longer-term solution, if clients are eligible for those services. Needs for shelter can also be dire, especially for those who have left their residences due to the toxic residues left over from meth-manufacturing activities. It is very difficult to be successful in substance abuse treatment without access to food and shelter. If parents retain custody of their children, the need for clean clothing, diapers, and developmentally appropriate playthings for the children would also be considered hard services.

Linkages to other systems (besides child welfare and substance abuse treatment) can assist clients in meeting other needs that they might have. Appropriate child care is critical in assisting parents to attend substance abuse treatment, as well as other required appointments such as court hearings, mental health appointments, and medical appointments. When parents are trying to put their lives back together again as sober people in recovery, they have many additional service needs, such as mental health, nutrition, medical and dental services, and frequently domestic violence treatment. One promising practice that has emerged has been the development of systems of care within communities that formalize the communications and functions of community service providers so that families have easier access to services to meet their needs. For more information, see the Administration for Children and Families Web site at nccanch.acf.hhs.gov/profess/systems/index.cfm.

CHAPTER 7

Community-Based Treatment for Methamphetamine Addiction

Nicolas Taylor, Ph.D.

> Nothing is as simple as we hope it will be.
>
> *—Jim Horning*

To say that addiction to methamphetamine is a complicated problem is an understatement. Across the country (and now even throughout the world), treatment providers and human service professionals alike are discovering the complex web of behavioral disruption, criminal lifestyles, collusive and insidious relationships, neurological damage, and psychological mayhem that characterize the overall picture of a meth-using community (Anglin et al. 2000). However, complex problems don't always require complex solutions; but they do require solutions of some kind. Community awareness, with perhaps the exception of first responders in law enforcement, lags months, even years, behind actual community problems. Because of the nocturnal and underground nature of the meth community, general awareness of the chaos of the "crystal kingdom" can often go unrealized until it has spread like a cancer through a community and has started to dangerously affect innocent victims like children of meth users and victims of property crimes, theft, check fraud, identity fraud, and damaged rental properties; to say nothing about public exposure to environmental toxins because of local meth production.

Perhaps the most vulnerable population in the community is its adolescent young women who, either because their parents are too busy to be involved enough in their lives to know what is happening to them or because their parents are meth users themselves, are enticed deep into the dark underbelly of the meth-using community by promises of romance from older men, slender figures, unrestrained energy, and an endless high that pot using or just drinking can't match and that other teenagers will never achieve or appreciate.

Meth was great! I loved it from the first time [41-year-old boyfriend] got me high. It was cheaper than pot and easier to get than alcohol. Plus it kept me thin, and I know that made him happy.

—16-year-old female meth user

The complexity of meth addiction and "the speed of speed" (meaning how quickly use of this drug acts to completely disrupt the life of a user and how quickly it spreads through an unsuspecting community) make community responses reactive for those who do attempt to address the problem. First solutions always involve a law enforcement response, mainly because, as was mentioned, they are the first to find out about it. Dutiful peacekeepers do what they know how to do best. That is, they find those who perpetrate crimes and arrest them so a just legal system can balance their "debt to society" with a rehabilitative effort so that the person does not return to the criminal behavior. Very quickly, however, the inadequacy of these solutions becomes apparent as law enforcement officers and judicial leaders alike become frustrated when they see the same people again and again. It is as if the users don't learn their lesson, or as if the kinds of tools that work to teach other people their lesson don't seem to work with this population.

It drives me nuts. We arrest a tweeker, send him to jail and then think, "yeah there we go, I just did my job," but then it seems like before you can blink he's out, doin' the same things he's always done and hurting the same people he's always hurt. The system sucks!

—Police officer with 15 years' experience

Inevitably, then, public attention turns to treatment professionals and the thinking reaches a brief moment of compassion in which it is figured, "If this person can just get the help they need, then they will stop doing this." The question hardly ever asked by those attempting to corral the scared, although unenthusiastic and often unwitting, addicted offender into treatment is, "So, exactly what *is* the help this person needs?" That is seen as someone else's concern, and since effective treatment programs seem to mask their skills and interventions behind a veil of patient confidentiality, it is as if the public *can't* know exactly what treatment entails even if they did want to make it their concern. But the problems are too involved, and, as was mentioned, too complicated for one treatment professional or one treatment agency to really do much about. The tide of the using community and the pull of the psychological and physical addiction to the drug are so powerful that they overwhelm even the well-intended or well-trained treatment professional. Short-term gains, made perhaps when the user was still in a state of shell shock from having been caught, fade quickly. Long-term change begins to seem much more unrealistic, and the addicted patient's case seems much more hopeless and the prognosis much poorer. So myths are perpetuated. "Once somebody tries meth they can't ever stop. They end up either killing themselves, killing somebody else, or brain dead." And, "Treatment doesn't work, because once people are out of treatment they just go right back to using." Myths, however, by definition are untrue. Of course it can't be true that *everyone* who tries meth is addicted for life until death, and it can't be true that no treatments work and that treatment efforts are only a waste of time since meth is the one drug from which no one can ever truly recover. In spite of this, the pessimism of those working with meth addicts continues to grow, and the mounting need for theoretically sound and effective treatment emerges as the headline issue upon which all other community efforts rest.

The purpose of this chapter is to present important issues to be considered in the community-based treatment of meth addiction. The focus of the material presented here will be on the development of effective treatment plans that make use of sound theoretical treatment principles and empirically validated treatment methods. Throughout the chapter three guiding philosophies permeate. First, as was mentioned, effectively treating meth dependence requires more than just one individual or agency. Collaborative efforts involving multiple disciplines and resources are necessary not only to make a difference in the complicated problems of users, but also to prevent overwhelming and burning out one community resource. The workload, and often the financial burden involved in helping someone distance themselves from the drug and from the meth-using community, is more than can be shouldered by just one community player. Medical complications, unemployment, unstable housing conditions, a lack of social support, and childcare needs can all potentially surface as issues needing to be addressed through treatment that will require a team of professionals and community resources working together. The unfortunately widely abused adage that "It takes a village to raise a child" is especially applicable to the treatment of meth addiction, although perhaps it should more appropriately be stated, "It takes a town, city, or community to treat a meth addict."

A unique aspect of groups of people who abuse meth to be discussed throughout this chapter is the powerful social forces that act to quickly adopt and consume new peripheral users deep into the using community, and that also prevent individuals seeking help from distancing themselves from the drug and from other drug users and high-risk relapse situations. Because of these social forces it is often as if the person seeking recovery is caught in a tug of war of sorts in which the using community has hold of one of his sleeves and the sober community has hold of the other. Who wins, of course, depends mostly on the individual him/herself; however, the around-the-clock influence from the meth-using community is difficult to compete with for helping professionals who have 40-hour/week jobs and who are dealing with their own lives. For these reasons, effective interventions for treating meth addiction must be multidisciplinary and community based.

It would be wonderful to be able to give these people [people addicted to metham-phetamine] what they need, but they need too much and no one has the money to pay for it. They are kind of like a hot potato that gets passed around to different people in the community. Everyone hopes that when the music stops they're not the ones who are stuck with them.

—*Addiction counselor with 10 years' experience*

Limited funds, understaffed agencies, and underdeveloped resources are the norm for communities attempting to address meth addiction. If the prob-lems in a meth user's life aren't complicated enough to deal with already, often added to the chaos are political infighting, finger-pointing and blame projec-tion of agencies within communities already overwhelmed with other social problems and perhaps not used to working together.

The second philosophy guiding discussion in this chapter is that of making do with a community's existing resources while at the same time, of course, pursuing every avenue to try to expand those resources.

Necessity is the mother of invention, it is true—
but its father is creativity, and knowledge is the midwife.

—*Jonathan Schattke*

Waiting for the ideal is not a luxury available to communities addressing meth problems. The reactive nature of their response, coupled with the fact that "the ideal" means the development of services and programs several years in the making even after elusive funding streams have been identified, forces communities into attempting much more immediate, and "make do with what we have" kinds of efforts. However, because, as Oliver Wendell Holmes said, "trouble creates the capacity to handle it," communities who do attempt at least something using existing resources find that there is little restraint on their level of ingenuity. Creativity replaces complacency, and austerity is exchanged for inventiveness.

The premise of the 1980s television series *MacGyver* (ABC 1985–1992), offers the example of an important guiding principle. Using science and sheer wit, lead character Angus MacGyver created solutions to almost any prob-lem mainly because he was able to step beyond the functional fixedness that prevents most people from perceiving many uses for just one thing. A paper clip can become a high-voltage fuse or an inescapable finger cuff, a birthday candle can become a complicated timing device, and duct tape . . . well, duct tape has a million uses.

In community-based interventions for meth addiction, a sobriety-oriented Bible study group becomes an important social support system, the local jail becomes an intake screening/assessment/triage/detox site, a local hiking club becomes a treatment tool for reorienting pleasure responses, and volunteer community service becomes vocational training. Because the destructive influences of meth and of meth-using/producing/distributing communities move so quickly, and because of the trail of destroyed lives and human refuse they leave in their wake, urgency breeds necessity, which can then breed originality and resourcefulness.

The third guiding philosophy has to do with shared ownership of treatment plans and accountability of treatment providers. In community-based interventions, treatment planning involves all participating individuals and agencies who are currently working with the methamphetamine-addicted individual, as well as those needing to participate. These include human service agencies such as county caseworkers, vocational rehabilitation counselors, nonprofit as well as for-profit treatment providers and hospitals, drug-screening providers, sober friends and family, housing authorities, physicians and health-care providers, neighbors and landlords, and mutual support group members (AA and NA) and religious leaders. While the theoretical approach about how people recover from methamphetamine use and get better may, of necessity and training, need to be dictated by the primary treatment provider, the resulting treatment plan, including how specific tasks and agency involvements fit into it, needs to be developed by all those participating. For these reasons, treatment providers must be accountable for how they envision treatment unfolding, and they must also have a treatment model in mind, preferably one with research support, which they use to help orchestrate the efforts of everyone working together to help effect change in the life of the meth-addicted individual. In this way, the treatment influence is broadened beyond the agency or office where the person attends their treatment sessions, and it encompasses the efforts of everyone working with the person. The treatment specialist then becomes the captain of the ranks for these professionals, guiding initially the development of the blueprint for the treatment and then leading the efforts to follow through with the proposed directions. All the while, the treatment model is transparent and obvious to all involved, and each participant is able to see how their individual piece fits into the broader treatment design.

WHAT IS SO UNIQUE ABOUT METH?

Traditionally, as can be seen in the differentiation of Alcoholics Anonymous and Narcotics Anonymous, substance abuse has been divided down the line of alcohol versus other drugs. In spite of this differentiation, principles of addiction are applied equally to understand and treat chemical dependency to both broad substance categories. That being the case, a chapter written specifically about the treatment of meth addiction may be unduly specific. Indeed, treatment programs across the country more commonly encompass all forms of substance abuse (drugs and alcohol), and even in some cases addictive behaviors as well (for example, gambling, sex, or spending) as opposed to having a focus on one specific chemical of abuse. The one possible exception to this would be programs designed to prevent withdrawal symptoms and dangerous drug-seeking and drug-using behaviors such as methadone clinics.

Why then focus on treatment of meth addiction specifically? The answer to this question lies in the unique aspects of the drug that truly set it apart from all others. The unique properties of meth discussed below are included because they create significant barriers to treatment and because they help to account for meth's epidemiological rise in use across the country and its devastating effects on the lives of users (Anglin et al. 2000; Pennell et al. 1999). Treatment programs that are successfully treating meth addiction are not necessarily exclusive to only meth, and they may employ traditional substance abuse treatment interventions (Hser et al. 2005). What is unique about them, however, is the individualization of their treatment plans, which allow counselors to tailor their treatments to meet the specific biological, psychological, and social needs of their clients addicted to meth.

PHARMACOLOGICAL EFFECT AND ADDICTIVE PROPERTIES

Like most psycho-stimulant drugs, meth is characterized by its powerfully rewarding direct effects on mood, pleasure, sense of power, and increased energy, as well as by the subsequent decline in mood and psychomotor energy when use is discontinued, leading to dysphoric states of anhedonia in which the user craves more of the drug. Meth is a sympathomimetic drug in that it mimics the effects of the sympathetic response from the autonomic nervous system. It does this by increasing the release and blocking the metabolism of the neurotransmitters classified as the "catecholamines" (epinephrine, norepinephrine, and dopamine) as well as serotonin. The sympathetic (flight/fight/fright/freeze) response involves an initial increase in heart rate, respiration, blood pressure, and muscle tension with increased blood flow to muscles and increased blood sugar, which results in hyperalertness, euphoria, excitement, wakefulness, motor activity, speech, and elevated energy output with a concurrent decrease in appetite, fatigue, and sleepiness.

The exact pharmacological effects of meth on human beings have not been clearly identified, but animal research has suggested that meth damages vesicles, the storage sacs for dopamine specifically, which then causes dopamine to be leaked into the cytoplasm of the presynaptic neuron. Meth has also been shown to damage neurons' axonal endings, such that the integrity of the presynaptic membrane is compromised, causing dopamine to then leak uncontrollably into the synaptic cleft. Excessive dopamine in the synaptic region overwhelms neurotransmitter recuperation and degradation processes (reuptake and enzymatic breakdown) (Rawson 1999).

Exact effects of neurotransmitter activity depend not only on the specific neurotransmitter but also on the region of the brain where the changes in neurotransmitter activity take place. Three brain regions have been identified in animal research: the striatum, the prefrontal cortex, and the parietal cortex. The striatum (made up of the caudate and putamen) and the prefrontal cortex systems most effected by excessive exposure to methamphetamine use dopamine as the primary neuro-messenger, while the effect of meth in the parietal lobe involves nondopaminergic systems, which likely involve more serotonin.

The specific part of the striatum affected by the abuse of highly addictive psycho-stimulants, such as meth and cocaine, is that intriguing region of the mesotelencephalic pathway called the nucleus accumbens. In the 1950s, neurophysiologist James Olds discovered dopamine pleasure pathways within the basal ganglia and the limbic system when he placed an electrode near the nucleus accumbens in the brains of rats and then allowed them to self-stimulate by pressing a level that activated the electrode (Olds and Milner 1954; Olds 1973). The experience of pleasure was inferred from the reinforcing properties of the lever pressing. In many cases the animals would lever press to the point of exhaustion and they never seemed to satiate. Further experiments showed that the rats would sometimes choose self-stimulation of the nucleus accumbens over other instinctive primitive behaviors including eating, sex, and maternal proximity-seeking with recently delivered litters. Even when the expense of lever pressing was increased by requiring the animals to cross an electrified floor that would deliver a very painful electric shock to the feet to get to the lever, the animals continued to choose self-stimulation of the nucleus accumbens over the other motivated behaviors.

Animal research models have been criticized for a number of reasons. First, of course, is the question of ethics when it comes to causing pain in animals. Another criticism has been the question of the validity of generalizing animal behavior to humans. While this broad philosophical issue is more than could be managed within the topic area of this chapter, it is important to highlight similarities between the self-stimulating behavior of the laboratory rats and the behavior of people addicted to meth (Baumeister 2000; Heath 1963, 1972; Heath and Mickle 1960). Among these similarities is the tendency of meth addicts to experience pain and self-punishment in order to receive the reinforcing experience of using meth. Loss of parental rights to children, the risk of incarceration, infectious diseases, and violent interactions with other users are all unpleasant and self-punishing behaviors often experienced as the cost of getting high on meth. This is to say nothing about self-punishing cognitive factors, including loss of self-esteem, shame, fear of addiction, and reduced self-efficacy.

I don't know what it is about these people [those addicted to meth], especially the women. It's like they'll choose the drugs over their kids . . . over anything . . . no matter what the cost!

—Human services child protection caseworker with
eight years' experience

In addition to its effects on the nucleus accumbens, meth also disrupts the functioning of dopaminergic neurons in the prefrontal cortex (Seiden and Sabol 1996). As a result, chronic use, especially, has the effect of diminishing higher executive functioning, such as the ability to develop and carry out a plan and the ability to remember and execute complex behaviors such as budgeting money, paying bills, parenting, and following through with orders from a judge or caseworker, or even homework assignments from a treatment provider.

Meth also affects serotoninergic activity in the parietal cortex (Bonhomme et al. 1995). Disruption of functioning within the somatosensory cortex of the parietal lobe may be what accounts, at least in part, for the tactile sensations and nonpurposeful fine motor hyperactivity, which lead to repetitive picking at skin sores and the resulting dermatologic diseases commonly found among people who abuse meth.

INCREASED ENERGY AND LENGTH OF EFFECT

The attraction to energy increase along with the euphoric sense of competency and accomplishment make meth, like other psycho-stimulants, uniquely appealing to people accustomed to the high demands of a fast-paced lifestyle. Meth is unique even when compared to other stimulant drugs like cocaine, nicotine, and caffeine because of its long half-life. A typical user can experience the desired effects of the drug after a single dose of $^1/_4$ gram for up to 16 hours. Given that the cost per amount of meth can be comparable to cocaine, individuals who desire a longer high and who wish to prolong the inevitable crash see meth as a cheaper and a superior drug to cocaine.

Perhaps with the exception of heroin, meth is also unique from other drugs of abuse in that people who start using it drift toward using meth exclusively, whereas prior to initiating their meth use they may have had a polydrug-use habit. Certainly the reinforcing properties of meth affect this, as do the social aspects to be discussed later in this chapter. Other drugs consumed by someone using meth, especially marijuana, alcohol, and prescription benzodiazepines, are often used to help regulate the affects of the meth as opposed to use being consumed for the system-suppressing properties of those secondary drugs themselves.

NEUROTOXIC EFFECTS

Meth is also unique in that along with alcohol and inhalant drugs, its neurotoxic affects are well known and well established in research studies and the specific mechanics of them have been identified. As was mentioned, meth affects vesicular integrity in the presynaptic neuron, causing neurotransmitters such as dopamine to leak into the cytoplasm. As this occurs, deactivating enzymes work to break down the excess dopamine and then to "repackage" it again for future use. The process of breaking down dopamine, however, is harmful to the health of the neuron in that it changes the cytoplasmic chemistry in a way that causes the affected neuron to atrophy and eventually die (Seiden 1991; Seiden and Sabol 1996). This process has been well demonstrated in research studies looking at changes in brain metabolism with prolonged meth abuse (Amen 2004), and changes in brain function mirror the accompanying neuropsychological deficits observed in people who have abused meth. Recent research has focused on the possibility that adaptive changes in brain function and structure can occur over time with ongoing abstinence from meth use, making normalization possible with the passage of long-term abstention. But the findings are still very preliminary (Nordahl et al. 2005). Other studies point to evidence for long-term neuronal damage in abstinent meth users, particularly in frontal white matter and in the basal ganglia (Ernst et al. 2000).

LIFESTYLE DISRUPTION

Meth is also unique in the speed at which involvement in use of the drug and involvement with other drug-using individuals act to completely disrupt basic lifestyle patterns of the addicted user, something that perhaps could be termed the "speed of speed." The reasons meth is unique in this way relates, in part, to the addictive properties of the drug itself. It also is related to the specific effects of it on sleep, energy, and sexual patterns. Changes in basic circadian patterns such as sleep/wake cycles and cycles of fatigue and wakefulness disrupt and change previous lifestyle patterns such as employment, parenting, education, and nonusing social activities. The net effect of the changes in lifestyle patterns is that an individual newly involved in use of the drug and newly acquainted with the social network of other users drifts quickly away from nonusing social groups and then becomes unable to maintain basic nonusing social role functioning.

CRIMINAL DRIFT AND SORDID SUBCULTURES

Several factors unique to meth and to the using population create a characteristic social network that people working with meth addicts are able to quickly recognize and discuss. The network of users is insidious as well as self-consuming, yet also self-protecting. There are often established norms and values within the networks about such things as feigned support and intimacy, "in groups and out groups," care of children, and loyalty, or "ratting out."

The fact that meth can be illegally synthesized, locally and with locally procured products and substances, creates a continual preoccupation among using populations about where the drug is being made, about who has more of it, about the quality of the drug that is available, and about how to get it. Individuals involved find themselves quickly drifting deeper into the sordid subculture of meth use. Days and nights are often blurred into one continual stream of using experience, and the using person often loses the ability to differentiate between periods of time and experiences. The criminal element is always involved not only because of the illegality of use and possession themselves, but also because of the illegality of manufacturing and distribution and because of illegal behaviors engaged in to obtain the money to support the addiction.

METH ABUSE AMONG SPECIAL POPULATIONS

The demographic characteristics of meth-abusing populations are worthy of note because of what they suggest about the drug itself. For example, a drug known on the street as "poor man's cocaine" or as "redneck heroin" says something about the population of people who abuse it. There are three specific populations mentioned throughout clinical research on meth that appear to be drawn to meth use because of the match between the effects of the drug and their specific culture or social organization. These three groups are women, lower-social-economic-status (SES) Caucasians (particularly those in rural areas), and gay communities.

The attraction of women to meth has been demonstrated in demographic research looking at treatment admissions, coroner's reports, drug-related emergency room visits, and hospital discharges. Unlike other drugs of abuse—with the possible exception of smokable forms of cocaine, or "crack"—among urban ethnic minorities, meth use is equally represented in both genders, often split almost perfectly down the middle, leading clinicians to conclude that meth is an "equal opportunity destroyer" that shows no favoritism based on gender. Reasons for meth use among women, of course, vary tremendously case by case, but several helpful generalizations can be reached that, of course, will not be applicable to every case (Blume and Zilberman 2005; Ross 2001). The appetite suppressant or anorexigenic effects of meth relate to its activation of the sympathetic nervous system; subsequently, meth is abused by some women because of its weight-reducing properties. In fact, meth abuse has appeared in eating disorder cases, particularly those involving diagnoses of bulimia nervosa (Matsumoto et al. 2001). Bulimic women who manifest poor impulse control in their eating and sexual- and substance-abusing behaviors are attracted to meth, and it then meets their demand for a rapid and extreme measure for weight reduction, perhaps in lieu of other, more widely known excessive weight loss behaviors such as self-purging through forced vomiting or abuse of laxatives.

An interesting correlation can also be drawn between increasing sociological demands placed on women and their increased use of meth, perhaps because of its energy-producing and sleep-reducing effects. Over the last 50 years in the United States, the expectation of shared economic responsibility for women has increased as average American households are quickly requiring dual incomes to meet financial demands. The expectations for men of shared domestic responsibility, however, have not increased as dramatically. It seems that women are expected to do more with less time.

As with other substance-abusing behaviors, women sometimes are drawn into the addiction because of a close association with a substance-abusing man who invites, introduces, and then supports their habit. This may be for many reasons including for heightened sexual activity, as a form of abusive control, or because of simple relationship enmeshment, in which each partner desperately clings to the one other person closest to them whose life has become just as forlorn and desperate as theirs has. As demonstrated in social psychological research, misery not only loves company, but misery loves *miserable* company.

Abuse of meth among poor, often rural, Caucasian populations occurs for a variety of reasons, most of which have to do with the match of the drug with specific characteristics of this population. Financial strain and general hardship may contribute to a sense of despondency and draw people from this population to seek greater thrills, excitement, and productivity via the use of meth.

Extreme sexual acts, sometimes to the point of violence and injury, are a noted feature of meth couples and social groups (Semple et al. 2004). Meth use in gay communities has also been a topic of interest in clinical research because of the growing use and because of the association between the use of meth with unprotected sexual activity and sexually transmitted diseases, especially HIV (Hirshfield et al. 2004). Excessive sexual behaviors are attributed to the heightened energy and arousal associated with the use of meth and with the dramatic increases in alertness with accompanying decreases in cycles of fatigue and sleeping. A recent study of meth use among gay couples concluded that that the drug itself attracts hypersexual, risk-taking gay people who, regardless of their use, engage in risky sexual behaviors (Halkitis and Martin 2005).

WHAT ISSUES SHOULD BE CONSIDERED IN THE TREATMENT OF METH ADDICTION?

Need for Alternating and Collaborative Levels of Care

Because of its relevancy to ongoing and long-term basic living habits, outpatient treatment is a preferred modality to best assist addicted individuals in making the needed transitions in their own world in order to begin living sober, non-drug-using lifestyles. However, inpatient treatment and detoxification are often needed in order for the outpatient counseling to be maximally beneficial. Unless an addicted individual is adequately stabilized in an outpatient setting such that they are able to abstain from drug use, attend treatment sessions, and avoid situations of harm or endangerment to themselves or perhaps to children or vulnerable adults under their care, then inpatient care or post-relapse detoxification are necessary to make outpatient treatment possible. For these reasons alternating and collaborative levels of care are often needed to meet the changing demands of meth-addicted individuals in treatment. One modality will often not suffice. Outpatient treatment, while preferred because the treated individual must apply the skills of sober living and use-refusal and relapse-prevention to their everyday experience, may in some cases be insufficient to provide the lifestyle stability and distance from drug-using contexts necessary for treatment to have any kind of impact.

Inpatient treatment, while helpful in that it does get the user out of the using environments and it does aid significantly in helping to stabilize eating and sleeping patterns, is still always a tall step removed from everyday experience. Subsequently, skills and therapeutic gains acquired in inpatient settings always face the challenge of never having been tried out in the actual day-to-day living context of the meth-addicted individual. The risk is that as soon as changes made in inpatient settings fail to stand up to the ever-changing relapse pressures present when the addict is back in their home environment, the individual generalizes this to mean that none of what was learned in inpatient treatment will work subsequently and abandons all drug-use cessation efforts. Varying levels of care are needed, especially a smooth transition from outpatient to inpatient and then from inpatient back into outpatient. Like passing the baton in a relay race, successful treatment really does come down to the "hand-off" between different levels of care. And, just as it would be difficult for one runner to run the entire race, it is often difficult for treatment to be delivered in just one setting with little or no titration into progressively less intensive treatments as the recovering individual approaches discharge.

Need to Treat Sociocultural as Well as Drug-Dependency Issues

The "sordid subculture" of meth addiction mentioned above suggests that effective treatment involves addressing the social disease of meth abuse just as much as it does the addiction to the drug itself. Whether voluntarily or involuntarily admitted into treatment, often the greatest challenge involved in treating the meth-addicted individual is that of helping them to distance themselves from the powerful forces inherent within the using community. These forces are fueled by several important aspects of the drug matched up with the using community. One aspect is the fact that meth creates a state of heightened paranoia in chronic and excessive users. Their state of paranoia makes them very leery of people who are distancing themselves from other users, even if they are sincerely trying to make a better life for themselves by discontinuing their use of the drug. The question asked subversively within the sordid subculture is whether or not a particular member of the network is "in or out." Addicts in treatment are potentially seen as moving to join the "out" group, and with the knowledge they have of the drug-using and criminal activities of the other users who are still very much involved in the using network, they are seen as a tremendous threat, again, in part because of the paranoia induced by the drug itself.

NEED FOR LIFESTYLE STABILIZATION

Effective treatment cannot occur when an addicted individual is continuing to live the lifestyle of meth addiction marked by irregular sleeping patterns, poor diet, excessive sexual or late night activity, and chaotic social contacts with other people continuing to use. For this reason, lifestyle stabilization, through effective case management, becomes a necessary groundwork that must be laid before treatment can occur. Table 7.1 lists case management issues in three domains of biological and psychological functioning and social issues.

Case management is a process of services coordination and accountability that was defined by Weil and Karls (1985) "as a set of logical steps and a process of interaction within a service network which assure that a client receives needed services in a supportive, effective, efficient and cost-effective manner" and can

Table 7.1
Domains of Biological and Psychological Functioning and Social Issues

Biological	*Psychological*	*Social*
Are the client's acute medical issues being effectively dealt with?	Are the client's withdrawal symptoms being effectively managed?	Is the client living with anyone who abuses drugs or alcohol?
Is the client eating three healthy meals a day?	Does the client have the skills to deal with cravings and to avoid relapse?	Is the client living in an environment that is safe for them and their family?
Is the client sleeping at least six hours each night?	Has the client been evaluated for anti-depressant medication if needed?	Does the client have regular contact with supportive and sober friends and family members?
Is the client getting in bed by 11:30 P.M. and getting out of bed by 8:00 A.M.?	If so, is the client taking the medication as prescribed?	Is the client being threatened or are they under any kind of duress from other people who are still using?
Has the client improved their self-care and grooming habits?	Is the client suicidal?	
Is the client taking all physician-prescribed medications as they have been instructed to do?	Does the client have sufficient energy in the morning to get out of bed and face the day?	Is the client interacting effectively with many people during the daytime hours?
	Is the client showing improvement in their cognitive functioning?	

Source: Developed by Dr. Nicolas Taylor, Taylor Behavior Institute, Montrose Colorado 2004.

take many forms, including teaching life skills and creating situations of accountability and follow-through. Case management is also unlikely to be completed at any one point throughout treatment. Instead, the addicted individuals will likely need ongoing support and direction to stabilize their lifestyle. Treatment sessions themselves may even be used to assist in case management efforts, especially since other interventions designed to address the addiction to meth itself are not likely to have an effect if the individual is continuing to experience lifestyle chaos and instability. Case management or life skills sessions can include any of the following topics, as well as others:

- How to plan a day and how to keep a schedule
- How to go to sleep when you are not tired
- How to enjoy sex without being high
- How to plan your meals (grocery shopping, cooking, preparing, etc.)
- How to follow through on a commitment/promise
- How to show up to appointments on time
- How to manage an urge
- How to break habits of places you go to and people you see
- How to job hunt
- How to interview for a job
- How to find a place to live
- How to budget money
- How to enter into contractual agreements with other people
- How to access public assistance
- How to arrange transportation
- How to work with a judge or probation officer
- How to meet sober people
- How to distance oneself from using friends and family
- How to keep house
- How to take care of one's appearance

While treatment sessions may be offered by the treatment provider to the addicted individual to help guide them toward adequate lifestyle stabilization, effective case management is more likely to require a much broader effort that includes many different people and agencies involved with the addicted person, including county human service caseworkers, state vocational counselors, schoolteachers, and probation or parole officers.

NEED TO ADDRESS COGNITIVE ISSUES (DELUSIONS)

With adequate lifestyle stabilization via effective case management, treatment can then be attempted to address the psychosocial factors underlying the addiction to meth. One of these will often be illogical and faulty thoughts the addicted individual has about their drug use, which have served to support their ongoing use often in spite of the negative and unwanted consequences that have resulted. Cognitive behavioral interventions have been effective in treating many severe behavioral and personality disorders, because they are designed to address and help change the underlying automatic cognitive processes, which, often almost slightly outside the awareness of the individual, have created cycles of ongoing use. Direct challenge of these irrational cognitions and the use of cognitive restructuring enable the user to recognize and change thoughts that have had a deleterious effect on their attempts to change their patterns of behavior.

With meth abuse, the irrational cognitions underlying severe addiction are often so poorly founded in reality and so bizarre that they border on being delusional. Delusional or not, when the user allows these thoughts to predominate their expectations about the drug and their use of it they continue to use it. Examples of irrational beliefs about meth use include:

- The expectations that one will use the extra energy and sleeplessness from the drug to be more productive, when, in fact, productivity decreases because of the restless, poorly directed nature of the energy increase.
- The expectations that weight loss from meth use improves one's appearance when, in fact, the using individual's appearance is worsened by severe skin sores on the hands, arms, and face; thin, stringy hair; and severe dental problems.
- The expectations that one can make easy money by buying a supply of meth only part of which is to be used to support a personal habit, the rest of which is intended to be sold for a considerable profit. Instead, the individual ends up using more than was intended and/or other individuals share in the drug use without offering any compensation for the amount they use. The net effect is that the individual is no better off financially and may even be in more dire straits because of the money lost in the purchase of the original amount.
- The belief that other meth-using people have an unquestionable loyalty to the addicted individual simply because of the solidarity from sharing the same bad habit, when in fact the individual has repeatedly seen others do anything and unscrupulously use other people to maintain their drug-using habit. The individual has also likely experienced what it is like to be tossed aside by other users who found someone in the way of their use.
- The belief that as long as a parent doesn't use in front of their children or if they make sure their children are in the care of someone else (sometimes even other meth users) when they do use then they are a good parent and are not allowing their use to impact their children in a negative way.

NEED FOR INCREMENTAL AND IMMEDIATE SANCTIONS AND REWARDS

Principles of operant conditioning are especially applicable in the treatment of meth addiction because of the need for the user to experience, immediately, the negative effects of their use, and, just as importantly, for the user to experience positive results from even short periods of abstention and of having distanced oneself from other users. Consequences of each must be immediate and they must match the targeted behavior in strength. Because work with addicted individuals can often be difficult because gains are so small and infrequent, especially in the beginning stages of treatment, incremental and immediate sanctions and rewards are required to reinforce successive approximations toward the targeted behavior of full sobriety.

NEED FOR STRUCTURE AND SUPERVISION

Obviously, in order to have the level of responsiveness in which small gains or small setbacks can be immediately addressed through appropriate sanctions or rewards, a level of structure and supervision is required. For this reason, again especially during the beginning stages of treatment, high levels of structure are needed, which may necessitate more intensive levels of care. Structure, of course, is also inherent when an addicted individual is mandated into treatment by a judicial system. In these situations it would seem to make intuitive sense that because the individual is being coerced into treatment and perhaps into doing something that they do not want to do or do not feel ready to do, that they will benefit only minimally from the experience and certainly not to the degree of other people who refer themselves into treatment. However, a recent study found that with the exception of relapses during the treatment episode, individuals mandated into treatment for meth dependency faired equally well in all other measures of short- and long-term outcome including treatment completion, time to relapse, and percentage of days during which meth was used in 24 months following treatment (Brecht et al. 2005).

As has been a recurring theme throughout this chapter, the provision of adequate structure and supervision to be able to administer immediate consequences to targeted behaviors, both to strengthen drug abstention and to weaken relapse processes, requires a much broader involvement than just one substance abuse treatment professional or agency. These critical behavior-shaping responses must be consistently applied in a uniform fashion by everyone involved with trying to help the addicted individual.

WHAT ARE EVIDENCE-BASED TREATMENT MODELS FOR METH ADDICTION AND WHAT ARE THEIR "THEORIES OF CURE"?

Because incident rates of meth addiction moved so quickly at what have been described as "epidemiologic proportions," the development of adequate treatment responses has at times been more reactive than proactive, or even preventative, and has struggled to match the apparently ever-increasing demand for high-quality, effective treatment. Perhaps this is why the myth that addiction to methamphetamine is untreatable first began and has been perpetuated in spite of clinical research to the contrary (Hser et al. 2005).

Treatment for meth has, perhaps, been challenged with matching the unique demands of the drug, but it has not been ineffective. If anything, it has produced comparable outcomes to treating other forms of substance abuse.

The earliest treatment approach for meth with supportive research is the "Matrix Model" (originally referred to as the neurobehavioral model). The Matrix approach was originally an outpatient model developed during the 1980s in Southern California by Richard Rawson, Ph.D., and his colleagues at the Matrix Institute (Obert et al. 2000; Shoptaw et al. 1994). Although originally developed to treat cocaine addicts, the Matrix Model has been found to produce comparable positive responses, in terms of drug abstention, with meth-using individuals as well (Huber et al. 1997; Rawson et al. 2000). In outpatient settings the Matrix Model can be delivered as a 12-month program that consists of two 6-month phases, or as 8- and 16-week protocols. Treatment interventions are manualized and are a combination of individual, group, and family counseling sessions. Participation in mutual support groups (AA or NA) is encouraged and the model itself involves the integration of approaches from a number of other treatment strategies including motivational interviewing, relapse prevention, cognitive behavioral interventions, psycho-education, and family therapy (Rawson et al. 1995).

The theory of cure is based on addressing four components of stimulant addiction throughout five "stages of recovery." The four components are behavioral, emotional, cognitive, and relationship; and the five stages of recovery are withdrawal, honeymoon, the wall, adjustment, and resolution (Rawson et al 1991a). Table 7.2 shows the approximate occurrence of each of these stages throughout the recovery process.

Each of the four components is addressed differently during each of the stages of recovery in order to match treatment with an individual's progress in recovery. The needs and the treatment focus for the components during each stage are shown in Table 7.3.

A recent multisite comparison of the Matrix Model with "treatment as usual" (Galloway et al. 2000) interventions delivered in eight outpatient community settings revealed that the Matrix Model impressively produced

Table 7.2
Stages of Recovery

- "Withdrawal"—0–15 days post-use
- "Honeymoon"—16–45 days post-use
- "The Wall"—46–120 days post-use
- "Adjustment"—121–180 days post-use
- "Resolution"—181+days post-use

Source: Rawson 1991.

Table 7.3
Stages and Domains of Methamphetamine Recovery

Stage	Behavioral	Emotional	Cognitive	Relational
Stage 1 Withdrawal Primarily feels disoriented, depressed, and very fatigued; feels out of control and does not understand what is happening.	Increased sleep Impulsive and erratic Inconsistency	Depression Anxiety Self-doubt	Difficulty concentrating Cravings Poor short-term memory	Hostility Fear Maladaptive coping skills
Stage 2 Honeymoon Primarily feels the problem is over and there is no continued need for treatment. May return to alcohol or secondary drug and are likely to discontinue recovery activities.	High energy Excessive work Poorly directed behavior	Over confidence Optimism Feeling of being cured	Inability to prioritize Misperceptions of relapse Minimizing cause/cure	Family elation and denial Desire for normalcy Conflict: family vs. treatment
Stage 3 The Wall A primary hurdle in recovery and high vulnerability for relapse. Low energy returns and they experience very little pleasure in their life. Patients experience great difficulty with concentration.	Risk of drop out Relapse behaviors Insomnia	Boredom Anhedonia Irritability	Rehearsal relapse Euphoric recall Misattribution	Mutual blaming Fear of separation Seek out contacts

This is a period of increased irritability and loss of sex drive. Insomnia is common for most along with feelings that condition will persist indefinitely. During this stage, high rates of relapse and treatment termination occur. It has been suggested that biological healing of the brain is occurring. Physical exercise alleviates the severity of symptoms. Continued support and encouragement is crucial during this stage.

Stage 4 Adjustment During this stage, feelings of accomplishment occur. The patient returns to pretreatment normalcy. They begin to adjust to lifestyle and relationship changes.	Return to high-risk situations Abstinence behaviors decline Return to normal life	Reduced depression Reduced anxiety Continued boredom	Reduced frequency of using Thoughts and cravings Questioning addiction	Emergence of new problems Resistance to help with relationship problems
Stage 5 Resolution Patient has been clean for six months and is learning new skills to monitor relapsing signals. They are able to maintain a balanced lifestyle and develop new areas of interest.	Emergence of other excessive behavior patterns	Boredom with abstinence Long-standing emotional issues	Maintaining commitment to long-term abstinence	Individualized problems

Source: Rawson 1991.

better treatment retention, better overall attendance at treatment sessions, more meth-free urine samples while in treatment, and more days abstaining from meth use than did the agencies' standard treatment. However, the superiority of the Matrix Model did not persist at the time of discharge and six months following treatment. Follow-up measures indicated that both models produced significant improvement in their participants when compared to baseline functioning (Anglin and Rawson 2000; Huber et al. 2000; Rawson and Marinelli-Casey et al. 2002; Rawson et al. 2004).

In addition to the Matrix Model, other treatment approaches previously used primarily to treat cocaine addiction have also been used to treat addiction to meth. The community reinforcement plus vouchers approach (CR+V) builds upon similar models that focus on skill development (Budney and Higgins 1998). It is also a manual-driven approach, like the Matrix model, and it involves two 12-week phases. The first phase of treatment includes twice a week individual and family sessions and the second phase involves weekly individual sessions. One purpose of the approach is to help make major lifestyle changes in four areas—family relationships, recreational activities, social networks, and vocation. In addition, a voucher program is used to help alter conditioned responses by reinforcing periods of non-use (as verified by regular and random urine screenings) with vouchers to engage in enjoyable activities. The purpose of the activities is to help the addicted individual break the conditioned response of pleasure to drug-associated enjoyable events during which the individual's experience of pleasure is tied more to the use of the drug than to simply enjoying the natural pleasure-producing aspects of the experience.

Research into stimulant abuse and pleasure suggest that drug abusers demonstrate a deprivation of specific types of reinforcing alternatives to drug use. For example, Etten et al. (1998) found that cocaine abusers report consistently lower frequencies of nonsocial, introverted, and passive outdoor activities than do control groups. They speculate that this may be because of differences in the immediate or long-term compatibility between recreational activities and the behaviors required to maintain cocaine use. They also posit that it could be that stimulant abusers have an insufficient history of exposure to and experience with enjoyable activities and hobbies for them to function as effective reinforcers. Finally, they found that greater overall frequency of pleasant activities, especially those less social and more introverted (such as enjoying a hobby or craft by oneself), was associated with greater abstinence for addicted individuals in treatment.

CR+V along with contingency management and other behavioral reinforcement treatment models have impressive research support for treating stimulant abuse disorders (Rawson et al. 1999; Higgins et al. 2002) and offer a direction for treatment of meth addiction that is less about using punishment to shape behavior and more about utilizing reinforcement contingencies and relearning the experience of pleasure and enjoyment of sober, naturally pleasurable activities.

CONCLUDING COMMENT

Perhaps the most promising news to come from recent clinical research regarding the treatment of meth addiction is that treatment, even that provided in standard outpatient settings, can be beneficial, especially when many of the unique needs of people addicted to meth are adequately targeted and addressed. The point that this requires the involvement of every person or agency invested in the addicted individual's treatment cannot be overemphasized, since effective case management, supervision, and structure require many people and are powerful predictors of a positive treatment outcome. Communities with existing programs, such as a drug court, may find it easy to coordinate multiple agencies and disciplines. However, even communities without a central organizing unit like a drug court can utilize the components of drug courts that add to effective collaboration to effect community-based interventions (National Association of Drug Court Providers 1997).

CHAPTER 8

A Multisite Comparison of Psychosocial Approaches for the Treatment of Methamphetamine Dependence*

Richard A. Rawson et al.[1]

INTRODUCTION

Methamphetamine (MA) use is a significant and growing problem in the United States (Anglin et al. 2000; Galloway et al. 2000; Rawson and Huber et al. 2000). The use of MA has increased to epidemic proportions and has become the dominant drug problem in the western and midwestern portions of the country, most severely impacting rural areas and moderate-sized urban communities (National Institute of Justice 2000; Office of National Drug Control Policy 2003; Pennell et al. 1999). In spite of the growing epidemic, no consistently effective pharmacological treatment has been developed to treat the disorder (Rawson and Gonzales et al. 2002). Psychosocial and behavioral approaches constitute the primary treatments available for MA-dependent individuals. However, even in the arena of psychosocial treatments, little research has been conducted to pinpoint an effective treatment or distinguish between what actually works and what is delivered by default simply because it is part of "standard community treatment."

One promising psychosocial treatment model for MA dependence has been tested in open trials. The Matrix Model, a manualized outpatient approach for treating stimulant disorders, has been assessed in several large groups of MA-dependent individuals. Outcomes demonstrated that, in general, the treatment response of MA-dependent individuals was positive (Huber et al. 1997; Rawson and Huber et al. 2000). Additional support for the Matrix approach has been reported in treatment trials with cocaine-dependent individuals (Rawson and Shoptaw et al. 1995; Shoptaw et al. 1994) and in a

---

* Reprinted with the permission of *Addiction* 99, no. 6 (June 2004): 708.

controlled trial of the cognitive behavioral therapy group component of the Matrix approach (Rawson and Huber et al. 2002a).

The Matrix Model combines techniques and materials from the cognitive behavioral therapy literature to include accurate information on the effects of stimulants, family education, 12-Step program participation, and positive reinforcement for behavior change and treatment compliance (Rawson and Obert et al. 1991). The 16-week intensive treatment protocol is delineated in a detailed treatment manual; the content and rationale of the protocol have been described in detail in previous publications (Obert et al. 2000; Rawson and Huber et al. 2002a).

Although the empirical evidence cited above was uncontrolled and descriptive, the promise of the Matrix Model for the treatment of MA dependence (and the lack of any empirical evidence for any other methods) resulted in an announcement sponsored by the Center for Substance Abuse Treatment (CSAT) to conduct a multisite study to replicate and evaluate the Matrix Model with an MA-dependent sample. The resulting Methamphetamine Treatment Project (MTP) is the largest randomized clinical trial of psychosocial treatments for MA dependence to date (Anglin and Rawson 2000). The project was funded through the Substance Abuse and Mental Health Services Administration's (SAMHSA) CSAT as a cooperative agreement providing funding to seven investigative teams at eight treatment sites and to one coordinating center that was charged with designing, administering, and executing the study. The MTP compares treatment outcomes in participants randomly assigned to receive either the manualized Matrix Model of MA treatment or treatment-as-usual (TAU) at each of the sites.

STUDY DESIGN

Sites

In addition to the coordinating center at UCLA, seven investigative teams conducted the study at eight sites in Northern and Southern California, Hawaii, and Montana. Each site was expected to recruit 150 participants into the study. In each site, half were randomly assigned to receive the Matrix Model of treatment, whereas the other half of the participants received TAU as delivered at that site. Considerable program heterogeneity was documented across the eight sites. One site treated women clients exclusively, a drug court provided the context for one site, and two sites treated significant proportions of Asians and Pacific Islanders. The remaining sites provided care primarily to Caucasian and Hispanic urban, suburban, and rural residents.

Treatment-as-Usual (TAU)

Specific and detailed information describing the theoretical foundation, setting, duration and intensity, services offered, and clinician qualifications for the eight TAUs has been previously published (Galloway et al. 2000). All treatment sites employed outpatient treatment models, with the intensive phase of treatment ranging from 4 to 16 weeks across sites. Participants were expected to have contact with their treatment program from 1 to 13 hours per week. All aspects of TAU varied widely across sites. In addition to the services delivered during the active treatment period, participants in both conditions at all sites were encouraged to participate in continuing care activities following the completion of the designated treatment dose. Elements of TAU at these sites are summarized in Table 8.1.

No attempt was made to standardize or monitor the fidelity of the TAU conditions, as it was the intent of the project to compare the Matrix approach to the treatments delivered routinely by the program staff. All TAU clinical staff were supervised by each program's clinical director and were not involved in any aspect of training, supervision, or service delivery of the Matrix condition. It should be noted that as "comparison conditions," these TAU conditions represented a "best available option" and not a "minimal contact comparison" condition. A recent report on the effectiveness of standard substance abuse treatment demonstrated that a community-based approach was shown to produce superior outcomes to a minimal treatment control (Davis et al. 2002). Therefore, this design comparing the Matrix Model to eight other "real-world" service configurations represents an adequate test of the model.

The Matrix Model

The Matrix Model of outpatient stimulant abuse treatment was originally developed using data from cocaine-abusing participants in treatment at Matrix Institute offices in the Los Angeles metropolitan area during the 1980s. The multicomponent treatment approach was constructed using empirically supported interventions and treatment elements and was guided by an iterative process of pilot-testing diverse strategies and incorporating those that enhanced treatment attendance and decreased drug use as measured objectively by urinalysis. The resulting package of treatment elements has been organized into a manualized treatment protocol consisting of 16 weeks of cognitive behavioral therapy groups (36 sessions), family education groups (12 sessions), social support groups (4 sessions), and individual counseling (4 sessions), combined with weekly breath alcohol testing and urine testing for cocaine, methamphetamine, opiates, cannabis, and benzodiazepines. Weekly or more frequent attendance at 12-step meetings was also encouraged. All treatment sessions were delivered using a nonjudgmental, nonconfrontational style and employed extensive positive reinforcement by therapists and peers for behavior change.

In this study, staff trained to deliver the Matrix Model received an initial 40 hours of didactic and experiential training. Clinical supervisors, under the direction of the clinical director from the coordinating center, conducted booster training sessions at each site, led mandatory weekly teleconferences

Table 8.1
Treatment-as-Usual: Elements of Treatment

Site	Duration of Treatment (intensive phase)	Individual Sessions	Group Sessions	12-Step-Program Involvement
Site 1	8 weeks	One per week for 4–8 weeks; 30–50 minutes each	Four per week for 4–8 weeks; 3 hours each; families attend one per week	Required; one per week for 4–8 weeks
Site 2	12 weeks	One per week for 12 weeks; 1 hour each	Five per week for 2 weeks; three per week for 2 weeks; two per week for 8 weeks	Recommended
Site 3	12 weeks	One per week for 12 weeks; 1 hour each	None	Recommended
Site 4	16 weeks	One per week for 16 weeks; 10–15 minutes each	Three per week for 16 weeks; 1 hour each	Required; three per week for 16 weeks
Site 5	12 weeks	One per week for 12 weeks; 30–60 minutes each	Three per week for 12 weeks; 90 minutes each and two per week for 12 weeks; 60–90 minutes each	Required; one per week for 12 weeks
Site 6	12 weeks	One per week–two per month for 12 weeks; 1 hour each	Two per week for 12 weeks; 90 minutes each; families attend one per week for two weeks	Recommended
Site 7	16 weeks	One per week for 16 weeks; 1 hour each	Two per week for 16 weeks; 2 hours each	Recommended
Site 8	12 weeks	Two per week for 12 weeks; 1 hour each	One per week for 12 weeks; 2 hours each	Required; 6 meetings

with site Matrix clinicians, monitored clinician performance via a weekly activity checklist, reviewed a sample of tape-recorded sessions, and provided feedback regularly to ensure that the Matrix Model was implemented as designed.

Based on the Psychiatric Rehabilitation Fidelity Toolkit (Bond et al. 2000), two fidelity scales were developed to assess adherence to the treatment protocol. Data from year two of the study found that sites adhered to the Matrix Model protocol in implementation of critical elements. The average score of fidelity for structural elements was 4.15 (model mostly implemented). The category with the highest average was "utilization of manual," at 4.88 (fully implemented), and the lowest was the "group characteristics" category, at 3.02 (model satisfactorily implemented). The average percentage of fidelity to therapist-client interaction elements for all sites was 82.39 percent.

METHOD

Research Design

All sites obtained all appropriate clearances and approvals from the relevant institutional review boards (IRBs) and agencies prior to study commencement. All potential candidates for the study participated in informed-consent procedures as required by the local IRBs. The coordinating center operated under the approval of the UCLA IRB.

Research assistants from all sites were trained and certified for proficiency in research practices, standard operating procedures, data collection protocol mastery, and instrument administration. Continuing oversight was maintained through regularly scheduled mandatory teleconferences and periodic site visits by the coordinating center staff for inspection of data collection and research procedures. Full details of the research procedures have been previously published (Huber et al. 2000).

Participants

Participant inclusion and exclusion criteria were as follows: Candidates had to be at least 18 years of age of either gender; MA-dependent as determined by the DSM-IV checklist; willing to complete forms and provide urine samples; able to understand scales and instructions; able to understand and provide informed consent; able to understand English; and able to participate in all aspects of either treatment condition. Exclusion criteria included having a medical and/or psychiatric impairment precluding safe participation; requiring medical detoxification from opioids/alcohol/other drugs; not having used MA in the past 30 days (unless the patient had been in a controlled environment, such as jail or prison); having been enrolled in another treatment program in the past 30 days; and having medical, legal, housing, or transportation issues precluding safe and/or consistent participation.

Almost half the recruited participants were male (45 percent); 60 percent were Caucasian, 18 percent Hispanic, and 17 percent Asian/Pacific Islander.

Other participant characteristics at baseline included age (32.8 years on average); education (12.2 years on average); employment (69 percent); and married and not separated (16 percent). Participants were recruited through a variety of means, including media advertisements, referrals from community agencies (medical, substance abuse, mental health, and criminal justice) and word of mouth. Although the inclusion and exclusion criteria for the study may have precluded participation by the most severely disabled individuals, the characteristics of the participating cohort were consistent with clinical treatment samples studied previously (Huber et al. 1997; Rawson and Huber et al. 2000). Multiple substances of abuse were documented in participants' drug-use histories, but both self-reports and urinalyses confirmed that there was practically no use of substances other than MA, marijuana, and alcohol throughout the duration of the study. The participants had on average 7.54 years of lifetime MA use and 11.53 days of MA use in the past 30 days. The preferred route of administration of MA was smoking (65 percent), followed by IV-injecting (24 percent) and snorting (11 percent).

Written informed consent was obtained from each participant after the study procedure had been fully described. After providing consent, participants completed an admission form and an inclusion/exclusion criteria verification, as well as a baseline battery of assessments including the DSM-IV MA-dependence checklist, the Addiction Severity Index (ASI; fifth edition) (McLellan et al. 1992), and others, the results of which are not presented in this paper. Instruments were repeated periodically during the active treatment phase, at discharge and 6 months and 12 months post-admission. Objective assessment of substance use was obtained by urine samples collected once weekly from participants in both treatment conditions at all sites. Samples were analyzed for methamphetamine, amphetamines, cocaine, opiates, and marijuana at a central, off-site contract laboratory.

Attendance Data

Before examining the treatment outcomes, it is necessary to determine whether study conditions differed in the amounts of treatment received. The eight TAU conditions provided diverse combinations of services and prescribed different levels and types of attendance at clinical appointments each week (see Table 8.1). The sites did record the number of clinical sessions attended by participants, and these data can be aggregated to reflect the total number of clinical contacts for each participant. The overall mean number of clinical contacts made by participants assigned to TAU was about 13 (SD = ± 15). For the Matrix participants overall, the mean number of clinical contacts was approximately 27 (SD = ± 20). A detailed summary of the number of clinical contacts by treatment condition and site is presented in

Table 8.2
Summary of the Number of Clinical Contacts Made by Participants, by Treatment Site and Condition

Site (TAU length, weeks)	Matrix		TAU	
	Mean	SD	Mean	SD
Site 1 (8)	25.2	17.9	17.2	14.0
Site 2 (12)	26.1	17.3	21.7	15.7
Site 3 (12)	28.4	18.2	6.3	3.6
Site 4 (16)	31.5	20.0	22.8	15.4
Site 5 (12)	25.7	20.0	15.4	19.8
Site 6 (12)	25.2	24.7	2.1	3.1
Site 7 (16)	35.4	19.1	13.8	14.5
Site 8 (12)	22.2	18.6	3.9	5.0
Overall Summary	26.8	19.7	12.7	14.7

Table 8.2. Although variability in the amount of Matrix treatment delivered to participants across sites is evident, these data indicate that participants at all sites received substantial doses of the Matrix treatment.

Follow-Up Rates

Overall, 798 of 978 participants (81.6 percent) completed discharge interviews, and 841 of 978 participants (86 percent) completed six-month follow-up interviews. (At the time of this manuscript preparation, the 12-month data collection/analysis was incomplete.) There was no difference in follow-up rate by treatment condition.

Design and Analytical Issues

Analysis of the MTP data posed several challenges because the study's design differed from that of traditional multisite studies. All sites in the MTP implemented the Matrix treatment model as one arm of the study (condition A). The other treatment condition, TAU, was site-specific and varied widely between sites (conditions B1–B8). Thus, the broadest and most critical issue was the conceptual design of the statistical comparisons used to analyze the primary outcomes. Variation in program length provided another major analytical hurdle in this study. The main study outcomes were based on weekly measures (for example, attendance or MA-free urine samples), but the length of TAU and Matrix protocols differed at most sites. As such, the number of chances participants had to provide evidence of satisfactory performance differed accordingly.

Analytical Approach to Comparisons between Conditions

Due to the complexities of this study, several comparison methods were used to evaluate the primary outcomes. First, summaries of raw data reflecting the outcomes were presented prior to any manipulation of that data in an attempt to analytically "equalize" Matrix and TAU conditions. Next, comparisons were presented in which Matrix participants' data were truncated to reflect only the data collected during the number of weeks that data were collected in the TAU condition at the same site. Finally, logistic regression models were employed to elucidate the Matrix–TAU differences.

Statistical Methodology

Statistical methods applied to this data adhere to clinical trial standards. All tests are two-tailed. For all tests, alpha was set at the conventional level of 0.05. Results of statistical tests are provided for the comparisons of the truncated data and the data that resulted from combining the programs by treatment length and for repeated-measures analyses of substance use across multiple time points. Due to the complex nature of this project, all results presented here have been confirmed by at least two statisticians working independently at the coordinating center.

For the logistic regression models presented, binomial and multinomial logistic regression analyses were run using SAS v. 8.2 software (SAS Institute Inc. 1999). Outcome (dependent) measures included retention, program completion, and abstinence during the active treatment period. Treatment retention was operationalized as an ordinal variable with five categories in an approximate uniform distribution. A score of 5 indicates the longest retention, and 1 the shortest. Treatment completion was operationalized as a binary variable, with 1 indicating completed treatment and 0 indicating treatment not completed. Abstinence from drug use was operationalized as an ordinal variable having three categories: Category 1 represents those clients who had 50–100 percent MA-free urine results (30 percent); category 2 represents those clients who had less than 50 percent MA-free urine results, but more than zero (32 percent); and category 3 represents clients with 0 percent MA-free urine results (38 percent). The analysis focused on predicting a trend of the probability of providing MA-free urine samples.

RESULTS

Retention and Treatment Completion Data

Retention Rates through Treatment

Matrix participants were retained at a higher level than were TAU participants, except at site 4, the drug-court site. Five of the eight comparisons are statistically significant and indicate increased retention in the Matrix condition (see Table 8.3). Comparisons at sites 3 and 7 achieve marginal statistical significance, with the Matrix condition exhibiting increased retention relative to the TAU condition.

The results of multivariate modeling indicate that Matrix participants, compared to TAU participants, were 38 percent more likely to stay in treatment (odds ratio = 1.384). This analysis controls for treatment length by equalizing measures of treatment retention between the two conditions, ensuring that the significant effect was due to the treatment process, rather than the generally longer length of the Matrix treatment (16 weeks) as compared with the various lengths of the TAU condition (8, 12, or 16 weeks).

Treatment Completion Rates

Another way to compare participation in treatment is to examine the percentage of participants who completed the prescribed treatment program. For the purposes of this analysis, completion of the program is defined as the participant having attended at least one treatment session in his/her last scheduled week of treatment. This definition of completion has the advantage of being a simple and concrete endpoint for which all data from the study can

Table 8.3
**Comparison of Retention between Conditions within Sites,
with Matrix Truncated to the Length of TAU at Each Site**

Site	TAU length (weeks)	Log-rank	2	P
Site 1	8	−20.07	33.17	<0.0001
Site 2	12	−9.49	4.98	0.026
Site 3	12	−8.39	3.68	0.055
Site 4	16	1.64	0.26	0.610
Site 5	12	−22.30	28.74	<0.0001
Site 6	12	−17.46	17.87	<0.0001
Site 7	16	−5.01	3.34	0.067
Site 8	12	−10.59	7.99	0.005

be combined and analyzed with the full, intended statistical power. A simple χ^2 comparison across all sites indicates that the completion rate was 40.9 percent for Matrix participants and 34.2 percent for TAU participants. This difference is statistically significant ($\chi^2 = 4.68$: P $= 0.031$).

Controlling for the potential effects of demographics and the frequency and route of MA use, the multivariate logistic regression reveals that Matrix participants were 27 percent more likely to complete treatment (odds ratio $= 1.269$) than TAU participants. Additional analysis indicates that TAU participants at three sites were 85 percent, 74 percent, and 54 percent less likely to complete treatment. No difference in treatment completion was found between the two conditions at four sites. As with the retention data, however, an exception to this trend was documented at the site operating in a drug-court context. The TAU participants at this site were 2.17 times more likely to complete treatment than Matrix participants at this site. When program completion data from the drug-court site were not included in the overall analysis, Matrix participants were 38 percent more likely to complete treatment than TAU participants.

Drug Use during Treatment, by Site Assessed by Urinalyses

Because participants were required to provide one urine sample each week, regardless of their treatment assignment, one way to look at these data is to calculate the mean number of MA-free samples collected from participants in each condition during the treatment period. The criterion that defined a MA-free sample required that the participant go to the treatment program to provide a urine sample that tested clean for drug metabolites. Therefore, the total number of MA-free samples is a measure that incorporates the influence of retention together with objective drug-use status. Table 8.4 presents the mean number of MA-free samples during the treatment period by site and condition.

The raw data indicate that at all sites except site 4 (the drug-court context), Matrix participants provided more clean urine samples than did TAU participants. When the urine data are truncated (when data from the Matrix participants are included only for the number of weeks equal to the length of TAU at each site), the trend supporting higher rates of clean urine samples in the Matrix condition is sustained. However, the differences between the conditions are generally not statistically significant in these smaller comparisons, as illustrated in Table 8.4. The one exception to this is at site 5, where Matrix participants provided an average of 4.3 MA-free urine samples compared to 1.7 for TAU participants. In six of the remaining sites (all but site 4) Matrix participants provided, on average, one additional MA-free urine sample than did those assigned to TAU (4.6 versus 3.7).

Results of urinalysis data can be aggregated by treatment length and compared. Figure 8.1 summarizes the data in this way. Although those assigned to the Matrix condition provided a greater number of MA-free urine samples than those assigned to the TAU condition in both the 8-week and 16-week treatments,

Table 8.4
Summary of the Number of MA-Free Urine Samples Provided by Participants, by Treatment Site and Condition

	Raw data				Truncated data					
	Matrix		TAU		Matrix		TAU			
Site (TAU length, weeks)	Mean	SD	Mean	SD	Mean	SD	Mean	SD	t	P
Site 1 (8)	6.23	5.41	3.38	2.95	3.75	2.91	3.38	2.95	−0.76	0.45
Site 2 (12)	6.25	5.94	4.19	4.24	4.86	4.59	4.19	4.24	−0.94	0.35
Site 3 (12)	5.75	5.51	3.62	3.67	4.61	4.28	3.62	3.67	−1.52	0.13
Site 4 (16)	8.44	6.28	8.6	6.18	8.44	6.28	8.6	6.18	0.13	0.89
Site 5 (12)	5.19	5.90	1.72	2.88	4.30	4.65	1.72	2.88	−3.70	0.0003
Site 6 (12)	4.24	5.36	3.27	4.12	3.3	4.19	3.27	4.12	−0.04	0.97
Site 7 (16)	7.0	5.93	4.54	5.22	7.0	5.93	4.54	5.22	−1.50	0.14
Site 8 (12)	5.39	5.65	3.30	4.05	4.28	4.23	3.30	4.05	−1.23	0.22

the comparisons are not statistically significant. However, compared to TAU participants in the five programs that received 12 weeks of treatment, Matrix participants in those sites provided significantly more MA-free urines in the first 12 weeks of their treatment (4.3 and 3.3).

After controlling for the potential effects of demographics and the frequency and route of MA use, the multivariate logistic regression indicates that Matrix participants, compared to TAU participants, were 31 percent more likely to have MA-free urine test results (odds ratio = 1.311). The equalized measure of urine test results ensures that the significant effect was due to the treatment condition rather than differences in treatment length.

Weeks of Consecutive Abstinence Documented by Urinalysis

Another way to address the urinalysis data is to calculate the longest period of consecutive MA abstinence by each participant by condition and compare the conditions across sites, for rates of abstinence as documented by urinalysis. Table 8.5 presents the mean durations of the longest MA-abstinent period by site and condition. As illustrated in this table, the Matrix condition is associated with longer mean periods of abstinence than the TAU condition. This finding remains regardless of whether the raw mean totals or the truncated mean totals are computed. The Matrix condition had statistically significantly longer periods of consecutive abstinence in two of the eight comparisons (sites 3 and 5) using the truncated means.

Figure 8.1
Mean Number of MA-Free Urine Samples, by Treatment Length and Treatment Condition (Matrix Treatment Length Truncated to the Length of TAU Treatment)

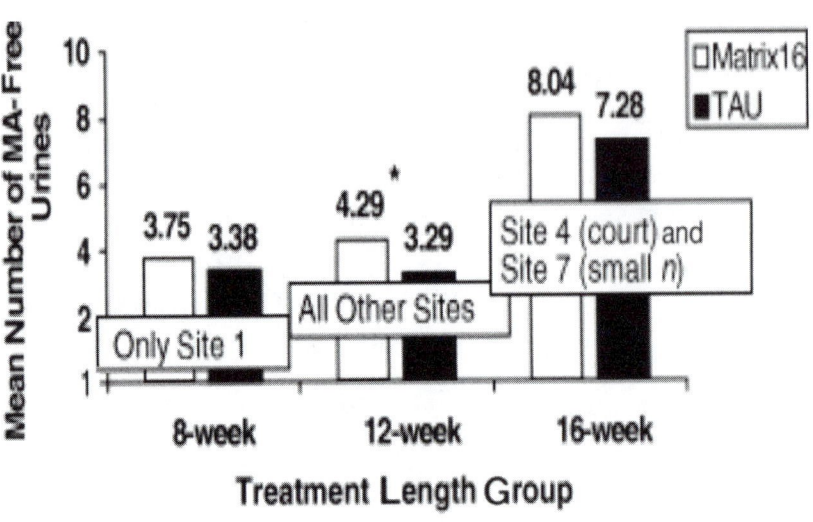

Table 8.5
Longest MA-Abstinent Period by Treatment Site and Condition

| Site (TAU length, weeks) | Raw data | | | | Truncated data | | | | t | P |
| | Matrix | | TAU | | Matrix | | TAU | | | |
	Mean	SD	Mean	SD	Mean	SD	Mean	SD		
Site 1 (8)	3.575	4.600	2.754	3.183	2.877	3.109	2.754	3.183	−0.982	0.328
Site 2 (12)	3.753	5.105	2.474	3.306	3.377	4.271	2.474	3.306	−1.47	0.144
Site 3 (12)	3.197	4.484	1.805	2.763	3.013	4.028	1.805	2.763	−2.16	0.033
Site 4 (16)	6.140	5.771	5.560	5.218	6.140	5.771	5.560	5.218	−0.546	0.586
Site 5 (12)	3.889	5.439	1.279	2.274	3.429	4.467	1.279	2.274	−3.393	0.001
Site 6 (12)	2.429	3.843	2.342	3.671	2.314	3.491	2.342	3.671	0.2	0.841
Site 7 (16)	4.682	5.056	2.542	3.978	4.682	5.056	2.542	3.978	−1.586	0.121
Site 8 (12)	2.833	4.705	2.130	3.448	2.519	3.879	2.130	3.448	−0.551	0.583

Results from Data Collected at Discharge and Six-Month Follow-Up

Self-Report of MA Use from Baseline to Discharge and Six-Month Follow-up

Overall MA use by study participants was substantially reduced during treatment. Using data from the ASI, the self-reported number of days of MA use in the past 30 days was reduced from approximately 11 days at baseline to slightly over 4 days at discharge, and this reduction was maintained through the six-month follow-up time point. Figure 8.2 shows the reduction in MA use by treatment condition and time. The magnitude of the reduction from baseline was consistent across sites and conditions. Repeated-measures analysis of variance results confirm that the effect of time was significant in the reduction in days of MA use ($F_{time} = 124.43$, $P < 0.0001$); however, no statistically significant differences by treatment condition were documented, nor was there a significant interaction effect of condition $\times$ time.

Changes in ASI Domains from Baseline to Discharge to Follow-up

Except for the medical scale, all ASI domains demonstrated significant improvement (reduction in the composite score) across the treatment period. At six-month follow-up, significant reductions from baseline were

Figure 8.2
Participant Self-Report of MA Use (Number of Days of Use during the Past 30 Days) at Enrollment, Discharge, and Six-Month Follow-up, by Treatment Condition

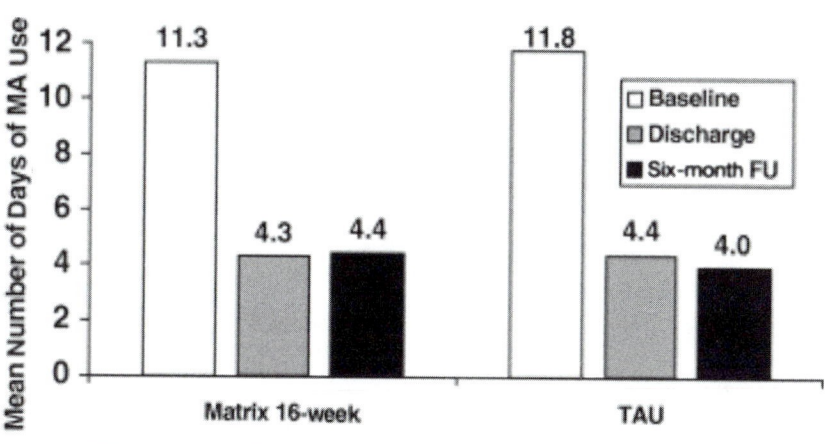

* Statistically significant two-group T-test, $P = 0.05$.

achieved for the drug, alcohol, psychiatric, and family domains. Analyses of these data indicate a significant effect for time. Overall and within each site, however, there were no treatment condition effects or time-condition interactions.

Urinalysis Results at Discharge and Follow-up

The percentages of the urine samples that were MA-free at the discharge interview were 66 percent for Matrix and 69 percent for TAU. At the six-month follow-up, both conditions had 69 percent MA-free urine samples. Missing samples, which were equivalent across conditions, are not included. There were no overall significant differences in these urinalysis outcomes across conditions, nor were any of the individual site rates significantly different across conditions.

DISCUSSION

This study was a large-scale, multisite undertaking to contribute to the knowledge about MA treatment. The study was designed to compare a multicomponent, manualized psychosocial treatment approach (the Matrix Model) with a variety of psychosocial treatments currently in use in several community settings. Because the study was funded by SAMHSA to be conducted in "real-world" treatment programs using the diverse collection of treatment approaches in existence in these community treatment settings, the study was not a conventional multisite study comparing identical treatment approaches at all sites (Rawson and Marinelli-Casey et al. 2002). The comparison of the Matrix approach to eight different types of TAU increases within-group variance, thereby increasing the difficulty of achieving statistically significant findings. Conversely, by comparing the Matrix approach to a variety of TAU approaches, increased knowledge about potential differences may be statistically detected. Because these treatment approaches represent "real-world" service configurations delivered by the organizations that developed them, rather than the "minimal service comparison" employed in many clinical trials, the Matrix–TAU comparisons represent a relatively good comparison condition.

Participant Performance during Treatment Period

Treatment attendance data suggest that it is very possible to deliver a substantial dose of psychosocial treatment to a diverse group of MA-dependent individuals. Across all eight sites, the mean number of sessions delivered to Matrix condition participants ranged from 22 to 35 of a maximum possible of 48. This across-site consistency of service delivery, as well as the data from the fidelity measurement procedures, reinforces the contention that there was appropriate consistency in the delivery of the Matrix approach.

Retention of participants in treatment has been shown to be an important correlate of successful outcome (Hubbard et al. 1989; Simpson et al. 1995). Because the Matrix approach was designed to be longer than six of the eight TAU conditions, the fact that the Matrix approach resulted in longer absolute retention in treatment is not surprising. However, the Matrix approach showed significantly better retention in treatment than the TAU condition, even when program length was controlled, except in the one site in which the TAU condition was conducted within a drug-court context. To the extent that retention in outpatient treatment is viewed as a key indicator of treatment efficacy, the Matrix approach appears to be superior to the other treatments (except in the drug-court locale).

Use of MA during treatment is another key dependent measure of the efficacy of treatment. Participants in the Matrix condition provided more MA-negative urine samples during the treatment period across all but the drug-court site. This is not surprising, as the Matrix approach is longer than six of the seven non-drug-court sites, providing more opportunities to give a clean sample. However, even when the length of the Matrix approach is truncated to the prescribed length of the TAU conditions, participants in the Matrix condition provided significantly more MA-negative samples in the five 12-week programs than those in comparable TAU conditions.

Participant Performance at Discharge and Follow-up

Certainly, measures of MA use and other areas of functioning at treatment discharge and at a six-month point following admission are of great importance in assessing treatment efficacy. The essential finding regarding treatment for MA dependence is that at the discharge and six-month follow-up data collection points, participants in both conditions demonstrated nearly a threefold reduction in mean days of MA use from baseline (self-reported days of MA use in the past 30 days) and a rate of 66–69 percent MA-negative urine samples at discharge and follow-up. More general measures of functioning at discharge indicate significant improvements in six of the seven domains of the ASI. (The medical scale did not show significant change.) At the six-month follow-up, four of the seven ASI domains showed sustained improvements across all sites. Statistical analyses of all discharge and six-month follow-up data indicated that the in-treatment superiority of the Matrix approach was not demonstrated at post-treatment measurement points.

Interpretation of Study Findings

The Matrix approach produces consistently better treatment retention and program completion than the TAU condition in overall analyses and delivers more treatment "events" than TAU at most sites. The Matrix approach also appears to result in more MA-free urine samples and longer periods of in-treatment abstinence than most TAU conditions during the active treatment period. The in-treatment superiority of the Matrix approach, however, is not reflected by measures of functioning collected at discharge or follow-up. These findings document that the use of the standard, accepted, dependent measures and statistical methods for measuring the efficacy of substance abuse treatment approaches can create less than uniform conclusions.

Is this demonstration that the Matrix treatment approach produces better in-treatment performance, but not superior outcome at discharge or follow-up, a meaningful advance in the knowledge about MA treatment? It could be argued that the only meaningful measure in a treatment comparison is the relative outcomes at study end and at follow-up points. The in-treatment differences are interesting, but not important, as the superiority of the Matrix approach is not detected at discharge or follow-up. From this perspective, the results of this study add to a number of large multisite trials in the substance abuse treatment literature that show that all treatment conditions are associated with comparable levels of improvement.

If the results of this study are viewed from the perspective that permanent behavioral changes are hard to maintain in many chronic illnesses, then the study data mark an advancement in the knowledge about treating MA users. First, the project recruited and treated almost 1,000 MA-dependent individuals who were, on average, using MA more than one-third of the days in the month before admission. At study discharge, the number of days of use per month had been reduced to about 4 of 30 days, and this reduction in MA use persisted until the six-month post-admission point for both TAU and Matrix participants. Secondly, the use of the Matrix manualized treatment protocol resulted in the achievement of multiple in-treatment goals to a statistically greater degree than did the TAU protocols, except in the drug-court program. Apparently, the drug-court intervention eliminated the difference between the Matrix and TAU conditions in this context.

The finding that the use of this manualized approach, employing many of the principles contained in the cognitive behavioral and motivational interviewing literature, produces better in-treatment performance than various community treatment protocols should not be unexpected. These specific therapies have solid evidence of efficacy in the treatment of cocaine users. The fact that the Matrix approach, which combines multiple components of these techniques into an intensive, structured protocol, produces significantly improved in-treatment performance is a significant advancement and is consistent with the increasing body of literature supporting these approaches.

NOTES

This chapter presents data collected by seven investigative teams at eight sites and organized by a coordinating center under a multisite cooperative agreement for research funded by the Center for Substance Abuse Treatment (CSAT), Substance Abuse and Mental Health Services Administration, and the U.S. Department of Health and Human Services (grant numbers TI 11440–01, TI 11427–01,

TI 11425–01, TI 11443–01, TI 11484–01, TI 11441–01, TI 11410–01, and TI 11411–01). CSAT is located at 5600 Fishers Lane, Rockwall II Suite 740, Rockville, MD 20857, USA; Tel: 301 443 5052. Contents are solely the responsibility of the authors and do not necessarily represent the official views of the agency.

1. The Methamphetamine Treatment Project corporate authors include the manuscript authors as well as the following: Joseph Balabis, Richard Bradway, Alison Hamilton Brown, Cynthia Burke, Darrell Christian, Judith Cohen, Florentina Cosmineanu, Melissa Donaldson, Thomas E. Freese, Vikas Gulati, Kathryn Horner, Martin Y. Iguchi, Russell H. Lord, Sam Minsky, Pat Morrisey, Norman Rodrigues Jr., Janice Stalcup, S. Alex Stalcup, Ewa S. Stamper, Janice Stimson, Sarah Turcotte Manser, Ahndrea Weiner, and Kathryn Woodward.

CHAPTER 9

Child Welfare and Methamphetamine

Herbert C. Covey, Ph.D.

THE SPECIAL CHALLENGES OF METH FOR CHILD PROTECTION

The Center for Substance Abuse Prevention/National Prevention Network (2006, p. 13) concluded, "The plight of children who live with meth-using adults or are at or near meth labs is a cause for real public concern." Most would agree that substance abuse by parents or other caretakers of children has serious ramifications. Children whose parents use drugs or alcohol are three times more likely than other children to be abused and four times more likely to be neglected (Wells and Wright 2004). For example, one recovering meth addict said this about her neglectful attitude toward her child while using, "My children were irrelevant." In addition to abuse and neglect, and the associated risks of exposure of children to chemically dangerous labs, there are other child protection concerns in meth-involved households.

Child welfare agencies working with meth-involved families face unique challenges. The family involvement in meth places children, families, and agency personnel at risk of serious life-changing and threatening harm. Because of the risks involved, the stakes are high for all, and special precautions must be exercised. Child protection workers need to identify signs of meth involvement and have strategies to ensure child, family, and worker safety.

CHILD WELFARE CASELOADS AND METH

The use and manufacturing of meth by parents or guardians has a profound affect on children. Nationally "We are seeing more children go into foster care because of meth, and for some of these parents, they abandon their children there" (Ray 2004, p. 31). This pattern is being experienced everywhere the drug is present.

Across the country, child protection administrators are well aware of the impacts of meth on the community and on child welfare caseloads. Where meth is available, many child welfare administrators report a large portion of their caseload growth can be attributed to its use by parents and guardians. In no instances have child protection administrators experienced a drop in caseloads with the spread of meth. Examples of the significant growth in child welfare caseloads include the following:

- In Del Norte County, California, two-thirds of the child welfare foster care caseload is associated with meth (Edwards 2005).
- In Merced County, California, between 67 percent and 75 percent of child welfare service cases are meth related (Edwards 2005).
- Hawaii, a state known for high use, reports very high percentages of children present in meth environments. Child Protective Services in Hawaii estimated that in 2003, 85 percent of its cases involved "ice" (meth) in some way (Honolulu Advertiser 2003).

Law enforcement, firefighters, and social service officials have known for years that meth labs place children in these settings at risk. We know that first responders find children living in or near meth labs. A number of child protection agencies report that labs are increasingly playing a role in the child welfare cases investigated. For example, the Colorado Alliance for Drug Endangered Children (www.colodec.org/) estimates on its Web site that 30 percent to 35 percent of seized labs are in homes where children live. Other states, such as Washington, report that children were or had been present in 35 percent of the labs law enforcement had investigated (Swetlow 2003). The North Carolina Department of Health and Human Services (2005) reported that in 2004 about 25 percent of labs had children present. The National Drug Intelligence Center (2002a) reported the number of children found in labs more than doubled between 1999 and 2001. Children are found in between 20 percent and 30 percent of labs (Drug Enforcement Administration 2005; National Jewish Medical and Research Center 2004). Meth use has had for some regions of the country significant effects on child welfare investigations and caseloads.

The El Paso Intelligence Center (EPIC) tracks meth lab–related incidents involving children in the United States. The data collected provide important but also incomplete information about actual lab incidents involving children, because reporting is voluntary. In spite of this shortcoming, the partial data provides an indication of how children are present in labs and are at risk. Table 9.1 shows some of the figures from the El Paso Intelligence Center, which reported (2003) that the number of children found in labs increased from 1,224 in 2000 to 3,474 in 2003.

EXAMPLES OF METH LAWS THAT RELATE TO CHILD WELFARE

Some states have enacted legislation and courts have made rulings that directly relate to child welfare and meth involvement. Laws have been

Table 9.1
Children Involved in Meth Lab–Related Incidents in the United States

			Number of Children				
Year	*Number of Meth Lab–Related Incidents*	*Present*	*Number of Meth Lab–Related Incidents[a]*	*Affected[b]*	*Exposed to[c] Toxic Chemicals*	*Taken into Protective Custody*	*Injured or Killed*
2003	14,260	1,442				724	
2002	15,353	2,077	2,023	3,167	1,373	1,026	26 injured; 2 killed
2001	13,270	2,191	976	2,191	788	778	14 injured
2000	8,971	1,803	216	1,803	345	353	12 injured; 3 killed

[a] Children included in this group were not necessarily present at the time of seizure.

[b] Includes children who were residing at the labs but not necessarily present at the time of seizure and children who were visiting the site; data for 2000 and 2001 may not show all children affected.

[c] Includes children who were residing at the labs but not necessarily present at the time of seizure.

Source: El Paso Intelligence Center, June 2003.

enacted that address situations when children are found in labs. References to many of these state laws can be found at the Drug Endangered Children Web site (www.nationaldec.org). Examples identified at this Web site include the following:

- Washington's statute (RCW 26.44.200) requires that the investigating law enforcement officer immediately contact the Department of Social and Health Services if a child is found in a meth lab (Swetlow 2003). Washington also has a law (RCW 13.34.050) that provides guidelines related to taking an endangered child into custody.
- Idaho has laws that require prosecutors to develop multidisciplinary teams to investigate child abuse and neglect referrals (Swetlow 2003).
- California's laws include sections on coordinating multidisciplinary response teams, preparing an annual report containing data on the number of children found in and removed from clandestine labs, and distributing funds (Swetlow 2003).

- California laws also focus on the possession of precursor chemicals with intent to manufacture meth. The laws allow for enhanced penalties when these chemicals are found in a structure where a child younger than age 16 is present. The California penal code requires people who are convicted of abusing a child or endangering a child's health while under the influence of drugs to abstain from drug use during probation and to submit to random drug testing (Swetlow 2003).
- In North Carolina, several new laws to fight meth were passed in 2004. These include increased penalties for making meth, additional penalties for making it in the presence of children, or if someone is injured while seizing a lab; if someone dies from using the meth, the manufacturer can be charged with murder (Eisley 2004).
- In California, the presence of a meth lab could result in felony child abuse charges. In other states, it may result in a misdemeanor (Herdy 2002).
- South Dakota enacted legislation that defines the exposure of children to labs or sales of controlled substances or drugs, such as meth, as child abuse or neglect.

PHASES OF CHILD PROTECTION CASEWORK

Child protection investigations involve making determinations on whether child abuse or neglect has occurred and assessing the risk of whether either may occur in the future. Given the powerful examples of children being raised in meth-involved homes, it is easy for caseworkers to jump to the conclusion that abuse and/or neglect have occurred. We know about the negative effects of meth use on parenting behaviors.

A comparison with driving under the influence "per se" laws seems appropriate. If we look at DUI models, "per se" laws came into existence so that officers wouldn't have to substantiate that an impaired driver was actually driving recklessly. It is assumed, of course, based on the voluminous research conducted on the effects of drugs and alcohol on driving behaviors that if someone has a certain blood alcohol level or if they are under the influence of mind/mood altering drugs then their driving behavior is dangerous whether they have been observed driving recklessly by an officer or not. The DUI per se laws have had a positive effect on alcohol-related traffic fatalities in Colorado. Because law enforcement officers were given the ability to do DUI check points and random stops under the per se laws, arrests for DUIs went up and there was a subsequent reduction in alcohol-related traffic fatalities that correlates with this timeline. The same could be said of a meth-using parent.

However, some would suggest that actual acts of endangerment must be observed by the child protection caseworker. They note that the exact negative impact of the parent's meth use on the children must be substantiated rather than moving forward based on assumption only. Parental substance abuse including meth does not necessarily constitute child maltreatment. When substantiating or finding a family in need of services, it is important to fully document the negative impact of parental behaviors on the children (North Carolina Division of Social Services and the Family and Children's Resource Program, 2005d).

Caseworkers who visit meth-involved homes often find children living in a world of chaos. Their parents may stay awake for days and crash into a deep sleep that can last for days. Children, especially small ones, are at high risk for abuse and neglect. The last thing on the mind of a "tweaking" or crashing parent is the well-being and care of a child. The net result for many small children is hunger, abuse, neglect, injury, emotional neglect, and other negative experiences. Small children who are neglected because of meth-involved parents often develop survival skills, such as seeking out food and drink. They, like their caretakers, develop a chaotic and altered daily schedule.

Meth-Exposed Children in School and Day Care

Children living in meth-involved homes may show signs of the drug in their homes while in school or day care. Exposure to the meth, as well as those chemicals used to produce it if it is being made in the home, may result in observable signs in children. Teachers and day care providers may notice any or a combination of the following outward signs of exposure: watery eyes, eye discharge, eye pain, burns, chest pains, diarrhea, headaches, fever, coughing, decreased mental functioning, hallucinations, irritability, or dark-colored urine. Some of these symptoms are similar to those of the flu, but if they persist, meth exposure may be the cause. Child protection workers may get referrals from day care providers or schools because of these symptoms in children.

The Issue of Meth Use during Pregnancy

Meth use during pregnancy is associated with prenatal complications, premature deliveries, and altered neonatal behavioral patterns (Wells and Wright 2004). However, research into the effects of meth on pregnancy and fetuses is just beginning. Researchers also have found evidence that prenatal exposure to meth restricts infant growth depending on the trimesters in which the fetus was exposed (Koch Crime Institute 2003; Smith et al. 2003). After observing an absence of research, Rawson and Anglin et al. (2002, p. 9) wrote, "However, it is known that meth use during pregnancy is associated with fetal loss and developmental defects, including developmental delay and possibly learning disabilities." At this time, however, the issue of what meth use does to the unborn is unresolved and requires further research. What is established is that there is no safe level of meth for pregnant women (SAMHSA 2006).

Children born to meth-addicted mothers go through painful withdrawal following birth. According to the July 26, 2005, congressional testimony of Dianne Edwards, the president of the National Association of County Human Services Administrators, the number of infants born and identified as being affected by illegal substance abuse has been increasing. Using Sacramento County, California, as an example, she noted that meth use has increased exponentially. For the most recent year (2003–2004), she reported that for those cases referred to court where substance abuse was the primary reason for the referral, 70 to 82 percent involved meth use (D. Edwards 2005). This pattern does not necessarily imply that newborns have negative health consequences resulting from its use before birth. More research is needed.

An important question is whether meth use by pregnant women should be defined as child abuse. Some states have passed laws that indicate it is. For example, in 2005, Colorado lawmakers passed a "Meth Baby" bill that made using illicit drugs during pregnancy a form of child abuse, but not before deleting a provision that would have given judges the power to immediately terminate the mother's parental rights. The intent of the law is to move women who use drugs like meth into the court system and treatment without fear of their losing their children. The bill defines meth or other illicit drug use as child neglect and would give the courts the power to quickly order mothers into treatment or to take parenting classes.

There is some evidence that if the mother continues to use at the same time she is breastfeeding her child there is a risk that the drug will transfer to the infant. Meth is believed to be transferred through breast milk, so in the opinion of some, use while breastfeeding is a bad idea. At least one case has made it to the courts on this issue. In Riverside California, Amy Leanne Prien, a meth addict, was convicted of second-degree murder after her three-month-old son died from a drug overdose from the drugs he received from her through breastfeeding.

In an effort to protect fetuses, infants, and children, some states have passed laws that focus on substance use by pregnant women. For example, in California, women who test positive for drugs can be referred to child protection services. This leads to an assessment of their parental fitness and possible challenge to custody of their children. Some states require medical personnel and other authorities to report suspected or known cases of drug use by pregnant women to child protection or law enforcement. Some states have implemented laws that require pregnant women found to be using drugs, such as meth, to participate in substance abuse treatment.

Opponents to such laws argue that addicted women will avoid prenatal care if they believe their children will be taken if they are prosecuted or forced into treatment. They further argue that prenatal care results in healthier babies than no care at all.

There are other policy and legal issues. For example, there are many laws that restrict disclosure of medical information. Some laws require that the individual must sign a consent form to release health-care and substance abuse information. In addition, the timing of when child protection and law enforcement can confirm child abuse poses difficult legal issues. The fetus is not legally defined as a person separate from the mother until after birth; thus authorities cannot consider a fetus a victim of a crime until after birth.

Irwin (1995) conducted an interview study of three groups of pregnant women who were using heroin, cocaine, or meth during pregnancy. She found the three different groups had different perceptions about the effects of drug use on the fetus. All three avoided or sought out covert prenatal care for different reasons. The study found the crack cocaine users were stigmatized, were concerned about the impact of cocaine use on their unborn fetuses, and felt guilty. Because of harsh social reactions to their use during pregnancy, they typically avoided prenatal care. Heroin users were less concerned about harming the fetus and more concerned about losing custody of their children. Pregnant women using heroin did not link its use with birth defects or problems. Some of these women also avoided prenatal care or sought covertly obtained medical attention. Finally, Irwin found pregnant meth users had little to no information about the effects of the drug on fetuses. Correspondingly, they were unsure about the effects of the drug. Irwin (1995, p. 628) wrote, "Outside of pregnancy, women viewed meth use as relatively harmless and did not feel that their drug use constituted abuse." Instead, they felt meth use had more positive than negative dimensions to their lives. Regarding child protection services, one interviewee commented:

I want to see them [Child Protective Services] sit there and do all the things they demand of me to do in the amount of time they give me to do them in without any kind of help. And I'm talking without any kind of drugs, 'cause I don't take aspirin for headaches and I can't afford a cup of coffee every morning, and this, that and the other thing. . . . no cocktail after dinner and no martinis and stuff. They'll find out it's just not that easy, when they can't just reach in the medicine cabinet and grab a sedative to go to sleep because it's prescribed by the doctor. It's still a drug, I don't care who it's prescribed by. (Irwin 1995, p. 630)

Wyoming enacted a child drug–endangerment law that allows for felony prosecutions for mothers testing positive for meth use during pregnancy. Some states, such as Hawaii and at least 16 others, have developed mandatory reporting laws that require medical doctors to report to law enforcement and/or child protection newborns that were exposed to illegal drugs, such as meth. In Hawaii, after the baby is tested and shows positive results, a report to child protection is mandated.

There are those who disagree with these and other legal mechanisms. The American Civil Liberties Union has taken the position that prosecuting mothers for meth use during pregnancy is a misuse of the law. Some authorities have focused on the medical effects of meth on fetuses and children. Some have concluded that most children with prenatal exposure to meth lead normal lives as they age, but some may have "subtle impairments" that negatively affect regulation of emotions and ability to concentrate, which could put them at risk for behavioral and learning difficulties (Mathias 2001). Not everyone agrees that meth use during pregnancy results in negative consequences for infants (Lewis and Millar 2005).

CHILD WELFARE INTAKE AND INVESTIGATIONS
WHEN A LAB IS SUSPECTED OR PRESENT

One of the fundamental considerations for child protection is when children are exposed to labs. We know that children found in labs test positive for meth. Carl R. Peed, the director of the Federal Office of Community Oriented Policing Services (Peed 2004, p. 1) wrote, "Children rescued from meth laboratories often test positive for toxic levels of meth and for toxic levels of the ingredients of meth." Peed (2004) summarized that 80 percent of children rescued from meth environments tested positive for meth or the substances used to make it.

Parents and guardians involved with cooking meth commonly expose their children to dangerous chemicals and unsanitary living conditions (Horton et al. 2003). In addition to chemical hazards, there are other risks associated with labs, such as drug traffic coming in and out of the home. Given the heightened effects meth has on libido, children of using parents may be at greater risk for sexual abuse (Swetlow 2003), either by parents themselves or by other adults coming in and out of the home. Children in labs are at significant risk for serious injury and neglect. For example, loaded firearms and other weapons are found in easy-to-reach locations in the vast majority of labs. Dangerous animals, such as powerful watch dogs, and booby traps designed to protect labs pose added physical hazards to children and caseworkers. First responders report that children living with labs in their homes have poor diets, lack adequate medical care, and suffer from respiratory problems (Peed 2004).

Often, cooks use and store dangerous chemicals in child-accessible locations regardless of the risks to children. Lab chemicals and equipment have been found in or next to baby cribs, diaper hampers, and toy bins. Cooks will locate labs and supplies in locations assuming that first responders or others, such as child protection workers, will not become suspicious. Cooks have a particularly dangerous practice of storing meth and dangerous chemicals in refrigerators and food storage areas where small children may confuse food or drink with chemicals. Plastic water bottles, baby bottles, and other seemingly innocent containers have been used or placed next to children's food and drinks. Baby hampers and children's toy chests have been used to store lab chemicals and equipment.

Setting up a lab (described in chapter 3) requires little more than a heat source and some pots. One method, called the "one-pot " method, uses a single container to cook meth. This means that the drug's toxic ingredients may be stored, left open, or spilled within easy reach of children. Tables, sinks, counters, and floors present opportunities for children to touch and taste chemicals and to inhale poisonous fumes. Children living in a lab or in the community are not aware of toxic wastes that have been dumped and may play in those polluted areas.

Besides the toxicity of chemicals, children are exposed to other risks. The production of meth involves and produces many toxic chemicals that contaminate surfaces, clothing, and toys. Small children frequently put things in their mouths and hence ingest whatever chemicals are on the surfaces of clothing, toys, and other household items. They also have greater risk because their skin in thinner and thus more easily absorbs chemicals (Mason 2004). In addition to hazards directly from the labs, it is important to note that those involved with production often live in filth. Homes with labs are usually unclean, cluttered, full of vermin and infestations of insects, and are generally squalid. Ironically, sometimes meth-involved parents perceive they are great housekeepers. According to the U.S. Department of Justice Report, *Children in Clandestine Methamphetamine Labs* (Swetlow 2003, p. 4), children in labs, in addition to abuse and neglect, face a number of risks, including:

- Fires and explosions—About 15 percent of all meth labs are discovered as a result of a fire or explosion. Children may be victims of fires and explosions in labs (SAMHSA 2001).
- Hazardous lifestyle—In addition to squalor, children in labs may live with booby traps, weapons, loaded guns, dangerous chemicals, unusable plumbing, meth in the air and on surfaces, and other hazardous circumstances.
- Social problems—Children may be exposed to dangerous individuals involved with meth, trauma from seeing their parents arrested and taken away, other substances being abused, and poor social relations to name a few.

Small children may accidentally ingest meth or other toxic chemicals left around their homes or dispersed during methamphetamine production. Research conducted by Dr. Martyny (Martyny et al. 2003) and his colleagues at National Jewish Hospital have found that children living in close proximity to labs are exposed and test positive for meth and other dangerous chemicals. The other risk is exposure to explosive, corrosive, flammable, and otherwise dangerous chemicals.

The response of child protection and other agencies to meth will differ greatly from routine procedures if a lab is present or suspected. Most of the professional attention has been focused on families and the associated risks of labs (Drug Enforcement Administration 2005a). Several state, local, and national agencies have developed protocols for responding to labs. The National Alliance for Drug Endangered Children's (DEC) Web site presents general protocols that can be useful for agencies considering developing interagency response procedures. The DEC Web site can be found at www.nationaldec.org. This site includes medical protocols, suggestions for developing interagency agreements, and other information on how to implement a local strategy. A number of states have implemented their own variations of the DEC protocols and policies. The Web sites are excellent resources because most are current with the latest information on how to appropriately respond. Examples of protocols can be found at these sites:

- National Alliance for Drug Endangered Children: www.nationaldec.org/
- Arizona Drug Endangered Children: www.azag.gov/DEC/index.html

- Colorado Drug Endangered Children Inc.: www.colodec.org/
- Drug Endangered Children Task Force (California): www.capc-coco.org/programs/drug-endagered-children-task-force.html
- Iowa Drug Endangered Children: www.iowadec.org/
- Kansas Alliance for Drug Endangered Children: www.ksmethpreventionproject.org/index.htm
- Kentucky Alliance for Drug Endangered Children: www.ca.uky.edu/heel/dec.htm
- North Carolina Department of Health and Human Services: info.dhhs.state. nc.us/olm/manuals/dss/csm-65/man/CSs1000.htm
- Oregon Alliance for Drug Endangered Children: www.oregondec.org/
- Riverside County Drug Endangered Children Program: dec.co.riverside.ca.us/
- South Dakota Alliance for Drug Endangered Children: www.mappsd.org/dec.htm
- Texas Alliance for Drug Endangered Children: www.dectexas.org/

These protocols generally require a HAZMAT Team to determine the degree of contamination and need for decontaminating occupants. Some response teams have portable tent or trailer showers that are used to decontaminate occupants (children) at the scene. Full medical exams are advised on all occupants, including children, either at the scene or within four hours to determine if there are needs for acute treatment. Included in the initial medical responses are pulmonary, skin, and neurological exams. Urine analysis or blood tests are recommended within 12 hours of identification of a child requiring such service.

Protocols generally specify that law enforcement should secure the scene, children, and offenders, in addition to collecting criminal evidence and jointly participating with child protection in forensic interviews of children. Child protection, following screening procedures, should assess the situation and begin securing court orders and the release of information; assess the children for injuries; and take pictures of dangerous surroundings and injuries. If a lab is present, members of the HAZMAT team or law enforcement in protective clothing should take photos in the lab area to ensure caseworker safety.

These protocols typically require children removed from homes containing labs to be decontaminated and dressed in new clothing before transportation in an emergency or medical placement. Contaminated clothing should be properly discarded along with any personal items, such as toothbrushes, toys, etc. It is not easy for children to understand why they have to leave their favorite toys or stuffed animals behind. First responders and caseworkers should be sensitive to the trauma children experience with the loss of their personal items, let alone separation from family members. The importance of the latter should not be underestimated. Lt. Lori Moriarty once shared a conversation where someone said to a child, "You sure have shitty parents." The child responded, "They may be shitty but they are my parents."

Many first responders have kits available for children and adults containing new clothing, underwear, backpacks, toys, and other essential items. Some exceptions can be made for eyeglasses, orthodontics, and other items, if they have been decontaminated by professionals. Locally, many individuals, non-profits, and businesses are willing to donate items or gift cards for this pur-pose. Some decontamination units have prepacked bags or backpacks that they take to all suspected labs. If labs are not present, children can keep their clothing and other items, but these should be cleaned.

Authorities need to conduct initial medical screenings before placement and full medical physicals on all children within 24 to 48 hours. First respond-ers and child protection workers may find lab-exposed children asymptomatic and appearing normal. However, these appearances may mask serious condi-tions; hence thorough medical evaluations are important. Caretakers should watch for respiratory problems, such as difficulty in breathing or excessive coughing.

The Importance of Having Multidisciplinary Teams

All of these drug-endangered children (DEC) responses involve multidis-ciplinary teams comprised of social services, medical, law enforcement, envi-ronmental health, school, and other local stakeholders. It is critical that these agencies work in concert to ensure the safety of children, families, agency staff, and the community, with an eye toward legal issues, prosecution, and law enforcement. In addition, the agencies must be sensitive to the traumatic effects of first responders on children and family members.

With meth, the rules of the game change for everyone. While many child protection procedures do not depart from normal practice, others will require different approaches to ensure the safety of the children and caseworker(s). For example, if a lab is discovered in the household, caseworkers need to take special precautions to ensure the safety of the children and themselves. However, many of the routine child protection practices will apply follow-ing the initial response. The procedures change for law enforcement as well, especially when children or innocents are also present.

From a traditional law enforcement perspective, a main goal is to get the "bad guys" off the streets. Thus, law enforcement agencies may be reluctant to work with other agencies, such as child protection, because they do not want them to hamper their investigations or ruin their criminal cases. In turn, child protection agencies want to protect children from abuse or neglect and do not have a criminal justice orientation in their work. Ideally, if a suspected meth-involved household (lab) is going to be raided, law enforcement should contact social services and find out if there are any known children, older adults, or other at-risk individuals in the residence. Social services will know if there is or has been an open case on the family. In addition, if law enforcement officers discover children during a lab bust or arrest, child protection agency involvement may be required. This does not always occur in all jurisdictions. Likewise, if child protection or caseworkers accidentally come upon suspected labs or meth-involved households that pose risks, they should report these situations to law enforcement. The key to addressing these issues and others is for agencies to plan and develop standing agreements or memorandums of understanding on how to work together to ensure public safety and child protection goals. Many experienced jurisdictions have developed agreements that specify how agencies will work together. Having this information can be valuable to law enforcement and social services.

When establishing agreements, it is important for local agencies to develop multidisciplinary response teams. Which agencies and personnel should participate in a DEC or multidisciplinary response team when children are involved? An adequate response to meth labs or meth-involved families requires a community response. According to a number of sources (www.nationaldec.org; Swetlow 2003), community response teams should include the following:

- Law enforcement to play a critical role in ensuring the safety of agency personnel, children, and others involved in a planned or unplanned lab seizure.
- Medical services to decontaminate, assess harm to health, and medically treat children exposed to hazardous substances and or who have been abused. Typically, medical staffs need to conduct physical examinations of children and others exposed to labs. Medical protocols can be found at many of the drug-endangered children Web sites identified in this volume. For example, timely urine samples and documentation of chemical exposure may play key roles in substantiating child abuse or neglect.
- Mental health services to address any presenting mental health issues and traumas experienced by children and others in the household.
- Child welfare/protection to ensure than children are safe and not at risk of abuse or neglect.

Multidisciplinary response teams should have established agreements (protocols) that address at a minimum confidentiality, roles, responsibilities, training, reporting, interviewing procedures, medical care procedures, evidence collection, and safety.

Accidental Lab Discovery by Child Protection Workers

During child protection investigations or home visits, child protection workers may unexpectedly find themselves in labs. For example, North Carolina reports that about 75 percent of the labs found were "stumbled upon" (North Carolina Department of Social Services 2005a, 2005b). The technology of cooking meth is such that small labs are relatively easy to set up and operate. Child protection workers may accidentally come across labs in infant rooms, kitchens, bedrooms, and pretty much anywhere in the household.

Child protection workers need to be aware that there are risks involved when even doing the simplest of child protection tasks. Child protection workers frequently open refrigerators to check on food and drinks in homes. The simple act of opening a refrigerator door where crystal meth is being made can cause an explosion. The Central Valley California High-Intensity Drug Trafficking Area (HIDTA) warns of one of the risks of crystal meth labs that should be heeded by all. Child protection workers and law enforcement personnel should exercise extreme caution when opening refrigerators and freezers found at crystal meth production sites. The vapors from the solvents used to convert powered meth to crystal meth are extremely volatile and can accumulate in a refrigerator or freezer during the evaporation process. These vapors may explode when the appliance's inside light activates as the door is opened. HIDTA recommends that law enforcement personnel should immediately unplug all refrigerators and freezers found at crystal meth laboratories to avoid this risk (National Drug Intelligence Center 2002). While it is not practical or realistic for caseworkers to unplug appliances every time they conduct a home visit, it is important to be aware of potential risks in possible labs and to immediately leave the site if production is suspected.

Most protocols direct child protection workers to leave the suspected lab immediately and contact law enforcement. This is to ensure their safety and engage the proper response agencies. It is critical for the child protection caseworker to have acquired the basic training on lab identification. Child welfare administrators need to train staff on meth lab identification and appropriate protocols. The Drug Enforcement Administration (2005a) recommends the following for anyone, including caseworkers, accidentally coming across a lab:

- Do not touch anything in the lab.
- Do not turn on any electrical power switches or light switches.
- Do not turn off any electrical power switches or light switches.
- Do not eat or drink in or around a lab.
- Do not open or move containers with chemicals or suspected chemicals.
- Do not smoke anywhere near a lab.
- Do not sniff any containers.
- Do decontaminate yourself and your clothing.
- Do wash your hands and face thoroughly.
- Do call your local authorities or Drug Enforcement Administration district office.

North Carolina Department of Social Services and the Family and Children's Resource Program (2005b) recommends that a caseworker who suspects a lab should take these steps:

- Remain calm. Give yourself time to think.
- Do not approach suspects. They are often armed and may be dangerous.
- Do not enter the lab area. Discarded containers, waste, and other materials remaining from a meth lab can be highly toxic and dangerous.

- Do not try to clean up the area. Evidence should remain undisturbed for investigation by law enforcement.
- If you are in the lab already, find an excuse to leave immediately. Never use touch or smell to try to identify unknown substances.
- Keep a safe distance. Hazardous materials may ignite, or the fumes may overcome you (Mason 2004; North Carolina Department of Social Services and the Family and Children's Resource Program 2005b).
- Promptly notify local law enforcement and follow all state policies regarding meth labs.

INVESTIGATIONS WHEN METH LABS ARE NOT SUSPECTED OR PRESENT BUT PARENTS OR CARETAKERS MAY BE USING

The presence of children in labs and the associated risks have garnered most of the media, public, and professional attention. A more common scenario is when children are living with meth caretakers or parents who are using on a regular basis, but not manufacturing. The absence of a lab does not ensure that children are safe and free from risk. To the contrary, while labs are clearly more dangerous, risks from use are still present. Parents and guardians who are using meth may, even if not intentionally, abuse and neglect their children.

Specifically, when parents routinely use meth, their children often do not have necessities such as food, water, and shelter, and they frequently lack adequate supervision and medical care. In addition, the cycle of meth abuse has a built-in phase when parents usually "crash" and are unable to look after their children (Wells and Wright 2004). Parents using meth often do not supervise children's activities and hygiene. Also, they may not provide enough food or good nutrition. In meth-involved homes, children may suffer malnutrition or go without appropriate medical attention. Parents who are in the "tweaking" phase can be abusive and violent to their own children (SAMHSA 2001).

Children in meth-involved families may also face hazards, such as used hypodermic needles and razor blades that are often found in the home (Swetlow 2003). For example, in chapter 3 Lynn Riemer recommends caution when sitting on soft furniture because needles and other dangerous paraphernalia may be present.

Because routine meth use reduces the appetite, parents or caretakers do not eat as much or prepare meals for children. The care and nurturing of children becomes unimportant to a heavy user compared to getting and maintaining a high. Addicted parents and caretakers lose track of time and their responsibilities. This results in children receiving inadequate nutrition (Rawson and Anglin et al. 2002). The children live in a perpetual state of malnutrition and hunger. Neglected children also have poor hygiene and grooming and display rapid mood swings and fatigue. Children being raised in settings where meth is being smoked have strong odors embedded in their clothing and may emit odors from their bodies. This does not always mean that meth-addicted parents do not love their children—the drug addiction simply interferes with their abilities to care for them. The North Carolina Division of Social Services and the Family and Children's Resource Program (2005) summarized:

Use of the drug for some becomes more important than caring for infants, children, and other vulnerable family members. Prolonged meth use takes over the whole person and becomes a way of life. A way of life that becomes more important than friends and family members. The drug is so addictive that using parents may seriously neglect and/or abuse their children.

With prolonged meth use, psychotic behaviors and mental illness may evolve. Heavy users become paranoid and violent. Too often, children are the targets of this violence. In addition, the withdrawal (crashing) from meth can precipitate emotional and physical abuse. The Drug Enforcement Administration claims there is a direct relationship between meth use and incidents of domestic violence and child abuse (Drug Enforcement Administration 2004a).

FAMILY ASSESSMENT

Following the investigation and determination that child abuse or neglect has occurred and the children's safety is ensured, the caseworker takes steps to assess the family or caretakers. Besides identifying strengths and needs of the family, an assessment of the factors that place the children at further risk of abuse or neglect is made. When meth is involved, a thorough assessment of the family's degree of involvement in use and or manufacture is critical, because the more extensive that involvement, the more time and resources it may take for the parent(s) or guardian(s) to recover and establish a safe household. There are numerous drug screening and assessment tools available for caseworkers and treatment specialists to turn to for guidance. The other basic component to the family assessment is for the caseworker to help the children appropriately cope with the maltreatment.

How to Spot a Meth User—Recognizing the Signs of Heavy Meth Use

It is useful for the caseworker, whether during investigations or in ongoing work with families, to know the signs of meth use. High-intensity (regular) meth use results in some dramatic changes in behavior and lifestyle disruption. While nothing can replace a full substance abuse assessment, it is possible to identify likely high-intensity use. A number of clues can help identify an individual as a high-intensity user. If you are a parent, friend, co-worker, neighbor, child protection caseworker, or associate, there are outward indicators of high-intensity use. High-intensity users may display some or all of these signs or behaviors that suggest use. For example, they only come out at night to shop, steal, or run errands; they may involuntarily twitch much of the time; they show drastic changes in personality or character; they have a distorted sense of time; they are characterized by incessant talking (rambling); they find ordinary things funny, when in fact they are not; they appear sloppy in appearance and behavior (a disheveled look); they may have sores up their nose or have open sores that scab over and itch; they have major deterioration or loss of teeth; and they have increased sensitivity to light because of dilated pupils.

These signs are important for child protection caseworkers and other professionals to be aware of for their safety and that of others. The North Carolina Division of Social Services and the Family and Children's Resource Program (2005a) makes recommendations for caseworkers to safely work with meth users. In addition to the signs of use listed above, North Carolina lists these possible danger signs that should be considered:

- Client is extremely irritable or argumentative, or there is an escalation of irritability
- Regular client does not appear to know who you are
- Evidence of paranoid thinking, delusions
- Client verbalizes implicit or explicit threat against you
- Presence of knife, firearm, or other weapon in the immediate vicinity

The North Carolina Division of Social Services and the Family and Children's Resource Program (2005a) recommends the following safety tips for caseworkers: Inform supervisor/co-workers you will be visiting a client with a history of making or using meth; follow agency safety protocols; and ask permission if you want to go to another area of the client's dwelling or look in cabinets (for example, to ensure food is in the house). In addition, North Carolina recommends that the caseworker look for symptoms of stimulant use—paraphernalia for using meth, such as glass smoking pipes, syringes, straws, and razor blades on mirrors or other surfaces; signs that the client is becoming upset, angry, or suspicious; scratch marks or scabs, particularly on hands and arms, (which could be evidence of tactile hallucinations and indicate a prior episode of stimulant psychosis); evidence of hallucinations; and strong chemical odors (which may indicate manufacturing) (North Carolina Division of Social Services and the Family and Children's Resource Program, 2005d).

Safety Tips for Approaching Someone High on Meth

Child protection workers may encounter situations when they come into contact with someone high on meth, and specifically tweaking. If they are crashing, they will not pose a threat. The National Drug Intelligence Center (2002, 2002a) offers suggestions for how to approach someone who is high on meth:

- Keep a social distance, preferably a 7- to 10-foot radius. Once a "tweaker" has been identified, contact law enforcement.

- Do not shine bright lights at him or her. The tweaker is already paranoid and if he/she is blinded by a bright light, he/she could run or become violent.
- Slow your speech and lower the pitch of your voice. A tweaker hears sounds at a fast pace and in a high pitch, and a side effect of the drug is a constant electrical buzzing sound in the background.
- Slow your movements. This will decrease the odds that the user will misinterpret your physical actions.
- Keep your hands visible. Because the user is already paranoid, if you place your hands where she or he cannot see them, she/he may feel threatened and become violent.
- Keep the person talking. A person who is high on meth who falls silent can be extremely dangerous. Silence often means that paranoid thoughts have taken over reality and anyone on the scene can become part of the tweaker's paranoid delusions.

CASE PLANNING/CASE MANAGEMENT

Chapters 6 and 13 of this volume address many of the child welfare case management fundamentals. Without being redundant, the outcomes of case planning should always address child safety, child permanency, and family well-being. Each of these goals should have corresponding plans. The safety plan for a meth-involved family poses challenges for the child protection caseworker, as it would for many substance-abusing families. The caseworker must determine whether the use in the home has stopped long enough to allow the children to be free of risk, maltreatment, or harm.

The case plan follows the assessment and must spell out what the goals are and how the family is willing to work toward reaching those goals. The permanency plan identifies the permanency goals for the children either with the family or in an alternative placement. The permanency plan identifies how permanency will be accomplished if reunification with the meth-involved family fails.

Regardless of the circumstances, the child protection worker must involve the family and community professionals, such as substance abuse treatment providers, in the development of the case plan. The substance abuse treatment provider must work closely with the caseworker to ensure that both are on the same page. With meth addiction, the caseworker should expect to see setbacks with the addict during the recovery process. If drug tests are part of the services provided to monitor progress, initially a positive test for meth use may occur. This does not necessarily indicate a treatment failure. Sometimes recovering addicts will self-medicate to cope with withdrawal symptoms, such as depression.

The Out-of-Home Placement Decision

One response to finding children in meth homes is to remove them from the home. In general, for all substances, the National Center on Substance Abuse and Child Welfare (NCSACW) reported that in cases where a child has been placed in custody, estimates of parental substance abuse range from

33 percent to 66 percent (NCSACW 2004, p. 1). The statistics for meth in some areas are likely higher. For example, Gibson et al. (2002) reported that in 2000 in the Central Valley of California more than 20,000 children were in foster care and 90 percent or more of the cases were meth related.

There is a correlation between substance abuse and permanency. Specifically, there is a greater likelihood that the permanency decision will be made sooner for substance abuse cases, including meth use. Children in meth-involved homes have a greater chance of being removed. The key question is when is this appropriate? The answer is that it varies with each situation. The caseworker and agency must be careful in not overreacting to meth use until a solid assessment of the situation is completed.

Some would argue that the parents or guardians must be engaged in treatment quickly. For a high-intensity user, this may not be possible. Some would also want progress or the lack of progress to be identified quickly. While this is desirable, for high-intensity users progress is measured in small steps. Just getting an addict to that first treatment may take several attempts. Meth addiction is similar to that of other stimulants in that it is not something that occurs over night.

Child protection workers, judges, substance abuse counselors, and others do not have standards for making decisions regarding the extent to which children are at risk in meth-using households. Removing young children from meth-involved parents is a critical decision that occurs at a time when children should be bonding with the parents, especially the mother. Foster care is not ideal, but neither is living in a meth-involved home, especially when the parents are heavy users. If the children are in a lab, they should be removed because of the health risks, at least temporarily, according to drug-endangered children protocols (health, safety, and so on).

The decision to recommend removal and out-of-home placement (foster care) is less evident if the parents are less involved in meth use and are cooperative with the investigation and authorities. Some parents may understand their inability to care for children and may want to turn over their children to authorities, at least temporarily until the child protection and substance abuse issues are appropriately addressed. Others will resist and become noncooperative.

Some jurisdictions have looked at creative ways to prevent the removal of children from suspected meth-involved households. For example, the Utah State Division of Children and Family Services child welfare investigators, in collaboration with law enforcement agencies, do "Knock and Talks," with families suspected of being involved with meth use. If the family is cooperative, the agencies work with the families on addressing drug-use issues and keeping the children in the home.

Know and Inform the Out-of-Home Placement

An important piece of information for child protection caseworkers is to know with whom the child or children are being placed. A common scenario in an emergency removal is to place children with immediate family members or friends while the parents are sent to jail. Because meth addicts' friends and relatives have a greater probability of also being involved with the drug, it is critical that children be carefully placed with guardians not involved with drugs. Caseworkers and placement agencies should check out relatives and friends to verify that substance abuse is not problematic with the placement. North Carolina authorities recommend caseworkers thoroughly assess kin and others before placing children, because meth use is sometimes a problem for extended families. Sometimes well-intentioned caseworkers or police accidentally make emergency placements with friends or kin in meth-involved homes. Consequently, the risk to the children remains. Sharing information between law enforcement and child protection can help prevent risky placements.

One drug enforcement agency, in a formal check of backgrounds of emergency relative or friend placements of children, found that over 80 percent of the placement homes had histories of substance abuse, sometimes of meth (Moriarty 2005). We know that meth use and manufacture can be multigenerational within the family unit. Morgan and Beck (1995) reported that it was not uncommon to find two to three generations of family members using meth. The bottom line is for the caseworker to be careful and not move the child(ren) from one meth-involved household to another.

Special Considerations for Foster Homes

If children are placed in foster care, it is equally important to train foster care providers in how to deal with children who have been exposed to meth. Children who have lived in meth-involved homes may act in inappropriate ways in foster care. For example, if a parent has a pattern of crashing for days, children placed in foster care may continue self-preservation behaviors, such as hoarding food or gorging or displaying strange sleep patterns. There is a good possibility that if the child or children have been living in a meth-involved household, they have learned a degree of independence to survive that may or may not be age appropriate. It is also likely they have developed survival skills that may or may not be positive.

Foster homes should also inspect or look over any items the children bring into care. Besides washing everything, foster care providers need to be aware that parents and others may hide drug paraphernalia, meth, needles, syringes, and other dangerous items in children's clothing, diaper bags, backpacks, or toys. Foster care providers should contact authorities immediately if anything looks suspicious.

Anecdotally, meth-exposed children may present special issues for foster parents. They have been raised under highly chaotic, violent, and disorganized living circumstances and often develop adaptive survival skills that make them more difficult to manage. The rules and structure provided by a foster home may seem difficult to understand or adhere to, at least initially. Foster homes may see any of the following behaviors from children coming from meth-involved homes:

- The children are both eager to please but also difficult to discipline. They have been likened to having Jekyll and Hyde personalities.
- They may hoard food and drinks.
- Their sleep patterns are anything but routine or normal. Infants that have been exposed to meth in utero are typically sleepy for a few weeks. They may eventually become irritable and jittery.
- They have poor diets and eating patterns. They may be behind nutritionally.
- Older children will take on parenting roles well beyond their years.
- They may act antisocially.
- They may distrust adults because they may have been sexually abused or exploited.
- They may display attachment disorder and act unemotionally or untrustingly, and be unable to form normal social relationships.
- They may exhibit low self-esteem or sense of shame.
- Long-term, they may mirror their parents' behaviors and be at risk for drug use, violence, teen pregnancy, criminal behaviors, and mental health issues.

According to an interview with Dr. Kathryn Wells (www.mappsd.org), some foster care givers provide lab-exposed children with sedatives, antihistamines, and other medications. Foster parents can be more thoughtful by having medical personnel diagnose whether or not the children are experiencing withdrawal from meth or other chemicals, then respond accordingly.

Ongoing Case Work with Child Welfare Clients in Recovery

Research indicates that brain cells that contain dopamine and serotonin are damaged by meth use over time (see chapters 4 and 7 in this volume). Prolonged use of meth may reduce levels of dopamine and cause symptoms similar to those of Parkinson's disease (Swan 1996). Two decades of research involving animals show that high doses of meth damage neuron cell-endings (Swan 1996). Prenatal exposure to meth has been found to have neurotoxic effects in mice, especially males (Martin 2002).

Summarizing recent medical research on the effects of meth use on cognitive and motor skills, Zickler (2002) found that long-term use by humans results in weakened memory and slowed motor skills two months after abstinence, but showed marked improvement after nine months. The bottom line for caseworkers is to acknowledge that the negative effects of meth will linger after the client stops using, but will eventually decline over time. Caseworker patience will be important to working with a meth-involved client in recovery. This can be trying if there are pressures from the court or child welfare agency to expedite the placement of the child(ren).

For the caseworker, family engagement can pose significant challenges. Caseworker attempts to engage meth-involved parents with social services and their families can be frustrating. Because the drug heightens energy and inflates self-esteem, some meth users feel so "on top of the world" that they are genuinely unable to see any reason for social service involvement with their family. But it is important to avoid prejudging or demonizing meth users. Assess each family individually. Families involved with meth also have strengths. The caseworker can help the family find these and build on them (North Carolina Division of Social Services and the Family and Children's Resource Program 2005d).

SERVICE PROVISION

There is much folklore and controversy regarding the effectiveness of treatment for meth addiction. If the child protection worker opens a meth-involved case with the assumption that nothing can be done to address the addiction, it is inevitable that the child or children will be permanently removed from the home. This assumption does a great disservice to meth-involved parents and their children. It cuts off the motivation for some parents to change. While it is true that some meth addicts will not recover, most research indicates that many treatment programs can work for most. The statistics indicate that meth treatment programs are at least as effective as programs directed toward other addictions (see chapters 6, 7, 8, and 14 for examples).

The actual implementation of the case plan is one of the most difficult and frustrating aspects of working with meth-involved families. Ideally, services are effectively matched with family and client(s) to address needs. However, client and family responses to the case planning and services will differ with circumstances, availability of appropriate services, and varying levels of commitment to change. Some clients and families will be responsive to services, but others will miss appointments or not be able to comply with sets of tasks. Much of this noncompliance is due to the long-term effects of the drug on their physical and mental functioning. Regardless of what is occurring, the child protection caseworker will need to rely on the professional advice of substance abuse specialists who have experience working with stimulant abuse.

Reunification and Keeping Families Together—Does It Make Sense?

Many child welfare professionals don't attempt to keep the family together or reunify them when they find children in a lab. Rather, they go straight for TPR (termination of parental rights). Opponents would say that children and previous meth-involved families deserve more. North Carolina (info.dhhs. state.nc.us/olm/manuals/dss/) has a policy that although the safety of the child is the primary concern, "The presence of meth use or a meth lab should be a signal to agencies to conduct a thorough, strengths-based assessment and to make a robust attempt to ensure family members receive the treatment and support they need to stay together or to reunify if at all possible."

Ongoing social casework with previous meth-involved families also poses challenges, because the time frames required to recover from intense meth use can be lengthy. In addition, many meth-involved families are involved with the criminal justice system and its requirements. The purposes and processes of the criminal justice system may run contrary to social services' objectives of family reunification and recovery. As North Carolina Social Services notes, it can be a challenge to achieve family reunification for meth-involved families within Adoption and Safe Families Act (ASFA) timeframes (North Carolina Division of Social Services and the Family and Children's Resource Program 2005d). Chapter 13 of this volume has a discussion and exhibit that compares the court, case management, and recovery time frames. They may not always be synchronized in a manner that facilitates family reunification. This makes drug court an attractive option.

FAMILY PROGRESS AND CASE CLOSURE

In child welfare, numerous agencies, policies, and laws promote periodic assessments and case closure. When assessing a family's progress, caseworkers routinely assess whether risk of maltreatment has been reduced, if the factors that led to the maltreatment have been adequately eliminated or reduced, whether the goals of the case plan have been accomplished, if the well-being of the family has improved, and if child safety can be ensured. The million dollar question is, "When can a child or children be returned to a previously methamphetamine-involved household?"

There are no set guidelines for making this important determination. Typically, the caseworker and other professionals meet with the family and mutually determine if progress has occurred and if the goals have been accomplished. If the household is free of meth use or manufacture over a prolonged period and case plan goals have been accomplished, this review is much easier. If a lab was present, it is important to detoxify the household before occupancy (North Carolina Division of Social Services and the Family and Children's Resource Program 2005c). However, if there have been setbacks or there is reason to doubt that true changes have occurred, the assessment and recommendation to the courts can be more contentious.

Dr. Nicolas Taylor (2006) has developed objective behavior benchmarks that can be used to establish whether or not a client is making progress and getting anything out of their treatment. He has been involved in many such cases when the effectiveness of treatment is measured by key decision makers, such as judges and caseworkers, by the length of time in treatment. He refers to this as the "Myth of Duration Expectations" that is to say, the false belief that if meth addicts complete x amount of time in treatment, that means that they are "all better." Courts love to order that the addict go to treatment for at least six months. If the addict goes and does a six-month "treatment sentence," then presto they're "fixed." He likes to compare this to believing that treatment is like sticking a cake in the oven and then setting the kitchen timer—30 minutes later (or six months later), "ding," the addict is fixed.

Rather than placing duration expectations, Dr. Taylor likes to talk about using objective behavioral benchmarks to measure treatment progress regarding the treatment the person is receiving. He believes that treatment can't be said to be working if the individual has not made changes in these areas, again regardless of the treatment they may be receiving. He has developed objective behavioral benchmarks, such as periods of thoroughly verified abstinence (say six months), verified periods of normal sleeping and eating patterns, verified distancing from key individuals, stable lifestyle, and others. If done adequately, the objective behavioral benchmarks can be used to help decisions regarding visits with children and then eventually even reunification. His approach forces the therapist to come up with verifiable objective behavioral benchmarks that make the therapist feel confident that the client is no longer using and has changed the things about the using lifestyle that place the children in danger. Using this strategy, Dr. Taylor reports that some clients feel empowered by this because they now know what they need to do, specifically, to "bind the court" into returning their children to them.

Some cases are closed because the client fails to cooperate with the case plan and or treatment. These situations require the caseworker to document the risks to the child or children and those specifically linked to meth use. If substance abuse remains a problem, the caseworker should encourage the client(s) to seek additional treatment.

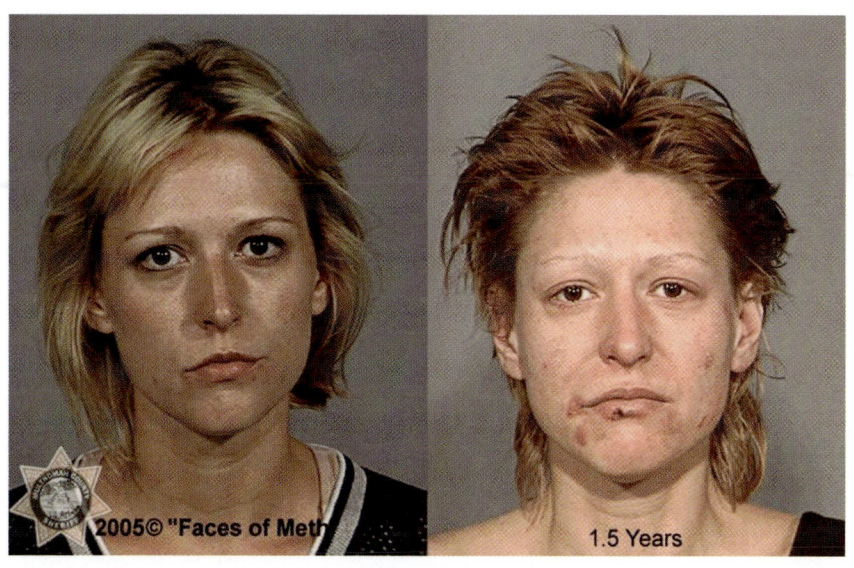

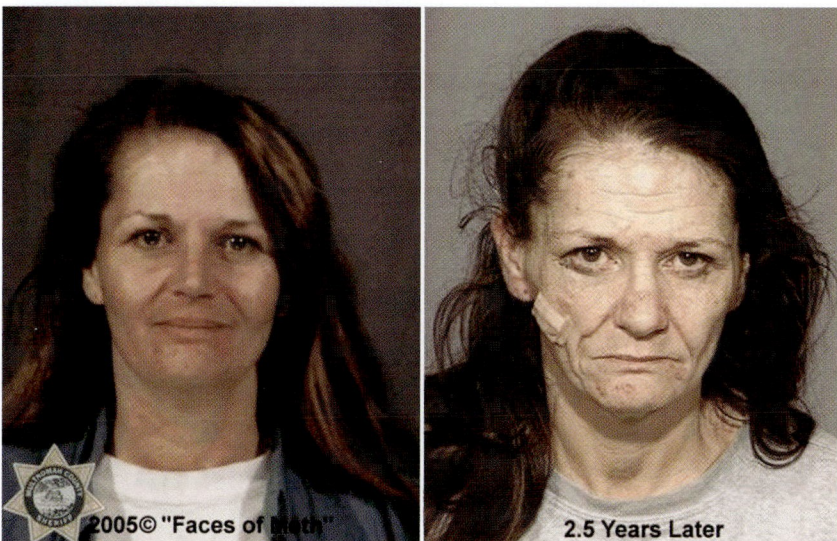

Examples of physical deterioration resulting from prolonged meth use.
Photos courtesy of the Multnomah Sheriff Office, Faces of Meth.

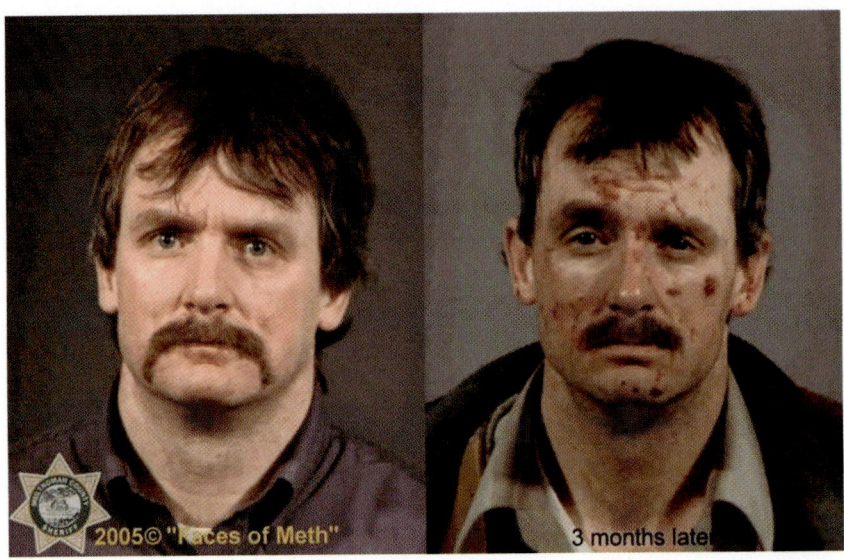

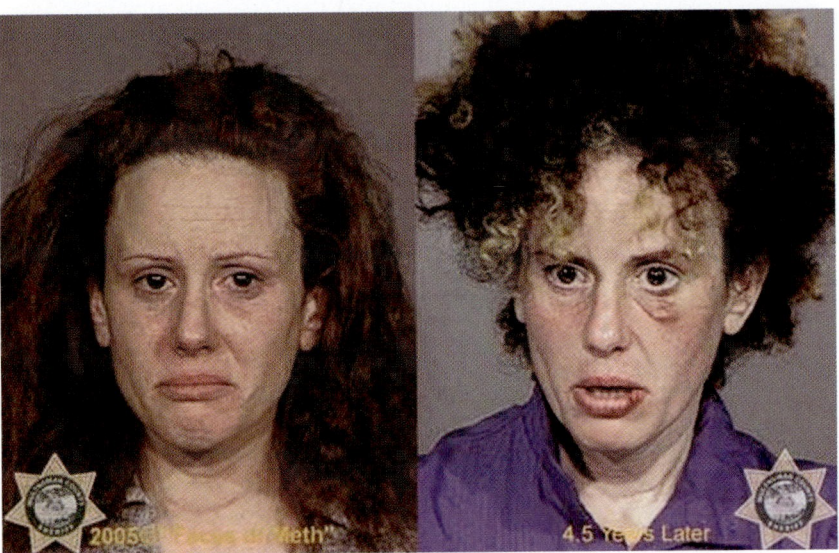

Examples of physical deterioration resulting from prolonged meth use.
Photos courtesy of the Multnomah Sheriff Office, Faces of Meth.

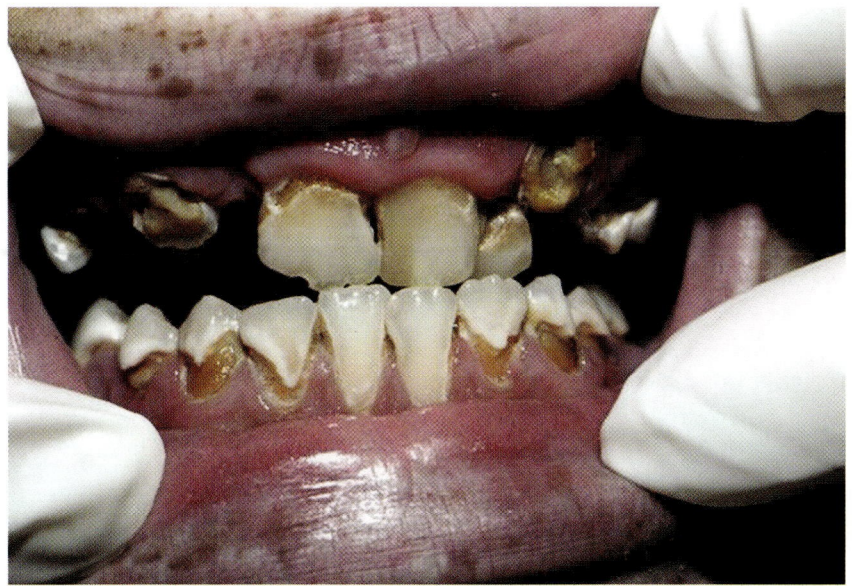

"Meth mouth" dental decay images. Photo by Bill Husa, *Chico Enterprise-Record.*

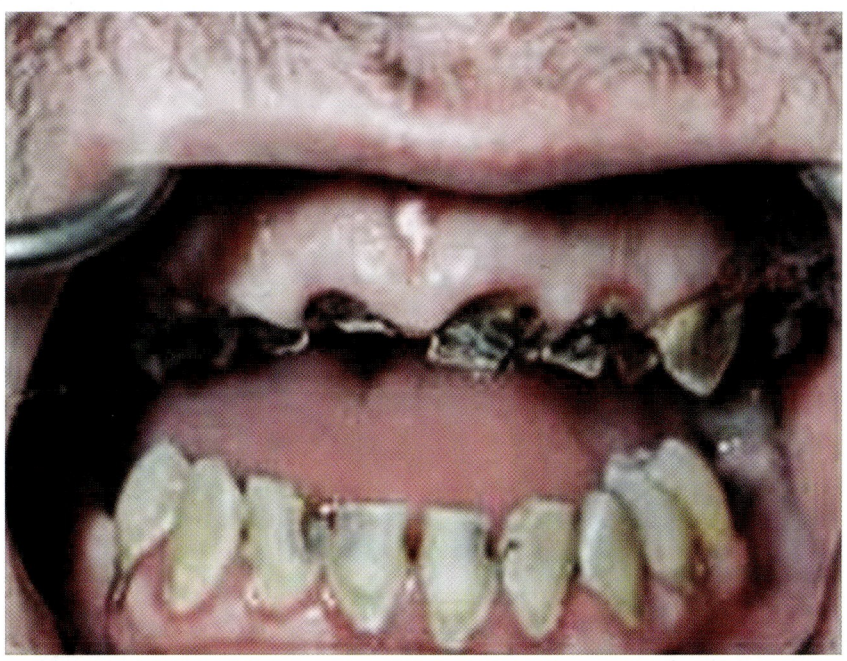

Photo by Dr. Chris Heringlake, The Minnesota Correctional Facility-St. Cloud.

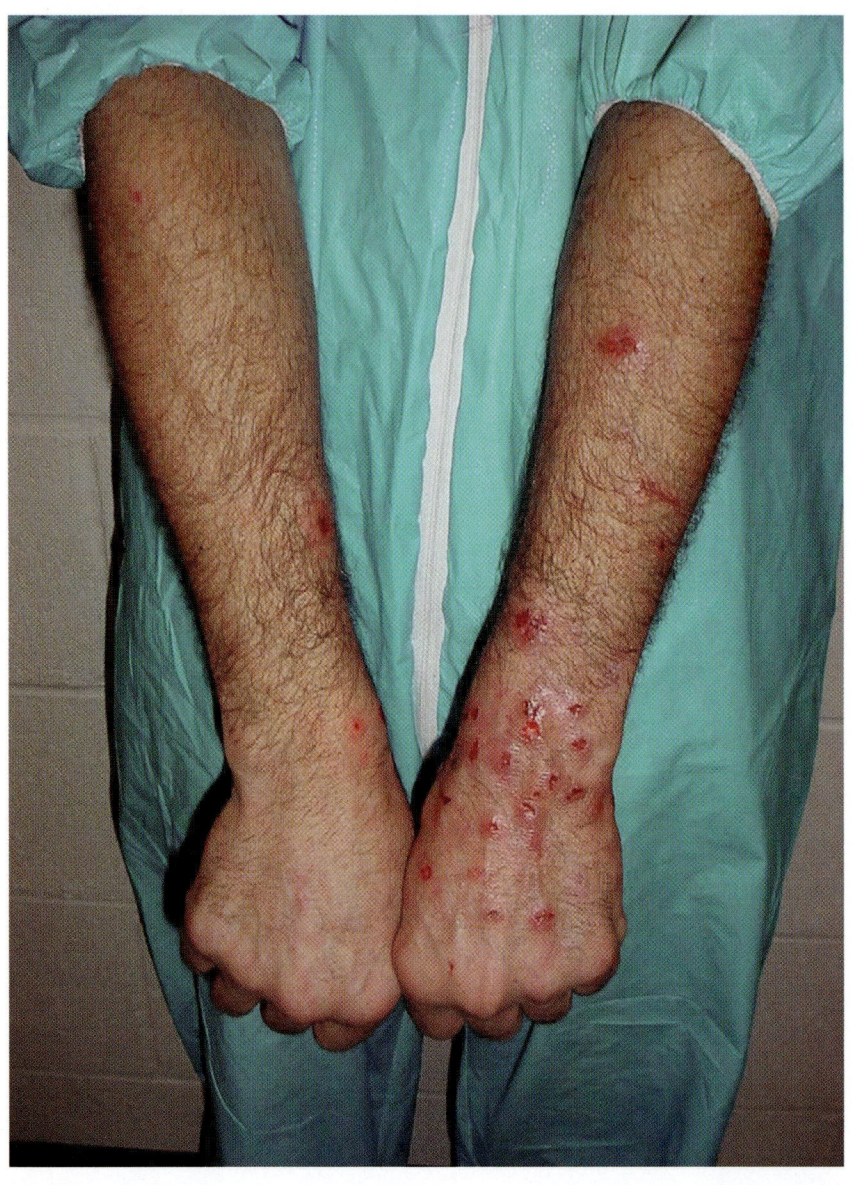

Example of crank bugs or meth mites. Photo courtesy of North Metro Task Force.

CHAPTER 10

Tonya's Story: Words of Experience from a Methamphetamine Addict in Recovery

Tonya Wheeler

As I sat on the edge of the bed that afternoon, a syringe full of meth in one hand and a bottle of Jim Beam whiskey in the other, I felt the hopelessness and helplessness of my addiction like I had never felt it before. A recovery book I had gotten when I was in treatment a couple of years back lay open on the bed. I read and cried and looked for the answer of how to stop this hell I was living in and praying for my life to end. That was about two weeks before I admitted myself into substance abuse treatment with the full admission that I was a drug addict and needed help if I was going to live.

My name is Tonya, and I'm an alcoholic and a drug addict. I have been clean and sober since May 23, 1990, and my life looks amazingly different today than it did on that miserable afternoon in March 1989. Today my life includes adjectives like happy, joyous, and free instead of hopeless, helpless, and miserable.

I was born in Plainview, Texas. My biological parents were married when I was born and they remain married today. I am the youngest of two children and grew up being Daddy's little girl. I can only say good things about growing up in my family. I was a happy child where family was very important, and my extended family spent a lot of time together. Both my maternal and paternal sides of the family were very close and we often had huge family gatherings where everyone was there. Love was everywhere! Some of my fondest memories I have include holidays where all of the family was together and times when my daddy would wake me up before dawn to take me fishing or hunting with him.

I was not taken to church on a regular basis, but it was obvious that my family had a belief in God. I was taught this principle at a very young age. My paternal grandmother would take the grandkids to church with her whenever we spent the night there, and she often talked to us about God.

My parents were both professionals. My mother worked for a large grocery store chain for many years and eventually became store manager. My father was a welder, and they made a sufficient living to support the family. As I look back, I can see that I had it better than a lot of kids. As years passed our houses got bigger and we always had the nice cars. My sister and I pretty much got what we wanted. By the time I was 11 years old we lived in one of the richest neighborhoods in town and had a concrete swimming pool in the backyard.

My father was an alcoholic, but not the kind that you usually hear about. He was a binge drinker and occasionally would start drinking and act out his own addiction for a little while, and then the chaos would stop and everything would return to "normal" again. I wasn't beaten as a child or sexually abused. I had both parents and an extended family that always appeared to me to be there for each other. I was taught about God and love and strong family values.

I realize the story I'm telling doesn't sound like the "typical" story of an alcoholic and drug addict. But one of the things I need you to understand is that even though I had all this love and all these wonderful things in my life there was something wrong. As a child I could not have told you what it was, but as the years have passed my recovery has helped me to identify it. I know now that my entire being was consumed by fear. What was I afraid of? Everything! I was afraid of the dark. I was afraid of being alone. I was afraid of dying. I was afraid of God. I was afraid of me and I was afraid of you. Of course, I never told anyone about all this fear. I just lived with it. I would lie in bed at night and cry myself to sleep because I was afraid that the "boogeyman" was going to get me or that I would die while I was asleep and never wake up and be with my family again. Most nights I would wake up in the small hours of the morning and go climb into bed with my parents, on daddy's side of the bed, of course. I would sleep there until morning. I could rest at peace sleeping beside daddy. I felt safe and protected from all of those wicked things that lived in my imagination. I would have never admitted I had all this fear to anyone, but it was always there. I believe this fear had followed me throughout most of my life, and my experience became such that when I used drugs and alcohol I could feel courageous and unafraid.

When I was 12 years old I had my first opportunity to drink as much as a wanted. I knew from the beginning of my drinking that there was no such thing as "enough," and I got drunk the first time. I had an alcohol blackout, vomited, passed out, and woke up with a hangover the very first time I drank. My response to this was, "Oh that was awesome and I can't wait to do it again!" I pursued that intoxication again, over and over, at every opportunity. I quickly discovered that when I drank the fear went away. I didn't have a need to tell anyone about it. I could sleep because I would pass out and I didn't have to lie awake worrying about all those horrible things that lived in my mind. At age 13, I was presented with the first opportunity to smoke marijuana. The effect was similar to that of the alcohol. The fear went away and I felt relaxed and at ease.

From the time I started using drugs and alcohol I wanted to be grown up. By age 14, I decided school wasn't the priority and partying with my friends was. I missed so many days of school at the public high school I attended my freshman year that I failed the school year. I convinced my parents that it was the school's fault because they wouldn't give me the credits even though I had made passing grades. My parents eventually agreed that the school was at fault and they allowed me to transfer to a private Christian school. I can best describe my experience at the private school as, "they (the school faculty) were not happy I was there." It didn't take long for me to teach my new friends how to skip school, drink alcohol, and smoke marijuana. At age 15 I became pregnant and was told by the principle of the school that I could not attend classes there anymore. I'm sure he must have been relieved to get rid of me. I can assure you that if I had been the leader of that school and was presented with someone like me I would have been relieved!

I convinced my parents that I was in love with the father of the baby, and they needed to sign papers for me to be allowed to marry him. They did, with reluctance. My new husband and I moved in with my parents. My mother gave him a job at the grocery store, and in my mind we were going to live "happily ever after." The drinking stopped during my pregnancy, because I was aware that drinking during pregnancy could be harmful to the baby, but I continued to smoke marijuana on a continual basis throughout my pregnancy. Back then (1984) I had even been told by the OB/GYN that smoking marijuana had not been proven to have harmful effects on the fetus. That information made for the perfect excuse for an addict to keep using! I delivered that baby on June 5, 1984, a beautiful, healthy baby girl. I just knew finally had my life straightened out and would be happy from then on.

I went to college as a business major. I was a mom, a wife, and a daughter. I thought my life was finally as I wanted it. During the first year of my daughter's life my parents opened a donut shop. They let me work there, and I also continued to attend college. The next year and a half brought ups and downs, especially financially. My husband didn't have the ability to hold a job for very long. I was working and going to school and trying to be a good mom and a good wife. I continued to use marijuana and alcohol on a consistent basis, without having any idea what lay ahead on the addiction highway.

In June 1986 I had become friends with a girl (I'll call her Donna) that my parents had hired to also work in the donut shop. Donna and I worked the same shift, which was all night long, making the donuts. One night before work she called me and said, "Why don't you come out to the house before work and we'll get high before we go in?" I believed she meant smoking pot. I went to her home where she and her husband lived, and when I arrived they began to tell me about the wonderful world of using meth. I listened intensely. I was skeptical about trying it. Not because I was afraid of this new drug, but because they told me "the right way to do it" was intravenously. I could feel my heart racing before I ever agreed to try it. Their excitement was overwhelming. They promised it wouldn't hurt and that I'd love it. I gave in. I believed that my IV meth use would be a one-time occurrence. I had no idea that I was about to embark on a journey that had the power to kill me, to destroy my life, to take away all that I loved.

I will never forget the first time I used meth. I was without a doubt in love. In love like I had never been in my life, fancied or real. I felt the warmth of the drug flow through my body like syrup and the feeling inside of me was almost orgasmic. I felt the rush and the high. I had the feelings of being so beautiful, happy, alive, and unafraid. Donna and I went to work that night after my experimentation with the drug. I had never had so much energy, ever! The illusion of feeling alert, in control, and satisfied was with me throughout the night. I laughed all night. We played the music loud and got our work done early. I was convinced I had found the answer to my happiness. I knew that this new drug, in combination with the way I had set my life up, would lead to a happy and fulfilling life. I WAS WRONG!

The desire to continue to get that high became my highest priority very quickly. I believe I was addicted to meth from the very first use. The false sense of awareness would have me believe that I did everything better—work, school, parent, clean, and function in my daily life. I used every day from the very first time. It seemed I couldn't get enough and I couldn't see the consequences that would come later down the road. One of my favorite things about meth was the enormous weight loss that happened immediately. I had always believed skinny equaled beauty. I had tried several different ways to obtain skinny during my adolescence. Starvation and binging and purging were my preferred way to become the "beautiful skinny girl," but with meth I didn't have to do any of that, not consciously anyway. I could use and I did not even think about food. I thought I had found "the answer."

It didn't take long for the drugs to start having so much of an effect that I started getting questioned from my family about what was different about me. I lost 25 pounds during the first 2½ weeks of my use. My parents started to ask questions about the weight loss. They asked, "Are you taking diet pills?" or "Are you not eating?" I did not have an answer for them about how I was losing all this weight. I would just ignore the question and change the subject. My husband wasn't happy about my drug use either. He would say to me, "Tonya, you have to stop this. You are going to be addicted." I would just laugh at him and deny the addiction and continue to use as much as a could, as often as I could. I could not understand why anyone could think that my using meth was a bad idea. I felt so alive.

I spent a lot of time with my new friend Donna and her husband. I started meeting their friends, and I liked them. Most of them were the "bad boy" types. They had stories and histories with jail. Their lives appeared so together and they were so cool. I met a guy that was friends with Donna and her husband. He seemed to always have his own supply of meth. I was so attracted to him from the beginning. He was gorgeous! He had money and was a college student with a very high grade point average. His parents were well known in the community, and I knew right away that I wanted to spend as much time with this man as I possibly could. He began to supply the meth for me. Some days it was free and some days it was not. It didn't matter; I just wanted to be around him. He had a strong sense of being in control. I thought he had his life together and I was tired of listening to my husband, at the time, bitch about me not being home and not stopping my drug use. He could not keep a job, and I thought if he really wanted something to change he needed to be changing himself. In August 1986, I told my husband to move out. I just woke up one morning, walked into the kitchen and said, "I don't want you anymore. Pack your stuff and leave." I had no explanation for my desire to be rid of him. Not an outward explanation anyway, but inside of me I knew. I wanted to be with the man who was supplying my drugs and who had his life together. My husband moved out that day and within a week he left Texas and moved to Michigan to live with his brother.

I immediately became involved with "the new guy." I wanted to spend every moment with him that I possibly could. We became very close very quickly. Joe and I moved in together by the beginning of September 1986. I rented an apartment in a complex where my parents also lived. I thought it would be a good idea to be close to them so that they could help me with the baby. She was growing, and I had a busy life. I needed all the babysitting help I could get. My daughter spent a lot of time with my parents or her father's mom. She was the joy of their lives, and at first they didn't mind having her with them as much as I would allow. But it didn't take long for that to become as often as I could. I began to not be able to get to work everyday. I quit school because, "I didn't have time for it." I continued to lose weight. My parents continued to ask questions about all the weight loss and I continued to avoid the subject. It did not take long for them to start asking me if I was using drugs. Of course I would deny that and would just laugh and say, "I'm fine," and "I'm just stressed."

My newfound boyfriend and I lived in my new apartment for almost a month before one afternoon, after a drug binge that had lasted about a week, I woke up and walked over to my parents' apartment. My intentions of going to see them were to get money or food, as it had been several days since I had eaten and I didn't have any money because I had used it all to buy drugs. I left Joe in our apartment and said to him on the way out the door, "I'll be right back." I would not see him or talk to him again for three days. When I arrived at my parents' apartment they were getting in the car. They told me they were going to the bank and asked me to ride along with them. At first I made a lot of excuses about why I could not go, but ultimately my dad said to me, "Just go with us; we'll be right back and we'll get you what you need while we are out." I climbed into the car with them, and we proceeded to the bank. I was quiet. The feeling that something wasn't right was inside of me, but I thought it was just because I hadn't slept much and hadn't eaten in days. When we left the bank my dad started driving out to the highway. He started to talk to me about his awareness of my drug use. He told me he knew I was using "crystal" and he knew I was using it IV. I denied it all. I swore he was mistaken and told him he was just making all this up. I claimed to have no idea why he would be so convinced about my drug use. I later learned he had been in my apartment and had found the spoons, the needles, and the other indications of my use. My parents and I pulled into the cemetery where my dad's parents were buried. We got out of the car and he began to say to me, "What would your grandmother think if she could see you like this today?" My father offered me a deal to clear my name and prove my lack of drug use, and I was convinced I would have to go through with this to show them I wasn't using. My dad told me that if I would go to a hospital and take a drug test and stay there until the drug test results were available that he would believe that I was not using and he would take me back home and never mention this again. I agreed. I forgot to ask about a few important details, like which hospital we would be going to and how long I would be at the hospital. When we all got back in the car my father headed toward the highway to Dallas, Texas. I became angry and suspicious at this point and started to demand my parents tell me where we were going. They told me they had made arrangements at a hospital in Dallas to have this drug test done and they continued to promise me that if there was no meth in my urinalysis they would take me home immediately. I knew that my drug test would not show any meth because I knew it had been about $2\frac{1}{2}$ days since I had last used any meth. I was convinced I was in a position where I would have to go into the hospital, pee in a cup, and within a few hours I would be allowed to go back home. That wasn't exactly my experience. My parents stopped and got me some food. I ate and then lay down and slept all the way to Dallas. When we arrived at Care Unit at Baylor University Medical Center I agreed to go in and talk to the staff. I agreed to do the urinalysis that my parents wanted and stay at the hospital until the results of that drug test were back. No one mentioned it would be three days before the test results would return. I signed myself into this treatment center under the absolute belief that my parents would be taking me back home soon. Back to Joe, back to my friends, and back to my life that I had orchestrated and loved. I got the drug test results three days later and they were negative for meth. I called my parents and told them and told them to come get me, "Now!" They were hesitant and said, "Just stay till in the morning and we'll come there and we'll talk about this." I explained to them that I would not be there in the morning, but they did not budge. They were not coming to get me. I called Joe and told him where I was and asked him to pick me up. Of course he said yes, and he arrived with some other friends early the next morning to take me home. I left that treatment center against medical advice and went back out into the world to pick up my addiction where I had left off.

When I arrived back in Paris, I was served with papers saying my parents had taken temporary custody of my daughter, Marcie. I was so angry. I just knew they had only taken me to that treatment center so that they could get her. The lie that my addiction told me said they just wanted her and they were not concerned about me at all. That was a lie I found out in later years. They were trying to save my life!

I continued to use drugs and drink with a new vigor after I lost custody of Marcie. I wish I could say that made me straighten up, but the truth is, what it did was give me more incentive to use drugs. I don't blame my parents for taking her. She was in a lifestyle that no child belongs in. They were saving her from me and the people that were involved in my life at the time. She needed to be away from me. I was not capable of loving anything except the drugs and alcohol at that time. I used daily, as much as I could, as often as I could, until February 1987. There was only one thing that could have stopped my use at that time, and it happened. The police came into our house and took us to jail. We had been watched by the police for some time apparently. They knew we were dealing drugs out of the apartment, but by the time they got in the door we had gotten rid of almost all of the drugs. Joe and I were taken to jail that night and booked on three charges: possession of a controlled substance, possession of marijuana, and possession of a prohibited weapon. I had never been arrested before and I was scared to death. I also knew that my parents would not come get me, so I didn't call them for two days. Mom and Dad had always said to me, "If you get arrested for something you couldn't help we'll be there to get you, but if you get arrested for something you could have helped don't call us to come get you." I knew this time they weren't coming. Finally, after two days, I called them. They were disappointed; I could hear it in their voice. They told me they loved me and they would come and see me and we would work on getting me out of jail, if I was ready for my life to change. I, of course, told them everything they wanted to hear. I promised to stop using, said I'd move in with them and be a good mother to Marcie. They got me released from jail after three days.

I had to follow up with my end of the deal, at least for a little while. I moved out of the apartment with Joe and moved back in with my parents. It was good to be around Marcie again. I had missed her and in my active addiction had not realized it. A part of me wanted to stop using meth. I could see that my life was out of control and I knew I did not want to live my life like that forever, but my desire to stop wasn't enough. I would occasionally use and I would see Joe without my parents knowing. I felt like I was 13 again. I had the desire to change my life, but I couldn't fight against meth. It would always win!

In April 1987, I found out I was pregnant. I thought surely this would be the thing that would make me stop using drugs. I told Joe I was pregnant, and we decided to get married. The hard part was going to be telling my parents, but I did it. They weren't happy about it, but they, like myself, may have had some hope that the pregnancy would make the difference. I continued to live with my parents until July 1987, when Joe and I moved in together again. We wanted to get married, but I had to convince my parents to return custody of Marcie back to me. When they had taken custody of her it had intervened in the divorce proceedings from my first husband, and the divorce could not be final until the custody of Marcie was resolved. They did return to custody of Marcie, and my divorce was granted in August 1987. Joe and I got married in September. I had the dream of having both of my children, a husband, and a normal life. I wanted that dream to come true. I was managing to get through the pregnancy without using meth, and believed that because I wasn't using then, I was cured! Little did I know addiction hides in the shadows waiting for us to drop our guard so it can take over again.

I was on probation at that time, and I was never asked by my probation officer if I thought I had a problem with drugs or alcohol, although I was sentenced on a drug charge. I was never asked to provide a urinalysis or asked if I was still using drugs. I just went into the probation officer's office, filled out a form, went in his office and talked for about two minutes and was told, "I'll see you next month." That was the extent of my probation. I had no real consequences from my probation.

I had Meagan on January 3, 1988. Joe was working at the hospital, and he was there when she was born. It was a VERY big day! That little girl was the most beautiful thing I had ever seen. She was born on my mother's birthday. I was certain I had my life back together and that I would never use meth again. How could I? I had everything a girl could want. But the disease of addiction is patient, and it waited . . .

I was a pretty good mother and wife for about 10 months after Meagan was born. I had managed to regain some semblance of normalcy in my life. I was a housewife who stayed home with the kids, cooked dinner, and cleaned house, and my husband brought home the paychecks to pay the bills. I thought I had my life back together again. I did, until that evening in October 1989, when I got a phone call from an old friend. He said he was coming to town and he had all the meth we could want for a long time. I felt my heart race immediately! I knew I was about to get back on the addiction road, and all I could recall was all the fun and partying I had been missing. I didn't care what the consequences were; I just couldn't wait for him to get there. He arrived sometime during the night. I'm not sure what time it was, but I know I didn't sleep. I just sat and waited, knowing he would be there soon. It was common in my past not to sleep if the dope was "on its way." That was my history. Don't sleep, don't eat, just pace the floor and look out the windows, waiting for it to arrive. I believe that the high started for me from the moment I knew the dope was coming. I have heard other addicts describe this feeling too. There is no sleeping or eating and nothing to distract the mind from, "It'll be here soon; I'll stay up and wait for it." Nothing would get in my way. I would wait until my friend arrived, believing I was headed for another good time and not having a clue that hell was about to be returned to me in full force.

I can't tell too much about what happened in my life from October 1988 to March 1989. I know that I left my house that night with that friend when he arrived from out of town, and everything past that point is a blur. I know that all I did was use. As much as I could, as often as I could, without thought of my kids, my husband, my responsibilities, my family, or my consequences.

I believe that's how much power meth has on an addict. I did not want my life to look like that, but it did. All it took was that one night to get me started again.

I remember a few significant events that happened during that time. One was a night in a hotel with a bunch of other addicts. I'm not sure who all was there. I'm not sure how long I had been there, how much dope I had used, how long it had been since I had eaten or how long it had been since I slept. I remember waking up lying on the bed in the hotel room and looking around. It seemed there were so many people in that room, but I'm not really sure how many there were. I sat up on the bed and looked around. I could see everyone, but I could not hear anything. I got scared and all of a sudden it felt as though I could not breathe. I jumped off the bed and ran for the door. All I could think of was getting outside so I could get some air. There was a guy sitting in a chair beside the door talking to another person. I was trying to get the door open, and it was jammed. It had been jammed off and on the whole time we had been there, that I remember now. But I thought this innocent guy sitting there was somehow keeping me from getting the door open. I shot him a fist in the right jaw and knocked him out of the chair and onto the floor. I desperately went back to trying to get the door open and finally I got it. I swung the door open and took off running across the parking lot of that hotel. It was dark outside, but I have no idea what time it was. I was screaming and crying as I ran through the parking lot. Finally, some of the people from inside the room got me and one of my friends stood there and hugged me and assured me I was okay. The people in the hotel room called Joe to come get me. When he arrived I went home with him and I remember lying on the bed and telling him, "I will never use methamphetamine again." I do not want to go crazy. I want to live. I fell asleep. The next day, when I woke up, I called my friend who had all the meth and asked him to come get me. He did, and I was off and running again.

The insanity of my meth use was so hideous that when I look back on those times now I'm surprised I survived. I had no ability to make rational decisions or to function normally. My use affected every area of my life including my ability to parent, my ability to work and play, my ability to love, and my ability to live. By March 1989, I found myself sitting on the end of my bed, reading that book, and wishing for the end. I couldn't go on like this anymore. I wanted to die!

I remembered my parents taking me to that treatment center on that afternoon as I sat there in tears. There was a smidgen of hope that lit through the darkness. I had to believe that if I could just get myself back to a treatment center they would teach me how to get my life back. I made my way into the living room. I was home alone and did not have to tell anyone what I was doing. I picked up the phone book and looked under addiction in the yellow pages. There it was! My glimmer of hope! A treatment center that was out of town, not too far away, that had an 800 number listed. I called the number and waited for an answer on the other end. Finally, someone responded. I told the person that answered the phone that I had a friend who had a drug problem and needed help. I explained that she was using meth and was in really bad shape. I was told that "my friend" could be admitted at any time. She just needed to show up, have a copy of her insurance card, and bring some clothes expecting to stay a while. The lady on the other end of the phone wanted me to give her my name and phone number, but I couldn't. I was just too scared.

I knew I couldn't get myself to the treatment center. I knew I'd chicken out if I didn't ask someone to help me, but who? Who could I trust to help me out with this task—my parents? No, I couldn't call them. They had been so disappointed in me for so long. I could not bear to drag them through this anymore. How about my sister? No, she would call my parents, so that wouldn't work either. I knew I could not tell my husband. He would just laugh at me and remind me that I was too weak to stop this on my own. I could not bear any more negativity. I had to have someone that would help me get there. I called a friend, Cindy. I was using with her, but she appeared to have a big heart and I was sure she wouldn't tell me no. I believed she cared, at least enough to help me get there. I called her and talked to her for a while, packed my clothes, and she came and picked me up. I felt a newfound hope for that moment. I believed I could get the help that I needed.

I'm not sure how long it was from the time I left my house to when I really did get to the treatment center. That situation itself was a drama, as well. I wound up at the drug dealer's house with my friend, Cindy. It seemed I always ended up at his house in times of dilemma. I must have told him about wanting to go to treatment. Either I did or Cindy did, but he knew. The next recollection I have of what happened was the drug dealer driving me to the treatment center. There were four of us in the car; the dealer, another friend of mine, Susan, her husband, and myself. We traveled down the highway, about 100 miles from where I lived. I was afraid, but confident that I was doing the right thing. We drank beer and smoked marijuana the whole way there and finally we arrived in Greenville, Texas. I was paranoid with fear. I was sure I wanted to go into treatment, but I was too afraid to walk in the door alone. I begged one of my companions to go inside with me, but of course, they would not. Why would another addict want to step foot inside of a treatment center? They were not the one who had decided to stop; I was, and it appeared I would have to find the courage to go inside alone. I couldn't! I tried, I swear I really did. I called a family member that lived in Dallas at the time and asked her to come meet me and take me in. She said no. I was crushed. At that time I did not understand how someone in my own family could say no, if I was looking for help. I was not capable of understanding at that time that she had a family to care for and for me to expect her to drop everything and drive an hour away, not even knowing if I would still be there when she got there, was unrealistic.

I told my friends I could not go in. I sat in the car and cried. Once again I felt the hopelessness flow in. The dealer told me he had a brother that lived in Greenville and if I wanted him to he could take me to his brother's house and I could call my sister and she could pick me up there and take me to the treatment center. I agreed with this plan, not having any better ideas of my own. I went to his brother's house and called my sister. Of course, she said she'd come get me. I explained to her that I wanted her to pick up my husband and bring him too. She reluctantly agreed. I called my husband and told him I was in Greenville and my sister was coming to get me. I asked him if he would come with her. Joe was furious! He was yelling at me and telling me what an awful wife and mother I was. He told me I was a useless drug addict and I didn't deserve to get help. He told me that the next time he saw me he would kill me and my drug dealer. I hung up the phone with him and called my sister back to say, "Yes, go pick up Joe. He wants to come with you." I did not tell her how angry he was.

About three hours later the phone rang at the house where I was. It was my sister. She said they had arrived in Greenville and wanted to know where to pick me up. She said she had Joe and her husband with her, and I knew I could not risk Joe being that angry and bringing him to the house where I was. I told her I would meet her at a store that was around the corner. When I arrived at the store my sister, her husband, and my husband were sitting in the car. My sister got out and walked up to me to give me a hug. I walked over to the passenger's side door and my brother-in-law stepped out to let me in. As he lifted the seat up for me, Joe grabbed my arm and pulled out a gun. He was trying to pull me into the car with him, and he was yelling at me, "I'm going to kill myself and make you watch!" I was terrified! All I could do was scream, wiggle, and to try and get away from him. My sister had a hold of my other arm trying to pull me out of the car. I felt like a tug-a-war rope, and I was not sure which side would win. I finally came stumbling out of the car and fell on the parking lot. I took off running into the night, terrified. I didn't know where to go, but I knew I had to run. I could see houses down the street. I don't know what time it was, but I was sure it was late. But up ahead there was a porch light on. I ran up to the door and started banging on it. I was crying and screaming, "Please help me. Please let me in!" A man opened the door with a suspicious look on his face. I started telling him what had just happened, and he opened the door and let me inside. He instructed his wife to call the police, which she did immediately.

The police arrived at the house and I told them the story. They promised me they would not let Joe hurt me. The police found my sister and the others on the parking lot at that store. They arrested Joe, took his gun, and took him to jail and then brought my sister to the house to pick me up. I was exhausted and could not imagine just going into the treatment center from there. I convinced my sister I needed to sleep a while before I went in. I made her promise not to call my parents. She and her husband took me to a hotel where I went to sleep, finally some sleep!

When I woke up the next morning and looked around the room the first thing I noticed was that my parents were there. I was so upset that she had called them. She promised she would not, but she did. I sat with my family that morning and something inside me said I wasn't ready to go into that treatment center. I was a mile away from it and I just could not do it. I tried to explain to my family what I was feeling, but they thought I was just telling a story again to not have to take responsibility. I can not blame them. That's how I had lived my life for a long time. I told my family that I needed to go back to Paris, just overnight, and I promised my mother that I would meet her back in Greenville at the treatment center the next morning at 10:00 A.M. My mother and I went to the treatment center together that morning and made me an appointment to be admitted the next morning at 10 A.M. Of course, I didn't tell them it was me that had the drug problem. I told them it was my sister. I have no idea if my mother was able to convey the message to them that I was the addict or if they just knew. But I could not admit I needed help that day, not then, not to them.

My sister drove me back to Paris and I had her drop me off at the dealer's house. I do not remember anything about that night, but I know I spent the night there and the next morning he drove me back to Greenville. Just before we got to the treatment center we stopped and I did what I thought would be my last injection of meth. When we arrived at the treatment center my mother was there waiting for me. She was crying. I think because she was both surprised and grateful that I had arrived. She took me into the facility and I met with a counselor. I completed all the admission paperwork and was taken into a room, where I was told I could lie down and rest. I remember very little about the inside of the unit. I do not remember meeting any of the people who were in treatment there. The only person I remember was the man who said he would be my counselor. I stayed at that treatment center for about two days. I think all I did was sleep. After a couple of days my counselor took me into his office and explained to me that I was going to have to leave because Joe's insurance would not pay for me to stay there. I was devastated! I begged him to let me stay there. I told him that if he made me leave I would die. I had no where else to go. I had worked too hard to get there. I wanted help. I wanted to live. He apologized to me and said it was not his decision and that administration had made the decision and he just had to give me the news.

I left his office with that same feeling of hope that I had become accustomed to. I knew I would die when I left there. I called the dealer to come pick me up. I did not have the heart to call my parents again and say I could not stay. All I knew to do was to reach back out to the drugs. The dealer arrived to pick me up that evening and we stopped at his brother's house again. He handed me the bag with the dope in it and assured me, "It's good shit and it'll make you feel better." I did the only thing I had known how to do for a long time. I used again. I sat on the toilet in the bathroom as I mixed up the injection. I did not want to shoot dope anymore. I wanted my life back and I had no idea now how to get it. I cried as I did that shot of dope. I felt the meth flow through my body and my brain and at the same time I felt another piece of my soul die. I could not live this way anymore.

When the dealer and I arrived back in Paris I had him take me to my sister's house. She opened the door in surprise. I explained to her that the treatment center told me I had to leave because I did not have insurance that would pay for my stay there. I cried as I talked to her and let her see the real fear that I had that I was going to die this way. She convinced me to call my parents and tell them what had happened. I called my mother and cried to her on the phone. I remember saying to her, "If you don't help me, I'm going to die." She assured me we would find the treatment I needed.

The next day my mother called me to say she had found a treatment center that would admit me into outpatient treatment. She said I could come to stay with her and my father in Marshall, Texas, where they had recently moved to, and attend treatment there. She said she had made me an appointment to be admitted the next morning and I just needed to get there. I called Joe, who had since been released from jail, and asked him to take me to my parent's house in Marshall. He agreed and came to my sister's house and spent the night with me so that we could leave early the next morning. When I woke up I called my probation officer and explained to him that I had a drug problem with meth and I was going to Marshall to my parents' house and checking myself into treatment. He thanked me for calling and asked me to keep him informed of my whereabouts. I agreed, hung up the phone, and Joe and I went to Marshall.

I was admitted into that outpatient treatment center on March 17, 1989. I went in there with a conviction to tell them everything about my meth addiction. What had happened, where it had taken me, what consequences I had suffered as a result of it, everything. I wanted to stop using it and I knew the only way they could help me was for me to be absolutely honest with them about my addiction. The one thing that I did not want to talk about was how alcohol and marijuana had played a part in my addiction. I insisted my problems had nothing to do with those two substances and there was no need to stop using those; I just needed to stop using meth.

I was admitted into the six-week intensive outpatient program, where I attended groups four nights a week for four hours a night. Wednesday was family group and Joe was in Marshall with me, but he didn't have any desire to attend the groups with me. He explained to me that he wasn't the one with a drug problem, I was, and he didn't need to be there. Marcie and Meagan were both at my parent's house with me and Joe. Joe's parents had been keeping Meagan and had filed for temporary custody of her, with Joe's agreement, just before I was admitted into treatment in Marshall. After we moved in with my parents, Joe's parents continued to try and convince me to let them have custody of Meagan for a while, but I wouldn't agree. My counselor in treatment kept saying to me, "Do not sign any papers; you're doing fine and you are a good mother." I refused to sign the temporary custody papers, and they eventually let the custody issue go and Meagan stayed with us.

I attended treatment as scheduled. I really liked having someone to talk to, and being in groups and with my counselor was a relief. Finally, I had people to talk to about my addiction, relationships, and my life that understood. Speaking of relationships, my relationship with Joe continued to be a struggle.

He continually told me that I was the drug addict, not him. That it was all my fault all this had happened in our lives, not his. He kept me under his control throughout the rest of our marriage. He said he wanted me to stop using drugs, and if I'd do that he'd stay married to me. He said I wasn't responsible enough to have any money. After I had been in treatment a while I got a job as an office clerk at the local newspaper; I was expected to put my check in the bank to help pay bills, but I was not allowed to have my name on the checking account. Joe did not usually attend any family treatment groups with me and he did not approve of me attending 12-step meetings. He would tell me I could not go to meetings in the car, so I'd have a friend, whom I had met in the meetings, to pick me up. Joe would insist I was not going to meetings, but instead I was having an affair with a man from the meetings. The accusations would convince me to not go sometimes and I'd stay home instead. Joe continued to smoke marijuana and drink alcohol daily in our house. I would try to fight the desire to use, but some days it would be too overwhelming. I'd wait for him to leave and then use the drugs he'd leave in the house. I wanted to be drug and alcohol free, but it just seemed to be too hard. I would convince myself smoking marijuana wasn't the same as using meth and my addiction did not include marijuana and alcohol; I was wrong. My life again felt like a tug-a-war. My counselor and my group members would talk to me about abstinence, total abstinence from all drugs and alcohol. My friends I had made at 12-step meetings would also tell me the only way to recovery was to stop all drug and alcohol use, and I believed that, but I just couldn't do it; not for very long at a time anyway.

In March 1990 Joe filed for divorce from me. He told me that I had not changed at all and that I was still a bad mother and a terrible wife. He told me I did not deserve to have custody of my children, and he filed for custody of Meagan when he filed the divorce. He told me he would prove that I was unfit and he would tell all the horrible things I had done in my addiction, like having affairs, being violent, and abandoning my children. He reminded me that his parents had plenty of money to hire attorneys to make sure he would get Meagan. I was so scared! I was afraid, again, that I was going to lose my little girl.

My friends in recovery rallied around me at that time and offered me the kind of support I had never known. They reminded me that I had done these things when I was using and not in sobriety and how my life was different now. Several of them went to court with me and were willing to testify in my behalf, if needed. The fear of losing Meagan was overwhelming. The fear of losing the man that I thought had brought me happiness was also overwhelming, and on May 22, 1990, just a few weeks before the divorce was final, I got drunk again. I can only say that I reverted back to all I had ever known; when living in fear, the only choice is to change the way I feel. The only way I had ever known to do that was with drugs and alcohol.

Something happened inside of me when I got drunk that night. Something that I still cannot fully explain, but I'm so grateful for. Upon awakening on

May 23, 1990, I realized nothing about my drinking was different over the past 10 years. I drank the same way this time that I always had, to oblivion. I lay on the bed that morning crying with a full knowledge that my addiction included meth, marijuana, alcohol, and all other substances that I had used over the years to change the way I felt. I wanted my life to change and I knew that the answer was abstinence. I knew I could not do it alone and I reached out for help to my friends who were living their lives clean and sober. Joe and I went to court for the finalization of my divorce and the outcome of custody of Meagan. I watched my new clean and sober friends file into the courtroom that day to support me. I felt confident and I knew, for the first time, that I was not a bad mother and I deserved to have custody of my daughter(s), both of them. It did not take long for the judge to reveal her verdict. I won, and I would go home and be with my girls, my friends, and my parents, the people who loved me unconditionally. Joe moved back to Paris with his parents, and Meagan would visit on occasion, but she lived with me, her mommy.

I decided about that time that I wanted to be a drug and alcohol counselor. I wanted to be able to help others, especially women, who had suffered the disease and its consequences the way I had. I went to my counselor and talked to her about my career choice. She smiled and said to me, "Tonya, you have to get your life together first. When you have two years of continuous sobriety you come and talk to me about this again. If you still have the desire to be a counselor I'll tell you how to get into school and make it happen." On my two-year anniversary date of my sobriety I went to her office and announced, "I'm here; now tell me how to be counselor." She gave me a hug and direction about how to make that happen. I started volunteering in a residential treatment center and starting taking classes at a college in Kilgore, Texas. I'd drive 70 miles, round trip, to school twice a week. My friends and family would care for the children while I went. I would get welfare and food stamps to pay the bills and I'd live my dream everyday, knowing that my life would not be this way forever. After six months of volunteering in that treatment center I was offered a full-time position, my first real job in a treatment center; I was ecstatic! This would be the beginning of a new career for me and a continuation of the successful life I had worked so hard for. It took a long time for me to get my license to be a counselor. Some days I thought I'd never reach my goal, but I'd be reminded by the people around me that I could do this and I'd keep trudging. In 1997, I became a licensed chemical dependency counselor in Texas. I remember the day I got the test results. I just sat and cried in gratitude. How could someone who had come from a life like mine have a success like this? I knew the answer; only the grace of God could make this kind of change.

The struggles that have continued throughout my sobriety have been many. Women, especially, are taught to rely on relationships to feel whole. I got married again when I was two years sober. I met this man in the office where I worked, and I believe this experience was my first at real love; to love someone without the distraction of drugs or alcohol. We got married in 1992, and about a year after the marriage he began drinking alcohol every day. I started finding out that he had been exposed to recovery in 12-step meetings in the past, but had no desire to stop his alcoholism. There were many affairs with other women during the marriage, and again I felt that I wasn't worthy of true love from a man. We got divorced in 1996. I was again on my own with my girls to make a successful life for the three of us. With the help of my friends and my family I learned more about taking care of myself and keeping the focus off of men. I rarely dated for the next four years. I worked on my career and taking care of my children, a gift I had no idea that I was even receiving.

My relationship with my children today is amazing, and I attribute that to my sobriety and taking responsibility for my own actions. Making amends to everyone I harmed during my addiction has been an important part of my recovery program. I can never go back and change the things I did, but I can change my behavior and not do the same hurtful things today. My children were most definitely harmed by my behavior when I was using drugs and alcohol. Thank God the harm was no more than it was. I learned how to be a responsible mother and how to care for my children's needs instead of them having to care for mine. I met other women who were in recovery and watched them parent their children. I believe watching them was one of my greatest teachers to improve my own parenting skills.

I say often, when I'm speaking, that my drug use never had anything to do with whether I loved my children or not. I always loved them. Even at the height of my addiction, my love for both of them was enormous. I understand today that meth addiction has the power to make anyone do things that they would never normally do when they aren't using. The days and nights that I sat in tears because of the way I was treating my children, my instability, my lack of concern, my inability to parent, all of those things were never about not loving my girls, it was about my addiction. When the drugs and alcohol were taken out of the equation, my ability to be a good mother returned. The real Tonya came back to life, and I was there for my girls!

My relationship with my parents has also improved dramatically. I have a relationship back with them that I thought I'd never get again. The pain that we cause our family is sometimes irreversible. I am so grateful that my parents stood by me and supported me, even when I believed I wasn't worth their support anymore. My relationship with the other people in my family has improved also. I have managed to set right the wrongs I caused in their lives as well. I believe it is much more likely for a person to get clean and sober and stay that way when they have a strong support system. I'm lucky to have the family I have; all of them!

In 1999 I met a man that lived in Colorado, who had also been clean and sober for a long period of time. We met at a recovery conference in Houston, Texas, and we were both clear that we wanted to spend time together and get to know each other better. He flew himself to Texas or me to Denver about every other week for the next three months, and in August I moved to Denver. We were engaged for the next year and got married in 2002. That marriage ended in 2003.

I have learned a lot from each of the relationships I have been in. I have learned more than I could have ever asked for about integrity and honesty. I'm a believer that nothing happens in God's world by accident and there is a purpose for all that we go through. I know that if I had not suffered from the disease of addiction that my life would not be where it is today. I know that I would not have had the values that I have in my life, had it not been for recovery. I'm sure I would not have had the benefit of working with others who suffer from this hideous disease and I would not have had the joys of meeting the people that I have crossed paths with in my life. Do you wonder if I would take it all back and change it? No! I would not change a thing!

ACKNOWLEDGMENTS

To my parents and my daughters, who have been my biggest fans, especially during my hardest times.

To my sister, who has loved me through my addiction and has always been by my side.

To my friends in recovery, who have always supported me and loved me.

To Mildred: I couldn't have made it without you. You were the one who gave me my most important gifts—a relationship with God and a relationship with me.

CHAPTER 11

Samantha's Story: Words of Experience from a Methamphetamine Addict in Recovery

Samantha Cameron

My name is Samantha. I am now 23 years old. I will begin by telling you the kind of person that I was when my life became a nightmare. I was a good kid with a huge heart. I always thought of others first and loved the satisfaction of a job well done. I knew right from wrong and was raised with love and good morals. I was a good student and loved school. I loved my family more than anything in the world, and they felt the same way.

I became pregnant when I was 15 and was told by my counselor at school that I would be like the rest of the teenage mothers and drop out of school and struggle through life. Well, I was the type of person that if you told me that I would fail I would work 150 times harder to prove you wrong. That is what I did. I contacted the state and they set up a tutor to help me while I was out of school. Three months after my son was born I returned to school with my head held high. I had not lost my desires to become someone and to do something with my life despite the rumors and laughs in the halls.

In May of 2000 I graduated with my class, and with my head held high I walked across the stage and received my diploma with the biggest smile that I have ever had. That happiness, however, was short-lived.

In the wee hours of the morning in June 2000 I wrote the following note to my best friend—my mom. It read:

Dear Mom,

I am sorry that I have to leave. I have some problems that I have to take care of. I will be ok. Don't worry. Sorry that I cannot take care of my son but he will be better off staying here with you. Thank you and love Sam.

I had only about 50 dollars to my name and was not even sure where I was going to go, but I knew that I could not let my family see me this was any longer. I had started using meth and was losing weight very fast and was treating my family like the dirt on the ground. Moreover, they deserved better than that. I thought that if I could just get away for a few days I could stop using and get myself together. Boy was I wrong. This was just the beginning of what was soon to be the biggest nightmare.

For the first few weeks that I was gone I would call my mom to tell her that I was ok, even though I knew in my heart that I was slowly slipping away. It is hard for me to put a very good timeline on my life back then, it is so foggy now. I think that a few weeks had passed since I had talked to my mom, and the phone calls home were getting further and further apart as the shame that I felt began to grow and the guilt sat heavy in my heart. I was living anywhere that I could, anyone that said I could stay for a few days that is where I was. I had stopped calling my friends because I had run out of lies to tell them, and the truth was too much for me to handle, let alone to tell to someone else. I felt as if I was in a room with no door or windows and my air was running out. I did not know how to handle the emotions that I was having. So instead, I started using more and more meth trying to cover up the pain. As soon as the high was gone I felt worse than I did before I got high, and this was the never-ending circle that my life became.

I would meet guys that had or could get large amounts of meth and I would sell it for them so that I could get money to support my own habit. I was living in dope houses, motels, and in my car pretty much wherever I could stay. I decided to get out of the area that I was living in and decided to go down south to a different part of town, I was staying in a long-term motel. Things were getting worse. Not only was I selling and using meth, a person along the way had showed me how to steal mail and make checks on the computer. So that is what I did. To explain how much of a fool meth can make of you and your ability to make good decisions: I was committing crimes all over town. I never thought about the consequences of getting caught, or the effect that it was having on the families that I was stealing their mail and writing checks against their accounts.

One morning I left the hotel room and the guy that I was staying with, to get some meth. I was gone about 12 hours, and that was not unusual for me to be gone that long. When you are high you have no thought process and you are distracted by everything. One simple task that should take an hour ends up being anywhere from 12 to 24 hours. When I returned to the hotel I found that the guy had gotten mad at me and locked me out. So I got back in my car and drove around and ended up at a local 24-hour store. I went inside and walked around. I was approached by two uniformed police officers, and they asked me if my name was Samantha. I was hesitant to reply, but I said yes. They had run my plates on my car and my mom had filed a missing person report on me. I had not talked to her in some time now. One of the police offices gave me his phone and asked me to please call my mom, that she was very worried about me. So I picked up the phone. My hands were shaking so bad it was hard to dial the numbers. This was a call that I had put off for so many weeks now. I knew that my mom would not be mad; however, I knew how disappointed in me she was. I would rather have her mad than have her be disappointed in me; that is far worse in my mind. As soon as she answered I started crying; just the sound of her voice made me feel the size of an ant. I knew in my heart this is not how things were suppose to be. I was a better person than this. But it just goes to show you that an addiction does not discriminate against anyone. I missed my mom more than anything, and I told her that I would come home. The police officer made me promise that I would go home, so I told him that I would, knowing in my heart that I would not. We both left. I did not think too much about it; I just went on shopping. The very next day in the same part of town I was pulled over by the same police officer. He said that the store had called him and told him that I had written a bad check yesterday. He then arrested me and put me in the back of his car. When they searched my car they found a bag of meth. At this point I had been up for many days and had not had anything to eat for as long as I can remember. They took me down to the police station and questioned me for hours. They finally called my mom and told her that they would release me to her with my charges pending. My mom and grandma came and picked me up and took me home. I must have slept for days. When I woke up all I wanted to do was go get high.

The addiction to meth is so strong you do not care who you hurt in the process of getting what you want. Every time that I would go home and leave again my son would cry, asking me, "Mommy don't go." I would turn my back and walk out the door. He would follow me outside on to the front porch crying, and my mom would have to run after him and hold him while I drove away. Still to this day that is one of the hardest things that I deal with on a day-to-day basis. I look into his beautiful little face and cannot image how I could walk out of his life.

So I was off again, this time to a different place. I had met this guy a while ago, and he called me on my cell phone and told me that if I wanted to get clean and get my life together that I could go and stay with him. I for some reason believed him, so I moved in. He told me that I would have my own room and that he would help me get in to counseling, and for a few weeks I did have my own room, and it seemed like he was trying to help me. Then one day I woke up and all that was gone and I found myself smack in the middle of the biggest mess, from meth to checks and everything in between. Everyone that I was trying to get away from was now living at his house. It had become a flophouse for meth users. When he turned my room into a check-making factory for all the meth users in the north part of town, I could not believe my eyes. Everyone thought this guy was God and walked on water. This guy was able to get very large amounts of meth. At first he would get me high all the time hoping that I would stay and keep my mouth shut, and I did. Up until this point I had been smoking and snorting meth; now I was shooting it. I was using about 3–5 grams a day, sometimes less and sometimes more. As time went on I was not allowed to talk to my mom. He would tell me that he just talked to her and everything was fine—I did not need to call. What I did not know is that he was telling her that I was fine and that I was in counseling and doing well and that he was doing everything that he could to keep me away from all the other people so that I would stay clean. This was the complete opposite. My mom started to get worried and would ask to talk to me. He would tell her that I was in the shower, sleeping, or that I had just left. This man was making me a prisoner in his home. When I would tell him that I wanted to leave, he would get violent and tell me that I knew too much and he would kill my family and me if I left him. I was so scared. I did not value my own life at this point; in fact most days I wish that I were dead. I did, however, value my family and loved them more than anything in the world. That was one thing that I did not lose and nobody could take away from me. I loved and missed my family. I stayed with him only for the fact that I was not sure what this man was capable of doing, and I thought that I was the one that got myself in to this mess, and if he ended up killing me when I was with him then he would leave my family alone.

Things progressively got worst. I now had felony charges in six different counties and was out on bond in all of them. Every time that I was arrested or got into trouble my mom would bail me out. Even though all this was going on, I was still out writing bad checks and getting high.

One night when the man was gone, I called my mom to come and get me. She and my dad came and picked me up. We put as much of my stuff in the truck that we could get and left. When he got home he was so mad. I can still remember the conversation. I was so scared to take the chance that he would hurt my family, but I could not take it anymore. I had to leave. He then started sitting outside of my mom's house all night long and calling 100 plus times a night. My mom would have to take the phone of the hook so that it would stop. Then he would walk around the house banging on the windows and door. I would go in my closet and curl up in the fetal position and rock back and forth in my closet for hours and sometimes days. My mom would bring me food in the closet hoping that I would eat something. This went on for a long time until one day my mom had had enough. She walked out front where he was sitting in his car and told him that if she ever saw him sitting out there again that she would call the cops, and that made him mad. Then she proceeded to tell him that better yet she would shoot him and drag his body in the house and tell the cops he was trying to break in. I still cannot believe that my mom did that. I guess that when you are pushed so far you will do just about anything. For the most part he stopped. I would go see him once in a while just to keep him away from my house.

However, this was far from the end. I was right back on the street. My mom and dad went looking for me one day and found me in a dope house, overdosed, passed out on the floor on a backpack of cold tabs. I was out for days, my lips were blue, and I was lying in a puddle of blood. No one in the house cared; they just walked over me. This is another part of the meth world. No one cares about anyone. Everyone is in it for themselves. No matter how much they say they care, they really do not. I can say that I had one true friend out of the hundreds that I knew at this point in my life. We still talk every once in a while to this day. He is doing well and has gotten his life together as well. It was so sad; when I was using I could sit in a room with a hundred people and still be all alone. I felt as if I was alone in this world with a thousand pounds on my shoulders. I was fighting a war in my own mind, a war that I thought would never end.

I was back and forth from my mom's, staying only long enough to sleep for a few days. I was going to court in one county and was suppose to be taking UAs. I knew that if I failed one more, the judge would make me spend a few days in the city jail. So the next time that I was to go to court, I did not go. This was on a Friday, and on Monday morning it was the beginning of the end.

For the last several months the Colorado Bureau of Investigation (CBI) had been watching my mom's house. They did not have anything to arrest me on. I had been making all my court appearances. They were working on building yet another case on me. Now, however, I had a warrant out for my arrest for not appearing in court, so as soon as my mom left for work, all hell broke loose. I was seeing a new guy, and he was at my mom's with me that day. I did not know at the time, but he was working with them and had helped set this up. He went out front and called me from their cell phone telling me to come outside. When I looked out the window they had my house surrounded from all sides. I lost it. I did not want to go to jail. I would have rather died. So I went into the garage and drank antifreeze, then went into my room and grabbed my gun from the closet and put it in my mouth. I was sitting on my bed thinking about how low my life had become in such a short period of time. My mind was racing so fast by the time that I had remembered that I had a gun in my mouth the CBI came busting in my room with their gun pointed at me. For some reason the Lord was watching over me, because as soon as they saw me with the gun in my hands they could have opened fire. Instead they threw me to the ground and put me in handcuffs. They could not take me right to jail because I had to go the hospital and get my stomach pumped. Then they put me in a mental hospital on a 72-hour mental health hold due to the suicide attempt. The police were to pick me up from there in 72 hours and take me to jail. However, they were not there, and they could not hold me any longer. So I was released and was on the run again, but not for long. The very next day I was at someone's house. I heard a knock at the door. I knew right away who it was. I tried to go out the back window but they had the apartment surrounded. This would be the last time that I was out on the street.

They took me to county jail where I sat this time without bond. I have never felt so powerless in my life. My life was now in the power of everyone but me, and I could not do anything about it. I was so angry with myself, but I took it out on everyone else. I could not even stand to look at myself in the mirror. Being in county jail is the worst thing in the world. I would look around in disbelief. I was not like the rest of the people in there, I would tell myself. I have a family that loves me, and a son that needs me. But I had no one to blame but myself. I sat without bond for about a month, and all I could think about is getting high when I got out. I finally got a court date and thought I was going home. Boy was I wrong. When I went before the judge he set my bond at $100,000 cash only. I was devastated, not because I wanted to get out and do the right thing, but because I thought that I would get out and be high by the end of the night.

The courts had also put together a grand jury case for racketeering against me, and all the counties that I had charges in agreed to lump it all together into one case. I think that the end result was 50-some felony charges for anywhere from Felony 6 to Felony 5 and then the Felony 2 for racketeering, which is only one below a Felony 1 for murder. This is when I realized how much trouble I was in. I went back to jail that night and did some serious soul searching. I decided that I had to change my life. I knew that if I went back out on the street I would die or I would spend the rest of my life behind bars. It took me awhile, but I found myself again. After about four months in jail, I knew what I had to do. I needed help bad, and not some 30-day dry-out rehab. So I started to talk to people and call around. I found one place that did not have a waiting list, and it was a long-term program. Everyone in jail said that it was the worst place to go. They would tell me horrible stories and tell me how mean they were. But I decided that was the kind of place that I needed to be. This was a 2½- to 3-year inpatient program. The next time that I went in front of the judge I asked him if I could go. He said, "I have yet to see anyone in my courtroom make it through that program and I have been a judge for a long time." Well being the person that I am, I was going to prove him wrong.

So the next day some people from the program came and picked me up. Boy were they right; this was one tough program. There were many days where I thought that I could not take another day, but then I would go to bed and wake up the next day and realize that this was not so bad compared to where I could be. So I pushed through, taking it one day at a time. When I had been in the program about a year, my son got to come and live with me. That was the best! I was a little scared at first; I did not know if I knew how to be a mom or not, but I soon found out that I did, and we began to bond right away. I learned so much in that 2½ years that I will forever be grateful to that program for all that it taught me. It taught me how to live a clean and sober life, as well as many life lessons that I would not have learned had it not been for that place.

While I was in rehab the grand jury case continued. I still did not know if I would be able to stay at rehab; jail was still a real possibility. I went before the judge and was expecting the worst. As I stood before him, I felt my whole body shaking. He said, "In my 30 years on the bench I have never seen the attorney general and a member of the CBI speak on someone's behalf, nor have I seen someone that has been in the rehab that you are in, make it this far." The attorney general asked for no prison time, but 10 years probation and $37,000 in restitution. The judge said that a crime like this required prison time; however, taking into consideration that I had a good family and had been in rehabilitation for 1½ years, he felt that I was sincere about changing my life. He read the following, "I must successfully complete the treatment program that I was in and do eight years on probation and pay off the $37,000 dollars in restitution that I owe." I felt a million pounds being lifted off my shoulders. On that day I felt 10,000 angels around me. As I walked out of the courtroom that day, I vowed to myself to never look back. This was a second in life that I will forever remember. I will be grateful for the rest of my life for all the people who stood by my side, walked with me, and never had a doubt that I could make it through this. To my family for never giving up on me and standing by my side, and for loving me no matter what. To all the people that prayed for me—they are my angels.

I went on to complete the program. I graduated in May of 2004. I am doing great and I have been clean for over 3½ years now. My son and I moved back home with my family where we belong. We are both doing great! If you would have asked me a few years ago what I thought my life would be like, I surely would not have told you that it would have turned out this good. I count my blessing everyday. I have so many goals and things that I want to do. I cannot wait to have a life full of happy times and wonderful memories.

CHAPTER 12

Mother of
a Methamphetamine Addict

Rhonda

It was a beautiful June morning—June 5, 2000, to be exact. Last week we had a graduation party for Sam, and it was extra special. Sam had Tanner when she was only 16, and her high school counselor told her she would never finish school. Well she showed them all, graduated on time, and walked with her class. Life was good, or so I thought.

I went to Sam's room and found the note attached to her door. It read, "Mom, I'm sorry I had to leave for a while. I have some problems that I need to take care of. Please forgive me for leaving Tanner with you, but I don't want him involved with this, I will call you, I promise." I stood at the doorway stunned. What problems could she possibly have?

Days went by with no call. I had called everyone I could think of and she was nowhere to be found. This was not at all like Sam. Finally, I received a phone call. It was short, and she said she was all right and not to worry, she would be home soon. She still would not tell me what was wrong or where she was.

Life went on like this for weeks, a call every week, no information. I looked for her every night, still calling everyone I could think of. Sometimes people would tell me they saw her here or there, but I could never catch up to her.

Finally, weeks went by with no call, I was frantic. I called the police department several times and asked to file a missing person report. Each time they told me she was 18 and probably using drugs, and eventually would be home; they refused to take the report. Finally after getting very persistent, I got an officer to take a report. It was now September . . .

November, early one Sunday morning I received a call from an officer in south metro Denver. He said he had found Sam sleeping in her car in a K-Mart shopping center, had run the plates, and saw the missing person report. Thank God they finally took that missing person report. She was standing right there with him, and he offered to let her talk to me on his cell phone. I could not believe it was her. She was crying and said she wanted to come home; I begged her to come home and told her there was not any problem that we could not solve together. She promised she would be home within two hours. Twenty-four hours went by and she never came. Finally, the next night at about 5:00, the same officer called and said he knew that Sam never came home because he arrested her that morning and told me I could come and get her; they would release her with charges pending. I felt like a miracle had happened; I was on my way to get her finally!

When I got to the police station, I did not even recognize my own daughter. She had lost about 50 pounds and looked like she had not slept in days. She did not want to come home with me, but finally agreed. They had impounded her car. They then advised me that they had found meth in her car and later went to a hotel room where they found stolen goods, and K-Mart had called the station, earlier that day, about a girl trying to pass forged checks. I could hardly believe my ears! This was not my Sam. From here, it just got worse, much worse.

When I brought Sam home, she stayed for about two days and disappeared again. This went on until right before the holidays. She would come home for a few days, say she wanted help, and then disappear again. When she did not come home after a couple of days, my mother and I went looking. I once found her at a well-known "crack" house; she had been unconscious for four days, people stepping over her, and they didn't even care. I picked her up, put her in the car, and brought her home again; she was worse than I had ever seen. She slept for days and was so weak that I had to take her in the shower with me and help her clean up. Denver had charged her with possession of meth, and now we had a felony court case. Once again, she left.

I finally got a call from "a man" who said she was with him and that he was helping her. He told me where he lived and that I had nothing to worry about; he was getting her help. I had to get to her; she has a warrant out and needed to surrender. I finally was able to pick her up at his house and we surrendered to the authorities; it was right before Christmas, and I bonded her out of jail. I just knew we could get a handle on this together, and I did not want her in jail at Christmas. Little did I know this was probably the worse mistake I could have made!

She refused to come home, so I dropped her off at that "man's" house. It was a nice house in a very nice neighborhood. He reassured me once again that she was safe and getting help. I was very uncomfortable with this, but at least I might now know where she was.

Well it was not long before lots of law officers were calling the house and coming over looking for Sam. I can only imagine at this point what my neighbors were thinking. Sam now had charges in several counties for fraud and theft. This was much bigger than I had imagined! I had tried several times for the last weeks to contact her, but each time this "man" would have some excuse as to why I could not talk to her. She would call every couple of days and leave a message for Tanner, Tad, and me, but I never spoke with her. Something was really wrong. . . .

In late January 2001, I got a call from Sam at about midnight one night. She was whispering and crying, begging me to come and get her. Needless to say, I took off right away, not really knowing what I might run into . . . did not really matter, I just wanted her home. In about five minutes, we grabbed about several garbage bags of her stuff, took off, and came home. The "man" wasn't there. It was then that I got the whole story about what had been going on for the past several months, and it was an ugly, ugly story.

I can't begin to tell you what our lives had been like. I had just received a new job, I was trying to provide as normal a life as possible for Tanner, and for several weeks my mother and I spent until the wee hours looking for her. I'm sure I looked awful as well, but it's amazing what you can do when you have too. Sam was involved in a life I had a hard time believing existed.

For the next several months, Sam stayed in touch, staying at home for a few days and then leaving, but always coming back. It was a really bad time for us; we had court dates weekly in one county or another, my son who was 15 quit school, and he was scared to leave the house and his sister. For as you see, at night when she was here, she would let all kinds of people in. I would wake up and kick them all out, only within a couple of hours to wake up and see them again. My son was scared and so was I, but we were working through the legal issues and hoping to get help for Sam.

In the meantime, I found out that the "man" was calling Sam several times a day and threatening her and her family if she didn't come back to live with him. During the day while I was at work, he would come here and threaten my son, telling him if he didn't sell drugs for him, he would kill all of us . . . this man was nuts, and after a conversation with an agent on the Colorado Bureau of Investigation (CBI), I found out just what this man was all about.

The CBI started watching our house almost 24 hours a day. Sam was deep in it with this "man" and they wanted her, but wanted him worse. Sam was making her court appearances, so they did not have a reason to arrest her. I know she was still using meth, because she continued to lose weight, act unpredictable and not at all like the little girl I knew.

One night this "man" came to our house in the middle of the night. He started banging on windows and demanding that Sam come out of the house. He told me that if I called the police he would have all of us killed. We were all so afraid of him. He finally left, but the next several weeks were worse. He called us sometime 120–125 times a day. He sat down the block and watched us all the time. The police said he had no outstanding warrants so they couldn't arrest him yet; the investigation was still being put together.

Sam was using heavily now and was beginning to have extreme paranoia. She would be in her closet sometimes for hours, I would have to bring her food in there, and she would only leave the closet to use the restroom. It was very frightening.

Finally one night I couldn't take it anymore—the phone had been ringing nonstop for hours. The "man" was sitting outside our house and calling from his cell phone. It was 2:00 A.M., and Sam was sitting in her room, curled into a ball crying, and my son looked like he was going to have a nervous breakdown. I told my son to get the phone and watch out the window and if this "man" made a move to call 911. I was going to try to talk to this "man." After all, he had been talking to me almost daily when Sam was living there . . . what was I crazy?

I approached his car and he rolled down the window and said "Hey Mom, what's going on?" I asked him to please never call me Mom. I begged him to leave us alone, let me have my family and my life back. He told me he couldn't do that because he was in love with Sam and needed her. I told him he was a sick person; he was 41 years old and she was 18. He just laughed and said, "So what are you going to do if I don't leave?" I told him calmly that I would go to the house, get a gun (I have never owned a gun), shoot him and drag him through the front door, call the police, and tell then that he forced his way into my house. He just started laughing, but drove away. I walked in the front door and nearly had a stroke. I think about this now and wonder what I thought I was doing; but I was desperate.

We saw him several times in the neighborhood the next couple of weeks and then I got a call . . . they had arrested him. I can't begin to tell you how I felt; unfortunately it was short-lived, because within a couple of weeks he was out, found Sam, and stole her car. However, a couple of days later he was arrested again in her car. The car was impounded, but at least he was behind bars. This time I left the car in the impound lot. Between the attorney fees and all the bonds I had paid at all the counties that she was in trouble with, I had nothing left.

It was now August; Sam was trying to do outpatient counseling, but it wasn't working. She was still using, but at least was home most of the time, would leave here and there, but always coming back . . . we made it through Thanksgiving and we were still appearing almost weekly for court dates. I was so thankful that she hadn't skip bail; my house was hocked up to the roof. The CBI was still watching the house, I'm sure partly because of the people that were coming and going during the day. My parents had recently retired, lived close, and came by at least twice a day to check on things. Most of the time they had to ask people to leave; fortunately, no one gave them a hard time. It was mostly the same people, but they continued to come back consistently.

December 1, 2001. Sam had been gone a couple of days, but I had talked to her every day; we had a court date this morning in Denver. She called at 4 A.M. to tell me not to worry; she would be home by 8:00. She never showed. I knew what this meant: They would put a warrant out for her. I was scared; this wasn't like her. As screwed up as she was, she always made her court dates. Sometimes we were flying down the highway barely making it, but she had always shown up. I was worried. Finally, on Sunday night she came home.

Her only explanation was she knew she had a dirty UA and did not want to go to jail. There was nothing I could do at this point but wait and see.

Monday, December 5, 2001. I left for work about 7:30 and waved to the CBI agent down the block; we had spoken several times, and I had offered to let them into the house anytime. I arrived at work about 8:15, and the phone rang. On the other end was an officer from the state patrol. He said, "We have just broken in your door and arrested Sam. She tried to kill herself. I think you better get here." I don't even remember driving home.

When I reached my neighborhood the entire cul-de-sac was full of emergency vehicles. They had Sam in the ambulance and had arrested another person who was in my house. I ran to the ambulance and talked to Sam. She was OK. She had drunk antifreeze and had a gun pointed to her head when they got into the house. They had talked her into putting down the gun, but she was going to need her stomach pumped. They told me to stay with the house. The CBI and state patrol then asked to search my house, and I allowed it. As far as I knew we had nothing to hide. They searched the house for about three hours and found a bag of stolen mail in the basement. There had been a "friend" of Sam's over to do laundry the night before, and I really think she left it, but at this point didn't really matter whose it was. Sam was released from the emergency room and sent to another ward and put under observations for 72 hours with strict orders that she was not to be released to anyone except the county sheriff. I went to visit, and as I was leaving I recognized two men that I had seen before. I asked what they were doing there and they said they came to see Sam. I tried to get them banned from seeing her—they were well-known meth users—but the hospital told me I could not control who came to see her; she was over 18. Big deal, like she was making rational decisions? Anyway, 48 hours later they released her to another "friend." When I arrived, I immediately called the detective on the case; the hospital had not read the orders, and she was gone again. Twenty-four hours later, they re-arrested her from the house of one of the "men" I saw coming to visit her that night. She was taken to the county jail.

Her first appearance was scheduled about 10 days later. I had talked to several people who told me to be prepared for a $2,500 bond, so I went to the bonds bailsman and had things ready to go. We showed up in court, Sam went before the judge, and the judge gave her a bond of $100,000 cash only. I about fainted. I could not understand why he would do that. There was no way I could afford that, so back to county jail she went. She continued appearing before this judge for the next four months. Finally, she started making phone calls to rehabilitation centers. The judge had told her that they were trying to find a place for her, but all the beds were full and it would probably be another six months before anything opened up. In the meantime, her trial had not even been scheduled. I cannot tell you what it is like to see your child brought into a courtroom in an orange uniform and shackles and chains. My heart could hardly stand seeing this. Then I would have to call a week in advance to schedule a visiting slot on Sunday to be able to see her, and visiting days were a whole other experience. The positive to all of this is I started to see her get well. She started gaining weight, her eyes came alive again, and that great bubbly personality she has was emerging again!

Sam continued to make phone calls and finally got an interview with a group called Cenikor. They interviewed and accepted her. Now she would have to clear it with the judge. This was not an easy decision. Cenikor was known as the toughest program out there, and it was a program of $2^{1}/_{2}$ to 3 years. I remember the weekend before our next court appearance. Sam must have called collect 50 times, and she was scared. She had seen several people returned to jail because they could not hack the Cenikor program. We talked for hours about determination and the want to have her life back. Finally, the next week we saw the judge. Sam explained that she had been accepted at Cenikor and the judge questioned her thoroughly, asking her what she knew about the program and if she was sure she was committed enough to be there. She finally convinced him that she was. The judge agreed to let her go, reminding her that if she failed or screwed up, it was back to county jail. Our attorney at that time felt this was not the right thing to do. He felt that Cenikor was too tough of a program for Sam; it was more of a program for habitual users, a last-chance type of program. I remember Sam saying, "Well, then this is the place for me, because I don't want to do this again." She added, "There is a reason I made the choices I did, and a 60- to 90-day rehabilitation center is not going to be able to help me figure out why." She then stated, "I want my life back, and I don't ever want to go back to this again." She was released to Cenikor about 24 hours later. I was a nervous wreck. This program is not a "lock-down," and the residents can walk right out if they want. I knew this was going to be hard for all of us, but especially for Sam. I did a lot of praying.

For the first three months of the program, she was not allowed to see any of us. Cenikor is a behavior modification program. They take all privileges away, and you have to earn everything back. First it starts with earning phone calls home, then come visiting on Saturday nights. It was a long three months. Cenikor is also different in the fact that they have a family reunification program. After a certain time and certain privileges are earned, the mothers can have their children live with them at Cenikor, providing they had custody when they arrived at Cenikor. Even though we could not see her, Tanner was allowed almost right away to visit every other Sunday. He had not seen Sam for quite a while. I did not take him to jail to see her. We told him that his mom was in a special school, and now he would be allowed to visit her. He was three years old now. Every day that she made it gave me strength to think she just might be successful at this. However, I wasn't fooling myself either; things could change on a dime.

Three months passed and we were finally allowed to visit on "Open House" nights, which were on Saturday evenings. Again, this was privilege and could be revoked at any time, which in Sam's case was a few weeks later. She was put in discipline for something she had done, and our visitation was cancelled.

Six months went by, and things were really starting to look up. Sam seemed to be getting better every day. Then another bomb dropped. The Colorado Bureau of Investigation showed up at Cenikor to arrest Sam. She had been indicted in a grand jury investigation. I could not believe this was happening, not now. Not just when things seemed to start getting better. They took her to county jail, not the same county as before. She was given a $50,000 bond. I went to family members and gathered up the cash ($5,000) to bond her out that night. She was making tremendous progress and needed to get back to Cenikor. They had agreed to let her come back if I placed the bond. We had her back at Cenikor that night. I think we really started to understand the trouble she was in. This was much bigger than I had ever thought.

She then started appearing in front of another judge for this case, and in the meantime was still appearing in several other counties on the charges in each of them. Finally a break—I guess you could call it that—two of the three counties had agreed to drop their charges and roll them into the grand jury case. This was huge because she was looking at several different felony charges in several different counties. She continued to appear in the last county, as well as in the grand jury county, for a couple of more months, when at that time, the last county agreed to drop their charges into the grand jury case. We now only had the grand jury case and the continuing case on possession, which she had been arrested for first. We continued to appear on the grand jury case; she did not have to appear in the Denver case as long as she was still at Cenikor.

Over the next several months, the state of Colorado continued to gather evidence in the case. Eventually, 10 people were indicted. They had the case on all the local news channels on the night they had arrested most of the people involved. I was sitting here by myself and on the 10:00 news there it was on every channel. How I hoped no one saw it . . . .

Sam was contacted by the district attorney's office and asked to come down and talk to them. They knew she was at Cenikor and wanted to talk to her about the case. Our attorney advised us to do so and that he would be there with us. It was now early 2003.

We continued to meet with the district attorney's office and made appearances before the judge when required. We were getting close to the end. Sam had been charged with 14 felony counts of theft and forgery and we were looking at 8–16 years in prison. Most of the other people involved in the case had already been sentenced to anywhere between 3 and 24 years.

Finally it was the "man's" time for sentencing; they contacted me and asked if I would want to make a statement at the sentencing. "Oh yes" was my reply. Sam was also asked along with a few others. We showed at the sentencing, and there he was. I had not seen him for over a year. I have never said that I hated anyone; in fact I cannot even stand the word, but this man I hated. I sat and listened to all the others make their statements about the things he had done to them in their lives. Sam then stood tall and told her story. I cried so hard I could hardly see. There were things that happened that even I did not know about. He sexually abused these girls, made them do criminal things to get drugs and protect their families. He was such a sick, sick man. Now it was my turn. I can't begin to tell you how nervous I was; he stared at all of us with no emotion as we read. It took me days to prepare my statement, and I felt good about what I said, and as the words came the stronger I felt and his eyes no longer bothered me. I wanted so badly for this man to go away forever so he could never hurt or steal from anyone again.

The judge listened patiently and then told the "man" to stand. He said, "I have seen a lot of really bad people in my career on the bench, but you Mr. ___ are about as close to the devil that I have seen. Your case carries a sentence of 16–32 years, and you will be serving 32 years." YES! It happened after all this time, all this pain. He was finally going away and we no longer had to fear from him. I was a huge relief to so many of us.

Now next to come was Sam's sentencing. It was about two months away. Cenikor was going well; Sam had done well in the program. Not that it had been easy, or that she did not have her ups and downs, but she keep working and slowly making a whole lot of progress. Then came the day when they told her that she could have Tanner come live with her. This was a bitter-sweet day. She had worked so hard for this, but with sentencing just a few months away, we didn't know where she would end up. We decided whatever time she had left, Tanner should be with her. Therefore, he moved in. He was so excited! I on the other hand was a little lost. He had been a part of my everyday life since he was born; however, there was no doubt in my mind where he should be.

My son had also made great progress. After a year of doing nothing and just kind of existing, he came alive . . . he took his GED and passed with flying colors. Shortly after that he enrolled in community college, found a job, and headed back to his sweet, funny self. Things were improving so well, but we knew we had the toughest day coming up.

Sam's sentencing was postponed—a good thing because it gave her and Tanner more time together, and gave us all more time with Sam; not such a good thing because it just put off the day we had all been dreading—it was now set for August. Sam continued doing well at Cenikor and now was granted the privilege of leaving the program for four hours once each month. We could pick her up and go to a movie or dinner, but she could not come to the house. We were thrilled just to be together.

August 2003. The day was here. We arrived at the courtroom, and I barely remember the drive. When we arrived our attorney who had worked so hard for us and Sam told us we needed to expect a sentence of at least four to eight years. He felt they would show some leniency because she had cooperated and had done well at Cenikor. I couldn't imagine how we were going to be able to say goodbye. . . . We were surprised to see the agent of the CBI there, the one that had arrested her twice. When the judge entered he asked if anyone was ready to speak. Immediately the agent asked to speak; what he had to say floored us all. He explained to the judge that this person before us was not the person he had arrested. He talked about how Sam came from a good family, had worked so hard at Cenikor to regain her life, and how proud of her he was. He said they don't see many success stories, and people like Sam why he did what he did everyday. I cried.

Next the prosecutors asked to speak. They talked a lot about how the things Sam did required jail time, but they too felt like she had worked really hard in the program and had cooperated with them throughout the case. They then asked the judge to give Sam 10 years probation. We were all so shocked, but again it was up to the judge.

The judge then started to talk and said that he too was proud of Sam, but the crimes she had committed did mandate jail time; however, this was a usual circumstance. He said he had never seen the people that were prosecuting the defendant stand and talk on her behalf. He then sentenced her to eight years probation, better than anything we had expected, along with the stipulation that she stay and complete the Cenikor program; she had about another year left. We were all in shock and overwhelmed with happiness. To think that these people could see who I knew in Sam, it was a wonderful day. She told them they would never have to worry about seeing her again. She accepted her restitution, which was about $27,000, and thanked everyone for giving her a chance. What a day!

Sam returned back to Cenikor and shortly earned the privilege to get a regular job outside the program. Tanner continued to live with Sam and was just a happy little boy. In the fall of the year, she was required to appear in the court with her initial case. This is the one that she was originally sentenced on. There was a graduation they wanted her to attend. She had been clean and drug-free for over 18 months and was being released from that case. She would still have the charge on her record, but they would close the case. We went to the graduation and were pleased to see the judge who sentenced her (who since had retired shortly after her case) there to celebrate the success of all of those there that day. After the graduation, I had an opportunity to speak to the judge; I knew that he was really a big part in her success. When I asked him why he gave her the bond of $100,000 cash only, he said, "I have done this for a long time, and pretty soon you start to be able to see the ones who really want help, who really have a chance, and I felt that Sam was one of them." He then added, "But, I knew if you bonded her out, she would be back on the street again. She needed time to get clean and do some thinking about where she was heading." Thank you, Judge. You helped save my daughter's life.

We were finally given a graduation date from Cenikor; she was to graduate on July 31, 2004. Things were going well. She was working 32 hours a week for a doctor's office, taking evening classes through the community college and spending time being a mother to Tanner.

In May of 2004, terrible news was announced on the television. Cenikor had been under investigation for food-stamp fraud, and their state license had been suspended. What did this mean for Sam? She had to finish this program or be sent to jail. For two days we waited to hear from her probation officer.

Most of the other residents were picked up and taken to other programs, sent back to the streets, or sent back to jail. This was truly a sad, sad day. My family and I had been very involved with the program; we donated time and money; my employer donated time, money, and furniture; I served on the board of advisors. How could something like this happen? When her probation officer called she said that Sam had satisfied her requirements and she should pack her things and come home immediately. We were so, so happy. She was coming home, but so sad that the Cenikor program was closing. This program had been in Denver for 37 years and had many success stories. This was another unbelievable day!

Sam and Tanner came home, and since then Sam and I have spoken to several groups about meth and the crazy world that goes with it. We are both so thankful every day that she is alive and able to be with us. We are also grateful that people are willing to let us try and help educate others, especially young people, on the dangers of this drug and the people that are involved with it.

I want everyone to know that it takes a tremendous amount of support to get where we are today. My family was unbelievable; they were there all hours of the day and night, they attended court hearings with me, held me when I cried, lent me money when I needed it, and drove the streets at night looking for her with me. My employer, what a wonderful group of people, they stood by me every inch of the way. My boss (our owner) allowed me to take time off during they day to be at court appearances with Sam (over seven weeks' worth in one year) and allowed me to work weekends, evenings, whatever I needed to do to keep my job. They now have employed Sam and continue each day to show their love and support. I have great friends who were always there when I needed them, and they are still there. One of my friends went to work for one of the metro drug task forces. She has taught me about the meth world and introduced Sam and me to a lot of wonderful organizations that we are proud to be associated with.

I don't know why God chose this path for us, but he did, and we continue to go down it. There have been many wonderful positives learned with this very difficult lesson. I am a much more compassionate person. I look at all people differently. They are no longer drug addicts or alcoholics; they are people just like you and I. They have a problem and they need help . . . help that maybe some of us can give, and that is not a bad thing to learn!

Sam now works at the same employer that I do. She interviewed and got the job on her own. I have never been more proud of her! Tanner is a happy six-year-old, and my son is finishing up his associate's of science degree in architecture. Things couldn't be much better—oh, except that Sam has meant someone wonderful, and we are in the process of planning a late-summer wedding. Tanner said to me the other day, "Nana, I am finally going to have a dad and a mom." And he deserves it!

PART IV

Community Responses to Methamphetamine Use and Manufacture

Agencies and communities within some regions of the country are addressing meth issues collaboratively. A collaborative community and agency response to meth is critical. The issues posed by meth use and manufacture require a community-wide collaborate response.

Chapter 13, Methamphetamine Addiction: An Integrated Approach to Case Management, Evaluation, and Treatment by Angela Mead provides ideas on how agencies and communities came together to address meth in the county. The county used focus groups and developed models of processing meth-involved families and children.

Chapter 14 by C. West Huddleston III is a previously published document on the use of drug courts as an effective community strategy to address meth addiction. Drug courts typically are more structured, demanding, and timely in their oversight of substance abusers. Drug courts always involve collaboration among law enforcement, the courts, social services, and treatment providers. Drug courts characteristically offer speedy sanctioning and consequences for the lack of compliance with treatment regiment. They have the ability to further restrict noncompliant addicts, should the need arise. Drug courts are also capable of rewarding cooperative addicts with incentives, such as visitation rights and fewer restrictions. Some would argue that these drug court features are exactly what is needed by meth addicts (Rawson and Anglin et al. 2002).

One example of a drug court is found in Maricopa County, Arizona, which established a court that has actively been involved with all substances, including meth. The drug court was established to give selected drug offenders a chance to erase their felonies, provided they meet the expectations of the court. Violent offenders or those found selling illegal drugs are not eligible for the court. The Maricopa court enters into contracts with the offenders that typically require community service, drug testing, counseling, treatment, and other structured requirements. Offenders completing the requirements receive diplomas in front of their peers and have their felonies erased. Similar drug courts operate in Sacramento County, California (Edwards 2005), and other jurisdictions.

The cost effectiveness of drug courts has been a central issue that decision-makers raise when deciding whether to implement a drug court. We do not know a lot about costs and benefits of drug courts, but do have some evidence from jurisdictions that have implemented them and then measured the costs and benefits. For example, Butte County, California, faced with a significant meth problem, instituted a drug court and then measured its cost benefit. Butte County officials reported that for criminal justice agencies over a four-year period, the system experienced about $1.4 million in savings through avoided costs, such as new filings, processing, convictions, arrests, and other costs (www.2stopmeth.org). Butte officials also reported that some criminal justice agencies had invested more heavily in the court, and these were not necessarily the ones that experienced the most savings (about $200,000 per year). They concluded that the drug court process was "well worth the initial investment." What is significant is that the calculations did not include other avoided costs, such as out-of-home placement for the children of meth addicts.

Chapter 15 provides an example of the development and operations of a drug court and how the court addresses meth-involved families and users. Some authorities have suggested that the criminal justice system may play a larger role in getting meth addicts into treatment compared to other substances (Rawson and Anglin et al. 2002). The development of drug courts may expedite addicts entering treatment. Meth addicts are known to enter treatment more slowly than the abusers of other substances.

Shirley Rhodus and Julia Roguski's chapter 15 describes the development of a drug court and how it works with meth-involved families. Their chapter provides an introduction to the establishment and operations of one example of a drug court. The Family Treatment Drug Court in El Paso County, Colorado, was created in 2002 to serve children who otherwise would be placed in foster care and their parents who abuse substances. The foundation for the program was begun prior to the phenomenon of the increase in the use of methamphetamine and its effects in the community. The program was then in a position to tackle the effects on children and families of the explosive, increasing use of meth by parents. This chapter describes how three major systems came together to develop an integrative and creative program with limited fiscal resources, the structure of the Family Treatment Drug Court, how to manage child safety and risk with the substance-abusing population, and developing, collecting, and using outcome data.

Methamphetamine Addiction: An Integrated Approach to Case Management, Evaluation, and Treatment

Angela Mead, MSW

Methamphetamine has been called the "equal opportunity destroyer." This powerful addiction tears at the very fabric of our society and presents a multitude of challenges for practitioners who are trying to manage the problem in their community. The abuse of this drug does not discriminate among gender, ethnicity, or socioeconomic status. Meth availability and production are being reported in more diverse areas of the country, particularly in rural areas.

Colorado has been greatly impacted by the insurgence of meth abuse, manufacturing, and distribution. Fortunately, the Colorado Alliance for Drug Endangered Children has made a statewide effort to broaden public awareness as to the depth of this problem and the threat it imposes on public health and safety. Larimer County has been taking this problem seriously and has organized to broaden community awareness and integrate their efforts toward managing the problems associated with meth abuse.

Child welfare is one agency that has been dramatically impacted by the abuse of this drug. The Larimer County Department of Human Services, similar to other agencies, has experienced a substantial increase in child maltreatment reports involving parents who abuse meth. Ten percent of their reports of child abuse and neglect indicate meth abuse as a primary concern. In 2005 (in the nine-month period of January–August), the department received child protection referrals identifying 388 children who were allegedly living in homes where parents were abusing this drug and who were being neglected or abused. Child and Family Services investigated more than 67 percent of those referrals and identified and substantiated findings of child maltreatment of 71 children; 60 children were identified in investigated cases with an inconclusive finding. Cases with inconclusive findings involve a significant level of risk and generally warrant some level of intervention. At least 52 children were placed out of their homes due to meth abuse, and 65 petitions were filed with the court in order to intervene on behalf of children and to ensure their protection and rehabilitation of their parents. Child maltreatment resulting from parental meth abuse involved physical abuse, sexual abuse, emotional abuse, and neglect. Neglect was the primary type of child maltreatment and involved 87 percent of the cases. The Larimer County Drug Task Force investigated 12 meth laboratory cases, and 4 of them involved the presence of children.

Due to the overwhelming concern of meth abuse by parents and the maltreatment of children, Larimer County Child and Family Services recently adopted a new model of intervention. The model includes an integrated approach to case management, evaluation, and treatment. It was designed to improve their ability to identify drug-endangered children and to enhance evaluation and treatment approaches that would ensure better permanency outcomes for children and rehabilitation for parents. This chapter describes the county's efforts to address meth abuse in child welfare. It also defines the underlying philosophy of the model and the integrated components. Components of the model include assessment/investigation, evaluation, and treatment approaches, family and community inclusion, visitation, support for care providers, permanency planning, and outcomes for measuring model effectiveness.

To understand the depth of this addiction, we must see it from the addict's perspective. A woman involved with the department whose children had been taken away because they had been sexually abused and neglected describes her experience and writes the following poem:

My Name Is Crystal Meth

> At first you think I'm really fun,
> But you'll find I'll hurt you till you're done.
> I'll sneak up on you when your life is whole,
> Then blind side you and pierce your soul.
> I'll make you lie, cheat and steal,
> Because you like how I make you feel.
> I can disintegrate the pipes in your drain,
> Along with your vital organs, flesh and brain.
> When it's me you need and seek,
> I'll be elusive, show you're weak.
> But if you try to walk away,
> I'll hunt you down and make you pay.
> You'll give up everything you've got,
> I'll tell you now, it will be a lot.
> I'm your new friend, "Crystal Meth,"
> And I'll make you miserable until your death.

This is all too familiar a story for people addicted to meth. So the question becomes, "Why is this drug so destructive to people?" First of all, it's important to consider its attractive properties. People are drawn to this drug because of the euphoria, high energy, weight loss, low cost, availability, and ease of manufacture (see chapters 1, 4, and 8 of this volume). Secondly, this drug is referred to as a psycho-stimulant. When an individual takes meth, the result is an accumulation of the neurotransmitter dopamine. The excessive dopamine concentration appears to produce the stimulation and feelings of euphoria experienced by the user. It has a much longer effect on the user than cocaine, marijuana, or other drugs, and a large percentage of the drug remains unchanged in the body. This results in meth being present in the brain longer than other drugs such as cocaine or alcohol, which ultimately leads to prolonged stimulant effects. Long-term use of this drug leads to dependence and dramatic changes in behavior that include violent behavior, anxiety, confusion, and insomnia.

Imagine you are a person struggling with this addiction and having to deal with the physical and mental effects of either abusing the drug or trying to get clean. Add to that the challenges of daily living and caring for children. It's no wonder child welfare agencies are inundated with child protection referrals. If you are a parent and abuse this drug, it will eventually lead to the abuse or neglect of children. As a parent abusing this drug, your priorities will go from caring for your children to only worrying about getting your high. Eventually with long-term abuse this drug will destroy parents' relationships with their children.

To manage meth cases in their child welfare system, child welfare caseworkers did what every child welfare agency did, and that was to apply traditional practices for treating substance abuse addiction. Little did they know that traditional approaches were not lending themselves to successful outcomes. Child welfare caseworkers frequently complained about how frustrating the cases were. They described the parents as not showing up for scheduled office or home visits and parenting time with their children. Treatment providers complained that parents weren't showing up for evaluation and treatment appointments. Removal of their children and court orders requiring them to participate in treatment were not motivating parents to stay off meth. Failure to complete treatment plans as ordered by the court was leading to termination of parental rights and an increasing number of children in need of permanency away from their birth family.

Substance addiction is not new to child welfare. In fact, 85 percent or more of cases in child welfare involve substance abuse problems by one or more parents. Traditional approaches such as drug and alcohol treatment, 12-step support groups, parenting classes, and mental health services are generally effective in treating most substance abuse cases and lead to successful reunification of the family. What authorities have found with meth addiction is that many traditional case management and treatment approaches are not as effective. Increase in cases, out-of-home placement of children, termination of parental rights, and practitioner frustration have led to evaluating and changing the ways caseworkers manage and treat this addiction. The Larimer

County team started with bringing practitioners to the table to discuss what was working and not working with these cases. Included in the discussion were the multiple challenges experienced not only by practitioners but also by clients themselves. They also started looking at system barriers that were preventing success. Through the discussions they came to the realization that they didn't really understand the addiction and knew they needed to learn more about the complexities of meth and examine other treatment approaches that have been effective. They also discovered that they were managing cases in a fragmented manner.

They failed to see the connection between substance abuse problems and mental health problems. Many of their parents who were suffering with meth addiction were also suffering with mental health disorders. Historically, drug and alcohol and mental health providers have managed and treated their clients independently of each other. Independent management of these cases lends itself to poor safety management and relapse. Becoming more aware of the physical and psychological ramifications of meth addiction, they knew that the two disciplines would need to integrate their efforts along with the case management facilitated through child welfare.

INTEGRATED MODEL FOR CASE MANAGEMENT, EVALUATION, AND TREATMENT

The integrated model for case management, evaluation, and treatment of meth addiction is built on the premise that parents are unlikely to be successful with their recovery efforts unless the caseworker and treating practitioners are integrating their efforts in the management of recovery and treatment. Along with treatment efforts there needs to be a level of accountability and structure that motivates parents to address the social and psychological problems associated with meth addiction. The model recognizes the value and importance of family and community inclusion. Parents who are addicted to this drug tend to manage the challenges with recovery better when they are supported by family, friends, and other adults who can identify with their experiences.

At the inception of a child welfare case, family unity teams are developed and made up of people who are directly involved in the efforts to support and rehabilitate an addicted parent. Members of the family unity team can be caseworkers, immediate and extended family members, friends, treatment providers, attorneys, guardians ad litem, probation officers, and other helping professionals. Involvement of recovery support group members plays a vital role in helping an addicted parent to stabilize during the initial stages of recovery. They are also quite effective in helping parents in recovery to sustain changes in their life. More importantly, the model recognizes the various stages of meth recovery and relies on behavioral intervention strategies developed and facilitated by members of the family unity team.

The model consists of four components addressing the life of a case in child welfare. Figure 13.1 is a diagram of the model for case management, evaluation, and treatment. The model identifies the stages of recovery and displays estimated time intervals of each stage. The model also displays the

Figure 13.1
Integrated Model for Case Management, Evaluation, and Treatment of Methamphetamine Addiction

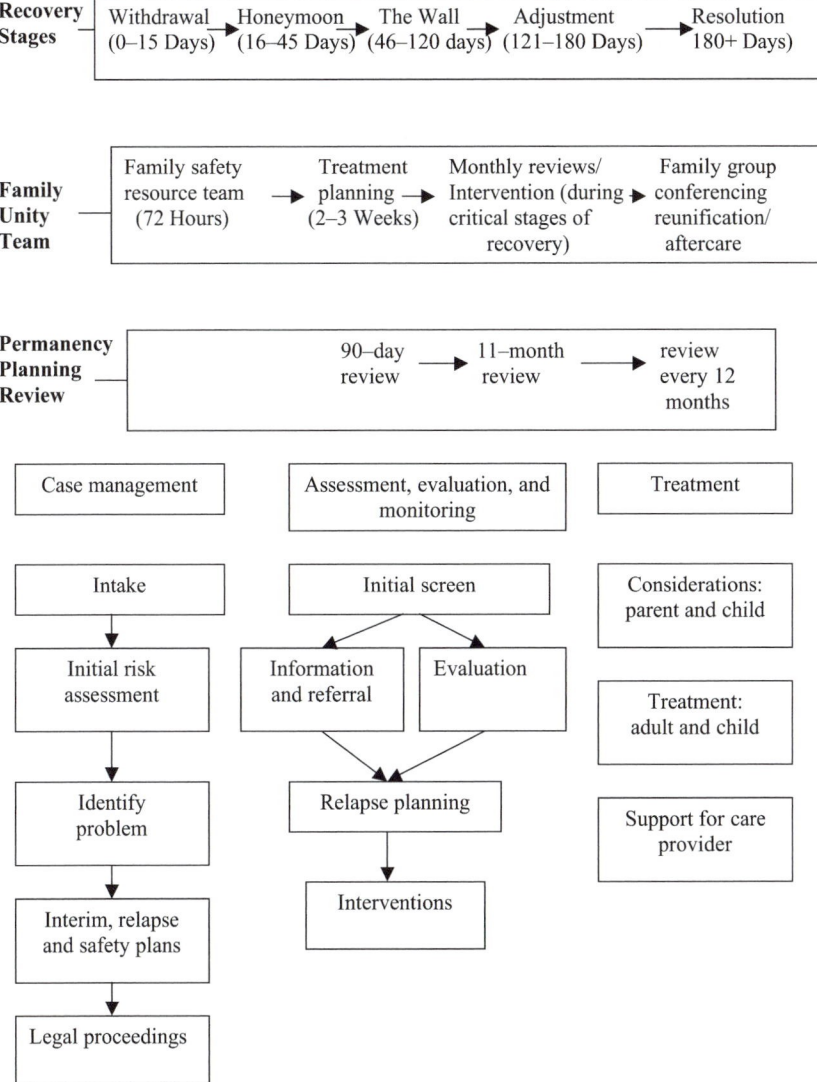

continuum of family unity team meetings and the time intervals associated with those meetings. The family unity teams are the forum for decision making as it applies to the case. Permanency-planning time intervals are also included and begin in the early stages of the case. The model has three primary sections: case management, evaluation, and treatment. Each section has multiple elements that influence decision making and case planning throughout the life of the case. Each component and section of the model will be described in subsequent paragraphs.

APPLICATION OF METH ADDICTION: FIVE STAGES OF RECOVERY TO TREATMENT

In developing this model they acknowledged the five stages of recovery for meth addiction as identified by the Matrix Institute and UCLA Integrated Substance Abuse Programs. The Matrix Institute is located in California and has more than 20 years of experience treating stimulant addiction. Table 7.2 in Chapter 7 identifies the five stages of recovery.

Each of these stages is critical to consider and helps to explain the challenges faced by the parent who is addicted to meth. As a practitioner (caseworker, mental health therapist, or drug and alcohol counselor), one must acknowledge changes and difficulties that are occurring for the client. Ken Minkoff, M.D., has published several articles on treating dually diagnosed consumers (Minkoff 2005; Minkoff and Cline 2004). He believes that effective treatment is based on empathic and hopeful relationships, and that treatment approaches should match the phase of recovery for each disorder. He strongly argues that mental illness and substance abuse are both primary diagnoses and should be treated as such.

Dr. Nicolas Taylor is a clinical psychologist currently working in the field of treating addictions with a particular emphasis on treating meth addicts. Through his work he has identified that within each stage of recovery the addicted parent experiences profound changes in the domains of functioning, behavioral, emotional, cognitive, and relational.

According to Dr. Taylor (chapter 7) and other treatment specialists, the different stages of recovery faced by a meth-addicted parent present many challenges for practitioners. The different stages of recovery experienced by meth addicts helps explain occasional low parent motivation, relapse, and failure to follow through with expectations. It is important to carefully consider each stage when setting treatment goals and expectations for the parent. This is not to say that a parent's tendency to make poor choices and failure to maintain sobriety should be excused. It does suggest that relapse and a slower response to treatment should not surprise caseworkers and treatment providers. It also speaks to the necessity of an integrated approach to evaluation and treatment. Caseworkers, mental health therapists, and drug and alcohol treatment providers should be gathering and exchanging information. Treatment goals should be carefully thought out by everyone involved and determined based on the parent's capabilities and resources. Those involved should also prioritize goals. Child welfare agencies have a tendency to construct treatment plans independently from treatment providers and do not take into consideration the inherent struggles of recovery. We are more likely to see favorable outcomes centered on reunification of the family when practitioners are speaking the same language and working together to manage relapse and preparing family members for various changes associated with recovery.

APPLIED PHILOSOPHY—FAMILY OPTIONS: RESTORING FAMILIES TO BUILD COMMUNITY

The Department of Human Services is committed to providing the best services possible for children and families in Larimer County. In doing so, the department implemented an applied philosophy called Family Options: Restoring Families to Build Community. There are core strategies within Family Options that directly influence the practice in relation to meth cases. The first strategy is the family safety and resource team meeting (FSRT). The FSRT is a meeting held within the first 72 hours of identifying a child in a drug endangered environment (see Figure 13.1). The meeting is held to share information that relates to the protection and safety of a child and to make decisions regarding any emergency placement. One of the goals of the FSRT is to ensure a network of support for the child and adults who care for him/her, while keeping safety as the main priority. Another goal is to do relapse planning for the parent to ensure the accessibility and timeliness of treatment services.

Within two to three weeks of the FSRT, a family unity team is established. These teams are comprised of people who are directly involved in either treating or supporting the family in meeting desired outcomes related to protection and permanency of the child. Members typically consist of practitioners who represent the departments of human services, mental health, and drug and alcohol treatment. Judicial representation is also included and typically consists of probation officers, court-appointed special advocates, and guardians ad litem. Care providers have a critical role as members of the team. They are foster parents, kin providers, or residential care facility treatment providers or child placement agency case managers. Immediate or extended family members are also involved. Parents are encouraged to invite people within their support system. These may include 12-step group sponsors, members of the faith community, and friends.

A critical first step in beginning family unity team meetings is the creation of the family service plan. The family service plan is mutually developed by members of the team and focuses on the safety and permanency of the child and rehabilitation of the family. Beyond the implementation of the family service plan family unity meetings occur monthly. Family unity meetings are scheduled to ensure continued consultation with the treatment team and review of progress or reevaluation of treatment needs. It is strongly encouraged that members celebrate milestones reached in recovery and successful completion of treatment goals. Family unity team meetings can also be called if a parent relapses and an intervention is warranted to assist the parent in getting back on track with sobriety. It's important that relapse is approached with a nonjudgmental attitude, and that feelings surrounding the relapse are validated. As the case progresses, family unity meetings can be helpful in planning and preparing children and families for transitions, reunification, or permanent care.

PERMANENCY PLANNING FOR CHILDREN

Permanency planning for drug endangered children is critical. Unfortunately some parents addicted to meth fail to sustain their recovery efforts and do not successfully complete treatment. For child welfare agencies, "The Adoption and Safe Families Act" (ASFA; P.L. 105–89) determines that child safety is the primary concern, and reunification of families is secondary. Provisions of the legislation mandate termination of parental rights for foster children within a limited time frame to ensure that children do not linger in temporary living situations. After a child has remained in out-of-home care for 15 out of the most recent 22 months, a petition for termination of parental rights must be filed in most cases. Parents are protected from potential consequences of ASFA. Exceptions may be made when termination of parental rights is not in the best interests of the child and when child welfare agencies have failed to make reasonable efforts through service provision that is necessary to return the child to a safe home.

The Department of Human Services views permanency of the child as a vital part of case planning (see Figure 13.1). Reunification is a goal of permanency for the child. Recognizing the limitations of some parents struggling with mental health disorders and substance addiction and the risk of termination of parental rights, concurrent planning for children is imperative. Concurrent planning requires practitioners to develop treatment plans with reunification as the first alternative and consideration given to other permanency alternatives in the event termination of parental rights occurs. Concurrent planning begins at the onset of the case and explores other permanent alternatives such as long-term foster care, guardianship, foster adoption, or adoption. Concurrent planning includes the pursuit of two potential permanency plans. The first priority is reunification. The second plan is to ensure that the child is placed in a home where the child can remain if reunification is not possible. Maintaining permanency in a placement and avoiding multiple subsequent moves is in the best interest of the child.

The Department of Human Services has implemented internal practices to ensure that the case stays on a permanency track regardless of the permanency goal. Permanency planning review committees have been established and monitor permanency decisions made on cases. The permanency planning committees are

ıbstance addiction, it's
ıtion of the substance
parents using motiva-
e intent of getting the

rranged as a means of
ıy analysis is set up on

g

aluation

ıl Assessment
Assessment

ıtal Development
ılopment Assessment Tool
ıth Assessment
ıl Evaluations
ıluations

Interventions

ncreased Supervision

Changes in Treatment

Probation Revocation

Contempt of Court

Negative Discharge

made up of practitioners in the field who are knowledgeable about children and private citizens who have a personal desire to advocate for the best interests of children. The permanency review process has shown many benefits to caseworkers and other practitioners involved in the case. The review meetings allow for opportunities for brainstorming and recognizing other permanency alternatives for children. The review process helps keep family unity teams centered and focused on the importance of permanency for children. Occasionally practitioners involved in the case experience roadblocks in the case and are discouraged about outcomes or lack of progress made by parents. Input from committee members who have not been directly involved often results in alternatives that may have been overlooked by the caseworker, supervisor, and treatment providers.

The review process can validate case plans and efforts made toward reunification. Permanency planning review committees ensure agency accountability and provide the necessary checks and balances for securing permanency for children (Figure 13.1). Permanency review meetings take place at 90 days and 11 months from date of placement. Permanency meetings are scheduled every 12 months beyond the first 11 months if the child remains in placement. Ninety-day reviews are scheduled to assess current placement of the child and associated plans for reunification. The department also identifies kin or nontraditional kin who may serve as a viable placement option. Eleven-month reviews are intended to prepare for the 12th-month judicial review. The review committee is particularly concerned about how the case is progressing toward reunification. If progress is not occurring at an acceptable rate, consideration is given to termination of parental rights or legal guardianship if children are placed with kin.

The first consideration is the response to child protection cases involving allegations of meth abuse and production. Early identification of children in drug endangered environments is crucial. Child protection employees must receive training regarding meth addiction and production if they are to have the necessary skills to recognize safety hazards and risk to children. Equally important to employees in child protection is personal safety. Investigating child abuse and neglect cases involving the production and manufacture of meth presents many occupational hazards. Caseworkers performing investigations in these cases must be fully informed on labs and first responder safety. In an attempt to handle the occupational hazards of managing these cases, the department implemented mandatory training on the following subjects:

- Meth 101—This training provides basic information about meth, acute and long-term effects of abuse, implications of use on parenting, and risks to children.
- Meth Lab Awareness—This training provides information on production and manufacture of meth, hazards to children and the community, and policies and procedures of investigating meth lab cases.
- First Responder Safety—This training provides information on physical and behavioral indicators of being under the influence of meth, indicators of meth labs, and safety precautions to take when dealing with someone who is under the influence or tweaking on meth.

Figure 13.2
Case Management

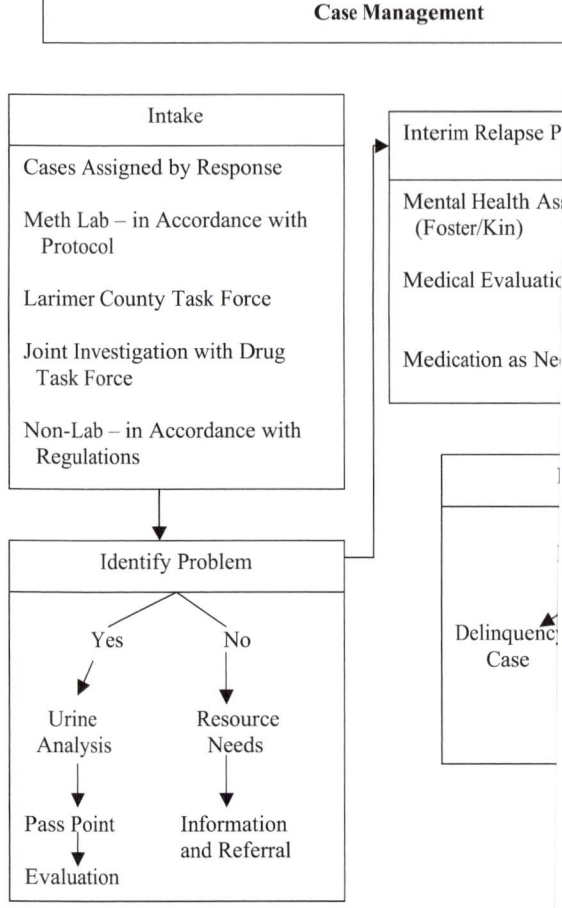

Joint Investigations between Child Pro
and Law Enforcement

To be more effective at identifying children i
ronments, law enforcement and child welfare ag
together. It is common for law enforcement and
respond to cases not suspecting parents who are al
Ensuring children's protection relies on identifica
both agencies. Collaboration between each agency
to be taken to protect a child and completion of
as to ensure successful prosecution and adjudicati
Law enforcement and child protection must be awa
sibilities of each agency and work in unison to ac

child and his/her family. As with any case invc
not uncommon to be faced with denial or n
abuse problem. Child protection workers int
tional techniques. They develop relapse plans
parent referred for evaluation and treatment.

Urinary analysis (UA) and Pass Point testin
monitoring a parent's commitment to sobriety.

Figure 13.3
Assessment, Evaluation, and Monitoring

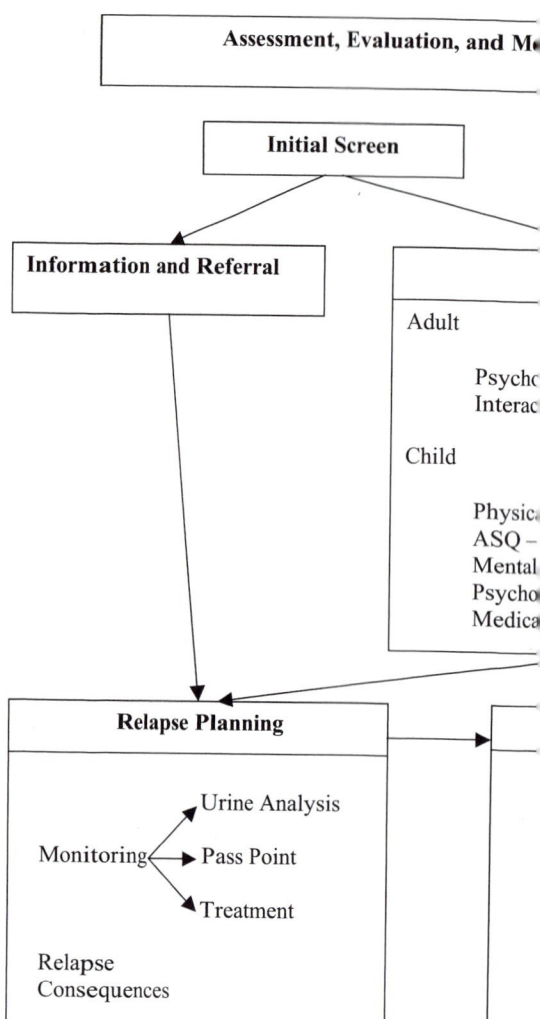

made up of practitioners in the field who are knowledgeable about children and private citizens who have a personal desire to advocate for the best interests of children. The permanency review process has shown many benefits to caseworkers and other practitioners involved in the case. The review meetings allow for opportunities for brainstorming and recognizing other permanency alternatives for children. The review process helps keep family unity teams centered and focused on the importance of permanency for children. Occasionally practitioners involved in the case experience roadblocks in the case and are discouraged about outcomes or lack of progress made by parents. Input from committee members who have not been directly involved often results in alternatives that may have been overlooked by the caseworker, supervisor, and treatment providers.

The review process can validate case plans and efforts made toward reunification. Permanency planning review committees ensure agency accountability and provide the necessary checks and balances for securing permanency for children (Figure 13.1). Permanency review meetings take place at 90 days and 11 months from date of placement. Permanency meetings are scheduled every 12 months beyond the first 11 months if the child remains in placement. Ninety-day reviews are scheduled to assess current placement of the child and associated plans for reunification. The department also identifies kin or nontraditional kin who may serve as a viable placement option. Eleven-month reviews are intended to prepare for the 12th-month judicial review. The review committee is particularly concerned about how the case is progressing toward reunification. If progress is not occurring at an acceptable rate, consideration is given to termination of parental rights or legal guardianship if children are placed with kin.

The first consideration is the response to child protection cases involving allegations of meth abuse and production. Early identification of children in drug endangered environments is crucial. Child protection employees must receive training regarding meth addiction and production if they are to have the necessary skills to recognize safety hazards and risk to children. Equally important to employees in child protection is personal safety. Investigating child abuse and neglect cases involving the production and manufacture of meth presents many occupational hazards. Caseworkers performing investigations in these cases must be fully informed on labs and first responder safety. In an attempt to handle the occupational hazards of managing these cases, the department implemented mandatory training on the following subjects:

- Meth 101—This training provides basic information about meth, acute and long-term effects of abuse, implications of use on parenting, and risks to children.
- Meth Lab Awareness—This training provides information on production and manufacture of meth, hazards to children and the community, and policies and procedures of investigating meth lab cases.
- First Responder Safety—This training provides information on physical and behavioral indicators of being under the influence of meth, indicators of meth labs, and safety precautions to take when dealing with someone who is under the influence or tweaking on meth.

Figure 13.2
Case Management

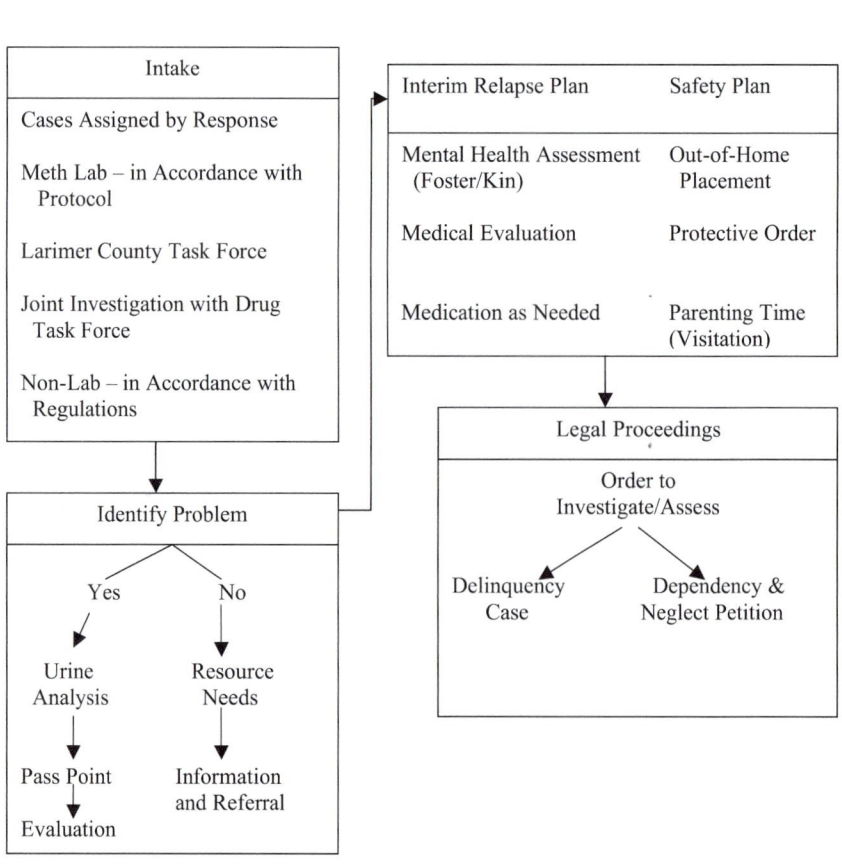

Joint Investigations between Child Protection and Law Enforcement

To be more effective at identifying children in drug endangered environments, law enforcement and child welfare agencies must work closely together. It is common for law enforcement and child welfare agencies to respond to cases not suspecting parents who are abusing or producing meth. Ensuring children's protection relies on identification and collaboration by both agencies. Collaboration between each agency allows for immediate steps to be taken to protect a child and completion of thorough investigations so as to ensure successful prosecution and adjudication of dependent children. Law enforcement and child protection must be aware of the roles and responsibilities of each agency and work in unison to accomplish the objectives of their case. Child protection's role is to assess child safety and risk, arrange for immediate substitute care if necessary, and rehabilitate the family. Law enforcement's role is to ensure the safety of children and the community in which they live. To ensure public safety they must investigate crimes and hold offenders accountable for the risk they impose.

The Department of Human Services and the Drug Task Force developed a memorandum of understanding to assist in the identification, investigation, and removal of drug-endangered children from hazardous drug-usage and manufacturing locations found within law enforcement jurisdictions. Both agencies agreed to make available specialized trained investigators, equipment, resources, and information needed for drug endangered environments. The agreement requires all law enforcement agencies in the county to report the discovery of minor children at laboratory sites to the department, as appropriate under Colorado statutes. In accordance with Colorado State Law 19–3-401(1) (a), the agreement indicates that children may be taken into protective custody by a law enforcement officer without an order of the court. When a child is abandoned, lost, or seriously endangered and immediate removal appears to be necessary for such child's protection or the protection of others, C.R.S. 19-3-102 (1) (c) allows the Department of Human Services to file a petition of dependency and neglect as long as the child's environment is injurious to his or her welfare. Under this agreement, the department agrees to provide the usual and customary services of its child protection services to peace officers handling minors involved in the seizure or closure of meth laboratories, including but not limited to:

- Response to the potential health needs of any minor at the site
- Taking the minor into protective custody unless the minor is criminally involved in the lab activities or is subject to arrest for other criminal violations
- Ensuring immediate medical testing for meth toxicity
- Arranging for any follow-up medical tests, examinations, or health care made necessary as a result of meth toxicity

Finally, the agreement ensures joint investigations in accordance with the "Investigative Procedures for the Handling of Minors in the Seizure or Closure of Meth Laboratories." Since the inception of this agreement, successful efforts have been made in identifying drug endangered children and ensuring timely response by child protection to make arrangements for their immediate care. Removal of children from these environments can be very traumatic. Through joint efforts by both agencies trauma can be minimized and immediate services can be made available to the child and family.

ASSESSMENT, EVALUATION, AND MONITORING

After children have been identified and emergency steps are taken to ensure their protection, immediate steps are taken to further assess the needs of the child and his/her family. As with any case involving substance addiction, it's not uncommon to be faced with denial or minimization of the substance abuse problem. Child protection workers interview parents using motivational techniques. They develop relapse plans with the intent of getting the parent referred for evaluation and treatment.

Urinary analysis (UA) and Pass Point testing are arranged as a means of monitoring a parent's commitment to sobriety. Urinary analysis is set up on

Figure 13.3
Assessment, Evaluation, and Monitoring

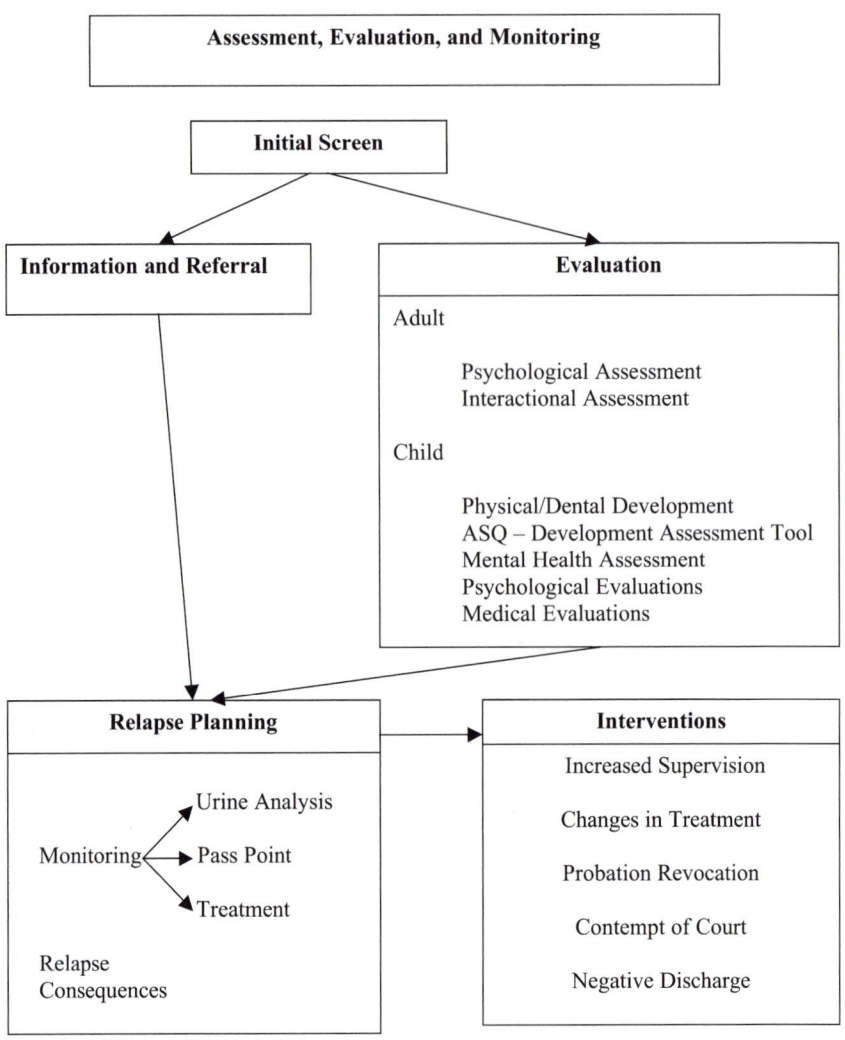

a random basis. Pass Point is an eye test that measures activity in the eye that is indicative of being under the influence of certain types of drugs. Both methods of monitoring are effective means of measuring sobriety as long as appropriate steps are taken to manage the risks associated with false positives or false negatives.

Relapse plans also include referrals for medical evaluations. Psychotropic medications may be beneficial to addicted parents during their early stages of recovery. The first months of recovery can be an extremely difficult time, and relapse is very likely to occur. Medication may help to manage the depressive side effects of withdrawal from meth and help to motivate a parent to participate in other elements of their recovery and treatment program. Mental health assessments are also very important to diagnose any mental illness a parent may be suffering. The recovery process for an addict can be hindered unless appropriate mental health interventions are in place. Many parents working with child welfare have experienced very difficult and traumatic lives, including surviving abuse as children and being raised in environments where substance addiction and domestic violence have occurred. Childhood memories may have been marked by very traumatic experiences and have significantly impacted their lives as adults. It is often the earlier life experiences that have influenced the choices they make as adults and explain their susceptibility to substance addiction and mental illness. Mental health and drug and alcohol evaluations are imperative and can assist practitioners as they determine appropriate treatment plans for parents.

Voluntary Services or Legal Interventions

First response can include voluntary agreements that include safety and relapse plans. Voluntary agreements for service are generally offered to families whose children have not been abused or neglected and still are in need of services to prevent maltreatment. Parents receiving voluntary services are capable of acknowledging the extent of their addiction and are highly motivated to receive treatment. For families who have abused and neglected their children and who are denying their addiction and are resistant to treatment or struggling with their recovery and compliance with treatment, legal interventions are pursued to ensure protection of the child and rehabilitation of the parent. Legal proceedings can involve court orders to investigate or assess a child's needs, dependency and neglect petitions, or the filing of a delinquency case. Dependency and neglect petitions are filed when a child has been abused and/or neglected, is in an injurious environment, or is beyond the control of his/her parent. Delinquency cases are filed when youths commit crimes. Legal interventions result in judicial involvement and oversight, thus providing necessary accountability for juveniles and adults abusing meth. Experts in the drug and alcohol field have recognized the value of accountability in managing successful recovery and treatment efforts with meth addicts.

TREATMENT AND EVALUATION

Treatment goals for the addicted parent have to be carefully prioritized and consistent with their primary diagnosis. Meth cases require emphasis on abstention and recovery in the early stages of the case. Mental health assessments or evaluations are important for parents exhibiting indications of co-occurring disorders. Access to treatment should begin as soon as possible, and there should be no arbitrary length of sobriety as long as the parent is capable of carrying on a reasonable conversation (Minkoff 2005). Medical evaluations are strongly suggested, as there are indications that many parents will benefit from prescribed medications during the early stages of recovery. Prescribed medication has been known to assist some people with the emotional side effects of sobriety, such as depression and anxiety (Taylor 2004). Considering the emotional and behavioral challenges associated with early stages of

Figure 13.4
Treatment

Considerations	Treatment	Support for Care Provider
Parent	Adult	Information Sharing
Drug Education	Drug & Alcohol Treatment	Frequent Contact
Gender-Specific Goals		
Nutrition	Inpatient	Support Groups
Exercise	Outpatient	
Vocational Skills	Narcotics Anonymous	Inclusion Planning
Parenting		
Life skills	Mental Health Treatment	
Emotional Well-Being		
Communication	Individual	
Healthy Relationships		
	Couples Treatment	
Child	Family Treatment	
	Reunification	
Age of Child		
Trauma Impact	Child	
Developmental		
Capacity	Raft services	
Available kin	Play Therapy Group	
Permanency Goal	Individual	
	Family	
	Mentoring	
	Group Therapy	

recovery, it's important not to overwhelm parents with completing too many treatment goals too quickly. Parents are more likely to succeed with case outcomes if treatment goals can be completed within reasonable time frames and are expected in accordance with their capabilities.

Upon completion of necessary assessments and evaluations, treatment practitioners meet with members of the family unity team to discuss recommendations. Consideration is given to self-disclosure of the parent and family members, child protection family risk assessment, collateral information obtained in the investigation, pending court orders, criminal history, and social history information and evaluation results. During the first family unity team meeting, the treatment plan is formulated. For most meth-addicted parents, treatment goals are centered around drug education, gender-specific goals, nutrition, exercise, vocational skills, parenting and life skills, and building healthy and supportive relationships. Treatment goals for children are influenced by the age of the child, degree of traumatic exposure, developmental needs, sustaining attachment with birth parent(s), and the permanency goal. Treatment goals focus on the physical and psychological development of the child. Physical and mental health assessments, or psychological evaluation, may be indicated depending on the degree of trauma and exposure to toxic chemicals. Children, depending on their age and stage of development, will participate in a variety of treatment milieus. They may include play therapy, support groups, individual and family counseling, and mentoring programs.

Treatment Considerations for Parents

The Department of Human Services is fortunate in that child welfare services are integrated with mental health and drug and alcohol services. The department contracts with providers that provide services on site of the child and family services division. This allows for better collaboration between practitioners and makes services more readily available to the families that are served.

Substance Abuse Treatment

A private treatment center provides evaluation and treatment services to substance-involved adults and youths. Since a very high percentage of cases involve parents who are substance addicted, the county contracts with a center to provide these services. The department's child welfare division houses three full-time drug and alcohol treatment providers who are employees of the center. They only serve child welfare clients and have specialized services to treat meth addiction. They have arranged walk-in clinics that occur weekly for evaluations. This has helped to make their intake services more readily available and accessible. Services include support groups that are specific for gender and type of drug and for adolescents. They also provide an intensive outpatient program. This includes a combination of weekly support groups and individual sessions for up to 24 weeks. The frequency of contact with addicted parents is extensive during the critical stages of recovery and becomes less frequent over the duration of treatment. Relapse in recovery may change the frequency and duration of treatment. Families who have suffered with both substance addiction and domestic violence receive specialized services through the treatment center, as well. The department has managed a high number of cases involving meth addiction and domestic violence. The integration of mental health services and drug and alcohol treatment services has been very effective in treating both the addiction and mental health problems resulting in domestic violence.

The basic framework of drug and alcohol treatment applied to treating addicted parents is based on Prochaska and DiClemente (1992) stages of change and motivational interviewing. The stages of change model identifies six different stages. For each stage of change the drug and alcohol treatment provider has strategies to manage the emotional and behavioral challenges associated with the addiction. The first stage is identified as precontemplation, which is also known as "denial." The addicted parent essentially does not believe he/she has a problem with addiction. During this stage the treatment providers are focusing on building rapport and finding out what is important to the client. They manage varied emotions and relapse tendencies through giving choices and providing feedback. The second stage is contemplation. During this stage the addicted parent is beginning to recognize the possibility that there is a problem with abusing substances. The strategies for managing the emotional and behavioral responses include exploring ambivalence, showing empathy, changing extrinsic to intrinsic motivation, and developing self-motivating statements. The third stage is preparation, when the addicted parent acknowledges the addiction and has decided they are ready to change. Managing behavioral and emotional responses during this stage requires the treatment provider to help the parent enlist social support, confirm their readiness for change, repeat motivational statements, and with permission, offer expertise and advice. The fourth stage is referred to "action." During the action stage the addicted parent is more motivated and acting on his/her thoughts regarding change. It's during this stage that the parent and treatment provider are working on a treatment plan. The treatment provider reinforces the importance of remaining in recovery through acknowledging the difficulties in early stages of change and helping the client identify high-risk situations that may lead to relapse. The fifth stage is referred to as maintenance. This is a period in treatment where the provider is supporting lifestyle changes and working with the parent on maintaining supportive contacts. A plan is developed during this stage to manage any relapse if it occurs. There is more emphasis on long-term goals and aftercare. The final stage of the model is referred to as "relapse." Most meth addicts will experience relapse. The goals of the practitioner are to process the relapse with the client and indicate how to learn from it. It is important to reward self-efficacy and to assist the parent in finding alternative coping strategies. It is also necessary to revise the maintenance plan and to consider things that may have been overlooked.

Mental Health Treatment

Since the fall of 2002, the Larimer Center for Mental Health, the Health District of Northern Colorado, and the Island Grove Regional Treatment Center—the state-approved treatment center for alcohol and drug abuse— have partnered to have a single point of entry for persons with mental health and/or substance abuse disorders. This change is the result of the recognition that it should be the expectation, not the exception, that clients with mental illness also have a co-occurring substance abuse disorder. The screening process for new clients has been improved to better identify the presence of both mental health and substance abuse issues, regardless of the presenting problem. Larimer Center Mental Health therapists have shifted their approach from expecting sobriety for a period of time before receiving mental health services to supporting a philosophy of dual recovery. Therapists provide care coordination with other treatment providers to offer integrated treatment of clients with co-occurring disorders as well as evidence-based therapeutic services, such as psycho-educational groups, motivational interviewing, assertive community treatment, cognitive behavioral therapies, and psychiatric medication services. Throughout the treatment process, services are targeted to the specific stage of change for each disorder, the possibility of relapse is anticipated as part of the change process, and relapse prevention/recovery is incorporated into the treatment plan.

Treatment Considerations for Children

Treatment services arranged for children are determined by comprehensive assessment of their physical, psychological, social, and developmental needs. During the early stages of the case, caseworkers, care providers, and treatment practitioners carefully assess children who are removed from drug endangered environments. The assessment begins with physical examinations by a medical doctor. Children removed from clandestine labs are evaluated for toxic exposure to meth and other chemicals. All children receive acute and medical follow-up care, as necessary, by medical practitioners. The National Alliance for Drug Endangered Children recently adopted a protocol for medical evaluation of children found in drug labs. The protocol describes the prospective roles of first-responding professionals in ensuring the immediate evaluation and treatment of children. Professionals include law enforcement, child protective services, and medical personnel, specifically emergency departments at hospitals. The protocols contain guidelines of evaluation in time intervals of acute care, 72 hours, and follow-up care. The protocol also addresses decontamination and emergency activation. The Larimer County Alliance for Drug Endangered Children is currently conducting forums to introduce and promote the application of these guidelines in the medical community. Child protective services' role is to assist law enforcement in the collection and documentation of the scene from the child's perspective. Caseworkers will determine appropriate arrangements for substitute care and make immediate arrangements for necessary medical care. Medical histories are obtained and documented in the child's health record. Substitute care providers are instructed to arrange for subsequent medical follow-up and transport children to appointments as necessary.

Developmental Assessment of Children

Consideration must be given to prenatally exposed children. Children removed from labs or parents who abuse meth can experience a range of problems that warrant a variety of special services. The Ages and Stages Questionnaire (ASQ) is a developmental guide of children for parents. The questionnaire helps parents and care providers learn more about the child's development. ASQ simply involves parents or care providers answering questions about the child's development while playing with them. The questionnaire has an easy scoring system and will tell parents or care providers if the child may have a delay in development. If scores in the instrument suggest possible developmental delays, then appropriate arrangements are made for further evaluation by parents, care providers, or caseworkers. Infants and toddlers removed from drug endangered environments can be referred to RAFT. The RAFT program is an interagency service for families of infants and toddlers. It helps families learn about their child's development and links them to professionals who can evaluate their child. RAFT will help families of children with delays or disabilities find services to help their child.

Maintaining Family Connections

Along with treatment, a critical part of rehabilitating families involves sustaining family connections during a child's temporary removal from home and placement in out-of-home care. If a child is removed from home and placed in substitute care, the department of human services has a legal and ethical responsibility to arrange for continuous contact between the child and the parent. Many child welfare agencies refer to this contact as "visitation." The department refers to visitation as "parenting time." The words visitation and parenting time are used interchangeably throughout this paragraph. We believe this is a critical juncture in the case that allows parents to integrate and apply what they've learned in treatment to the relationships they have with their children. The department is committed to maximizing the effectiveness of safe parenting time with all child protection cases. Early and frequent visitation decreases the emotional distress children suffer when removed from their parents. Parents have better attendance in treatment if they have consistent and frequent contact with their children. Special consideration is given to cases involving substance-abusing parents. Conditions of parenting time, such as frequency, duration, and degree of supervision, are determined by the degree of risk, if any, a parent may pose to a child. Urinary analysis and physical and behavioral observation of parents by supervising agents are key processes in making determinations about visits. Recognizing the inherent risks that substance-abusing parents can pose on children, the department has taken the following precautions toward ensuring safety of all parties during parenting time:

- Training for department staff and supervising agents (foster parents, kin) is mandatory on drug recognition and first responder safety.
- Pre-check-in process with parents is required prior to visits to determine to what degree they are impaired by substances. Check-in process is facilitated by the supervising agent and includes behavioral observations and delivery of questions eliciting responses from the parent to determine degree of functioning.
- Urinary analysis testing is required on parents who are in the early stages of recovery and are actively using meth. Parents are denied visitation if they are actively under the influence of meth.

The process of parenting time begins as soon as possible after out-of-home placement is made. Visitations occur within 48 hours of out-of-home placement if the parent is not determined to be actively under the influence of meth. Interim parenting time plans are developed at the Family Safety Resource Team meetings. Parenting time will be conducted with "specific intent," utilizing coaching, goal setting, application of parenting skills, and continual assessment of parental strengths and progress. Visits are supervised initially by caseworkers or case service aides. As the parent progresses in treatment and associated risk is significantly reduced, the visitation plan will increase in frequency and duration. Structure, location, and supervision requirements change as the family progresses and safety concerns are diminished. Eventually visitation will be unsupervised and will take place in less controlled environments with the goal of overnight stays, and eventually, reunification.

For the management of parenting time in drug endangered children's cases, the Drug Endangered Children Drug Endangered Children Risk Matrix for Child-Parent Visitation was developed. The risk matrix is simply a level system that has been created to guide caseworkers and supervisors in the decision-making process. Decisions regarding structure, frequency, duration, and supervision are determined in order to ensure the safety of the child and the creation of parenting opportunities. The effects of meth abuse present many challenges for practitioners in making decisions about parenting time. The matrix was developed taking into consideration the inherent risks associated with meth abuse. Parents are introduced to the level system as they are beginning their relapse and treatment plan. As they acquire sobriety and sustain progress in treatment, they advance through the level system, eventually allowing them to have the least restrictive measures for parenting time. Initially, the parent starts at level four, the most restrictive level for child-parent visitation, which requires supervision of the visit at the Department of Human Services.

The Drug Endangered Children Risk Matrix for Child-Parent Visitation levels are described below:

Level Four—Most restrictive measure for child-parent visitation. Requires supervision at the Department of Human Services (applies to use of hallucinogens, stimulants, narcotics, and opiates).

Criteria

a. Early stages of case assessment and requires further evaluation and establishment of relapse plan.
b. Indication of violent and drug-related crimes.
c. Requires clean swab or urinary analysis on day of scheduled visit.
d. Requires supervision by agency personnel who are trained in drug recognition and intervening in behaviors that could emotionally or physically harm a child.
e. Supervising agent has the authority to suspend the visit if pre-check-in process determines the child will be unsafe.

Level Three—More restrictive measure for child-parent visitation, but still requires supervision and is located in a controlled setting (applies to use of hallucinogens, stimulants, narcotics, and opiates).

Criteria

a. Parent in early stages of recovery and becoming engaged in a treatment plan but still vulnerable to relapse.
b. May have experienced periods of sobriety but still experiencing relapse.
c. Case assessment has concluded that restrictive measures are necessary to ensure protection of the child. Child-parent visitations take place at the department or other settings that are secure.
d. During periods of relapse a requirement of clean swab or urinary analysis on day of scheduled visit.
e. After three consecutive clean swabs or urinary analysis, random testing is required.
f. Child-parent visitations are supervised by agents who are specifically trained in drug recognition and intervening in behaviors that may result in physical or emotional harm to children.
g. Requires a pre-check-in process with parent prior to visit.
h. Supervising agent has the authority to suspend visitation if the pre-check-in process determines the parent is unsafe to meet with child.

Level Two—Less restrictive measure for child-parent visitation, but still requires an element of supervision.

Criteria

a. Parent is actively participating in treatment and making progress and or complying with treatment elements.

b. No indication of recent violent or drug-related crimes.

c. Sustained evidence of sobriety as monitored through random urinary analysis.

d. Case assessment has concluded that safety of the children can be ensured through child-parent visitation in the community and supervised by designated party. Visits located in various community locations and supervised by foster parents, kin providers, family members, court-appointed special advocates, case service aide, or caseworker.

Level One—Least restrictive measure for child-parent visitation.

Criteria

a. Actively participating in treatment and making sufficient progress in meeting treatment goals.

b. Sustained sobriety for extended lengths of time.

c. No indication of violent or drug-related crimes.

d. No restriction on location of visit.

e. No requirement of supervision.

SUPPORT FOR CARE PROVIDERS

A significant part of treating children and parents is the role of care providers, who can be licensed foster care parents, certified or noncertified kin (family members), and nontraditional kin (significant adults with no familial relationship). The Family Options philosophy requires that care providers play a participatory role in not only providing care for children but also working directly with their parents. The extent to which they are involved in direct work with parents is dependent on goals and stages of treatment, safety, and risk factors inherent in the case, and the skill and comfort level of the provider and parent. Family Options recognizes the value of relationships not only between parents and treatment providers but also between parents and care providers.

It has been our experience that parents respond more favorably to and progress more in their treatment if they have supportive and trusting relationships with care providers. The change in the department's philosophy has not been an easy one and involved a significant degree of resistance in the beginning. The resistance came from care providers and department staff. Practitioners and care providers were operating under assumptions that in many respects hindered progress toward rehabilitation and reunification. It was assumed that treatment staff needed to protect children while in out-of-home care; doing so required separation, or minimal contact, between parents and care providers. Historically, the extent of contact may have included brief face-to-face contact during visitation exchanges, case staffing, or court appearances. Parents were never allowed to know the location of foster care residences or phone numbers. Information concerning the child was exchanged through the caseworker or treatment providers.

What has been learned over the years is that parents are less likely to appreciate or trust care providers if they don't have direct communication and involvement with them. The child has a lot less anxiety in placement if they know that their care provider and parents are working together and trusting one another. Currently, care providers are actively involved in these cases. Above and beyond providing day-to-day care of the child, they attend family conferences, family unity team meetings, and foster care reviews and supervise parenting time with children and their parents. The caseworker encourages direct contact between care providers and parents via phone contact or face-to-face meetings where they discuss particular things concerning the child, such as the physical and emotional condition of the child and progress with treatment. During supervised parenting time, the care provider can be a coach to parents as they are learning new ways to communicate or discipline their child. As care providers directly observe parents with their children, they can witness firsthand the progress of the parent and the improved relationships with the child.

Care providers have a great deal of anxiety about reunification of children. They worry about the child's safety and well-being. If care providers are directly involved in working with parents they can be reassured that those circumstances have improved and that the child will be all right. This new approach, although very valuable toward rehabilitating parents, can also create significant challenges for care providers. This approach requires more of the care providers' time, energy, and skills to deal with children and parents. The direct care of drug endangered children can be very difficult even under the best of circumstances. We know that many of these children present with a variety of special needs requiring constant care in managing their emotional and physical well-being. Some meth-exposed children suffer from health complications and emotional and behavioral problems. Care providers work very hard to manage the complexities of their care and then are faced with having to deal with parental actions and omissions that impact the children for whom they are caring. An example of this would be parents who don't show up for visits with their child or do something in a visit that is inappropriate, and they have to be confronted and redirected. Many care providers have other foster children and their own family as well. The demands on care providers in meeting the needs of these children and their own family make them vulnerable to a myriad of problems. If they are to be successful in caring for foster children and still manage their own families, they need tremendous support and resources.

Built into the matrix is a section referring to support of care providers (Figure 13.4). This is crucial if we are to succeed in stabilizing a child's temporary out-of-home care and prevent unnecessary moves in care. Recognizing that if care providers are going to meet the demands imposed on them by this model they need continual support, guidance, and resources, licensed foster care and certified kin providers go through extensive training orienting them to the department, legal system, applied practices in managing a variety of cases, and information that will allow them to be successful in caring for children with special needs and working with parents. Also available to all care providers are ongoing support groups. Clinicians and qualified department staff facilitate the support groups. The purpose of the group is to join them with other care providers who experience similar challenges and who are in need of information and support. Along with discussion about particular needs and concerns they have, they can review a variety of topics that are specific to caring for children.

The department's foster care unit also provides a monthly newsletter that highlights events and activities occurring in the community. Articles covering special interest stories, changes in departmental policies, and procedures are also included. Care providers of children removed from environments where parents abuse meth are provided with information specific to drug recognition, practitioner safety, and the science of meth, specifically the stages of recovery. This information is very helpful to care providers in that it will allow them to appreciate the challenges of addiction and the acute and long-term effects of the drugs on parents and children, if they are exposed. Care providers are more equipped in working directly with parents affected by this addiction. A key component of supporting care providers involves the working relationship between case managers and care providers. To avoid placement disruptions of children in care, there are practical steps a caseworker can take in maintaining effective working relationships with care providers:

1. **Keep communication open and honest**—Care providers need to have sufficient information that allows them to arrange for whatever the child needs while in their care. Special provisions and accommodations have to be made to ensure the child's comfort and physical and emotional well-being while in care. Care providers need to be continuously informed of developments of the case, particularly as it impacts the child. Caseworkers and care providers should be honest regarding their limitations in knowledge, experience, and skills.

2. **Listen with respect**—Caseworkers should listen to the opinions or concerns of care providers. Consideration should be given to their ideas or concerns or the struggles they are personally experiencing.

3. **Provide regular and frequent contact**—Care providers benefit from having regular contact with caseworkers. Care providers need ample opportunity to process their concerns and opinions with the caseworker. They routinely need guidance from caseworkers on how to handle a variety of things that are occurring, such as behavior management of kids, setting limits with parents, and de-escalation techniques to use with kids and parents that are upset.

4. **Have empathy for care providers**—Be sensitive to their feelings and struggles. Expect varied emotional responses stemming from the stress they're under in

providing care and in meeting other demands placed on them. Be open to processing their feelings and experiences and directing them to other resources that may be helpful to them.

5. **Maintain objectivity**—Avoid making assumptions and gather all pertinent information regarding a situation before reacting prematurely.

6. **In managing conflict, caseworkers and care providers should look, listen, and learn—** This simply means look at a problem from all perspectives and be willing to listen to different points of view. Be open to learning new ideas or ways to manage problems through the experience or expertise of others.

7. **In managing conflict, caseworkers and care provides should stop, step back, shift thoughts, and refocus**—Recognizing the complexities of these cases and the frustration everyone feels when things are not going as well as hoped, it's important to realize that conflict is likely to occur between practitioners, care providers, parents, and children. Each of us has to take responsibility for our contribution to the conflict. Generally conflict stems from lack of understanding, poor communication, and responses to emotional reactions. If we stop and step back to self-evaluate our role in the conflict and shift our thinking to consider other points of view, we are more likely to refocus our energy toward problem solving and resolving the conflict.

EVALUATING MODEL EFFECTIVENESS

Outcome measures have been developed to determine this model's effectiveness in rehabilitating parents addicted to meth and reuniting children who have been placed in out-of-home care. These same outcome measures are used to determine program effectiveness. The following outcomes are measured annually:

1. Negative Move—percentage of placements requiring a move to a higher level of care, for example, child originally placed in foster care who is moved to residential care

2. Positive Move—percentage of placements resulting in a lower level of care, for example, child originally placed in residential care who was moved to foster care

3. Reentry into foster care (within 12 months of last removal)—number of youths who were in out-of-home placement and returned home, and number of youths who reentered out-of-home placement

4. Reunification (within 12 months of last removal)—number of youths who were in out-of-home care prior to services and number of youths reunified within 12 months

5. No more than two placement settings within 12 months—number of youths who entered care during or after services and number of youths with no more than two placements

6. Exit to adoption less than 24 months—number of youths who exited to adoption in less than 24 months

7. Recurrence of maltreatment—number of youths associated with a substantiated finding of abuse or neglect, and number of those youths who had a recurrence of substantiated abuse or neglect within six months

8. Substantiated abuse or neglect to any youth during or after service—time intervals of 0–6 months and 7–12 months

CHAPTER 14

Drug Courts: An Effective Strategy for Communities Facing Methamphetamine

C. West Huddleston III

OVERVIEW

In recent years, methamphetamine, a highly addictive, easy-to-manufacture stimulant, has become one of the most destructive and widespread illegal drugs in the United States. The drug induces violent and erratic behavior in addicts, endangers children living in the vicinity of its manufacture, and jeopardizes the safety of communities in which it is present. Dealing with this epidemic has been extremely difficult for law enforcement agencies: Methamphetamine is often produced in vans and trailers that can be moved across jurisdictional lines, and only a small percentage of addicts have responded to traditional methods of treatment and punishment. To fight this scourge, many states and counties are sharing law enforcement resources through multijurisdictional task forces, which make manpower and expertise available to underserved areas. But the primary tool for fighting methamphetamine addiction and trafficking is the drug court, which combines intensive drug rehabilitation services for addicts with legal requirements to complete treatment. Drug courts offer longer treatment periods, an emphasis on addressing co-occurring mental health disorders, and intensive community supervision and monitoring. They are also helping children who are exposed to methamphetamine use by providing them with health care, educational, and child protective services. Positive outcome data and anecdotal evidence have created broad support for drug courts in communities, law enforcement agencies, and academia.

The methamphetamine crisis that began more than 20 years ago in the western and southwestern regions of the country has now spread to the central and southeastern areas of the United States (Drug Enforcement Administration 2004). Use of the drug has increased to epidemic proportions throughout the nation and poses a significant public health treat (Rawson and Anglin et al. 2002).

Methamphetamine is a toxic, illegal, and highly addictive central nervous system stimulant that can be injected, snorted, smoked, or swallowed. The drug can be produced using a variety of household chemicals and inexpensive over-the-counter ingredients and is often made in clandestine laboratories such as car trunks, hotel rooms, backyard garages, and kitchen cabinets.

The effects of methamphetamine on the user are destructive. Addicts suffer from post-use responses that range from violence, paranoia, and agitation to cognitive impairments such as memory loss, confusion, insomnia, depression, and boredom. Most alarming are the neurological damage and psychotic symptoms that persist for months or years after use has ceased. Therefore, to ensure that methamphetamine-addicted offenders are abstinent and progressing in their recovery, a long-term view of treatment and accountability is required.

The rise of methamphetamine is often compared with the crack cocaine epidemic of the 1980s and 1990s. Unlike crack cocaine, however, which affected primarily urban areas, methamphetamine has infiltrated unprepared rural regions of the country. Many, if not most, of these rural communities did not experience the crack epidemic and therefore did not develop resources to address the personal and social devastation cause by stimulant addiction. As a result, law enforcement, corrections, social services, drug treatment agencies, and courts in rural areas are overwhelmed with the management of the risks and needs of methamphetamine users and manufacturers.

Urban communities know all too well the strain these users and manufacturers create on health-care and dental services, mental health and drug treatment providers, child welfare, environmental protection, and even real estate markets. In addition to these effects, methamphetamine poses serious safety challenges to police and probation officers in rural areas, who often encounter toxic chemicals and violent behavior.

In many communities, the central response to this crisis is the drug court, which is unprecedented in its ability to effectively intervene with the methamphetamine-abusing population and unequalled by any other criminal justice response. This document provides state and local policymakers with information needed to build safer communities, reduce recidivism, reunite families, and promote abstinence from methamphetamine.

DRUG COURTS: A LONG-TERM RESPONSE TO A NATIONAL CRISIS

> We are 30 years deep in the methamphetamine epidemic in Butte County, California, and drug courts are the only thing that has worked with this population.
>
> —*Helen Harberts, special assistant district attorney and lifetime member of the California Narcotic Officers' Association*

For more than a decade, a number of drug courts have been extremely effective in stemming the tide of addiction in some of the most methamphetamine-affected areas of the nation. Federally funded drug courts in California, Oregon, Hawaii, Nevada, Oklahoma, and Kentucky have been using the drug court model—that is, pairing the coercive power of the justice system with effective treatment strategies—to successfully intervene and manage the methamphetamine-addicted offender. Drug courts tackling the methamphetamine epidemic have demonstrated that the following are among the most effective strategies for helping methamphetamine addicts:

- Intensive community supervision and monitoring
- Ongoing accountability with increased court hearings
- Longer treatment periods
- Treatment for co-occurring mental health disorders
- Implementation of evidence-based treatment

Drug courts provide the added accountability and service coordination that methamphetamine addicts desperately need to recover. Using these tested methods, drug courts are building safer communities, reducing recidivism, reuniting families, and promoting abstinence.

EFFECTIVE METHODS EMPLOYED BY DRUG COURTS

Added Accountability

To effectively address the methamphetamine user's potential for volatile behavior and deep cognitive impairments, drug courts apply increased accountability, supervision, monitoring, and structure.

Drug courts integrate public health and public safety to optimize outcomes for offenders. Substance abuse treatment assumes a central role rather than being peripheral to punitive ends. Responsibility for ensuring that participants attend treatment and avoid drug use and criminal activity is not, however, delegated to treatment personnel. Rather, the court and law enforcement maintain substantial supervisory control over offenders and are thus able to respond rapidly and consistently to infractions in the program (Marlowe 2003). This added accountability from the court, probation, and law enforcement is central to effectively managing and treating a methamphetamine-involved offender.

Role of the Court

Drug courts bring to bear added accountability to the methamphetamine users. First, participants must frequently appear in court before highly trained judges. In many cases, the participant attends drug court weekly for at least the first 90 days of the program. During the hearings, the judge explores the participant's compliance with treatment, random drug testing, and other court requirements. The immediacy of sanctions for noncompliance and the repetitive reinforcement of target behaviors and requirements are especially important because of the cognitive impairments that occur in this population. In addition, drug courts have been able to expedite the bench warrant process; therefore, when participants fail to appear in court, law enforcement officers rapidly bring the offender before the judge for the appropriate sanction, continued treatment, and ongoing community supervision.

As a seasoned judge, I have found that frequent and immediate responses are the most effective way to deal with the methamphetamine addict. In addition, it is essential through treatment and court intervention to get to the underlying cause of the addiction and deal with the physiological and psychological reasons for the addiction. Drug courts are the most effective way to deal with these problems.

—*The Honorable Dennis Fuchs, Salt Lake City, Utah*

Finally, many drug court professionals throughout the nation have joined local and state methamphetamine action committees and task forces. In Oregon, a retired drug court judge chairs that state's methamphetamine task force. On a local level and as a central function of a community, the courts are often called on to educate the greater community about drug and crime trends. In that role, drug court prosecutors and police personnel volunteer to speak to community groups, churches, and business leaders about the dangers of methamphetamine and the precursor chemicals used to manufacture the drug. In Oklahoma City, Oklahoma, a drug court police liaison officer speaks to such groups to help citizens spot and report individuals purchasing large quantities of precursor materials at local retailers. In Washington, the drug court coordinator sits on a community methamphetamine task force and, together with other leaders, speaks throughout the community using a scripted media presentation about methamphetamine. These strategies are just more examples of how drug courts coordinate community resources to combat methamphetamine on the state and local levels.

Role of Probation and Law Enforcement

Participants are closely monitored by law enforcement and probation officers through creative and effective community supervision. Because methamphetamine addicts affect public safety and increase risk in the field for supervising officers, they are among the highest risk offenders and require intensive supervision.

Methamphetamine users are volatile, unpredictable, and often violent. More so than users of other drugs, they can misinterpret body language and become violent in response to a perceived threat. They demonstrate paranoia and seem fine, only to become agitated at a moment's notice. Clandestine methamphetamine labs also present real risks to officers. Breathing fumes from an active lab can be life threatening, and the risk of a chemical explosion is high. Coupled with the methamphetamine addict's belligerent and unpredictable behavior, clandestine labs place officers at great risk.

For these reasons, drug courts are proactive in their supervision of methamphetamine-involved participants. As the court's eyes and ears, law enforcement and probation officers are highly trained to work with this population and employ community supervision and community policing strategies to ensure safety and effectiveness. Proactive supervision requires probation and police officers to work in tandem and regularly visit the participant's home. While there, officers administer a drug test and canvas the property for signs of drug use and laboratory agents. When a participant is found in violation, he or she is immediately detained and brought before the drug court judge at the earliest opportunity. When a participant is "caught doing right," the officer gives the participant positive reinforcement before leaving.

In 15 years of law enforcement responding to situations that encompassed everything from methamphetamine labs to the methamphetamine addict, drug courts are the most effective criminal justice strategy I've seen to treat the offender, reduce criminal activity, and build safer communities.

—*Sergeant Vanessa Price, Oklahoma City Police Department*

Whether it is the judge, probation supervisor, or law enforcement officer, the drug court's coercive power is the key to providing what research characterizes as "closer, more comprehensive supervision and monitoring during the program than other forms of community supervision" (Belenko 1998, 2001).

SERVICE COORDINATION

To effectively address the chronic, acute, and long-term effects of methamphetamine abuse, drug courts implement comprehensive, long-term, and evidence-based stimulant-specific treatment protocols.

Effects of Methamphetamine on the Addict

The effects of methamphetamine addiction are both acute and chronic. When used in high doses, the drug can cause irritability, aggressive behavior, excitement, auditory hallucinations, and paranoia (delusions and psychosis). Mood swings are common; the addict's demeanor can rapidly change from friendly to hostile. Because of the long-lasting effects of the drug, withdrawal may be severe and protracted. Several hours after last use, the addict experiences a drastic drop in mood and energy and may sleep for days. On waking, the addict may experience severe depression that can last for several weeks or longer. Cravings are pronounced, and the addict is at increased risk of attempting suicide (Center for Substance Abuse Treatment 1999).

The chronic effects of methamphetamine addiction have been well documented. Prolonged use drastically disrupts brain function in fundamental and long-lasting ways (Swan 2003). Chronic use of methamphetamine significantly reduces brain dopamine and serotonin levels with ramifications that can last from one to four years. Some neurological impairments may be permanent. These impairments in brain functioning may underlie the cognitive and emotional deficits seen in many methamphetamine addicts (Center for Substance Abuse Treatment 1999). Thus, the treatment needs of the methamphetamine addict are sizable and distinct.

Keeping the Client Engaged in Treatment

To benefit from treatment, the client must attend treatment sessions as prescribed. Drug courts are uniquely suited to promote a positive treatment response in methamphetamine users because ongoing attendance and participation in treatment are assured. Research shows that the length of time spent in treatment is a reliable predictor of a client's post-treatment performance. The longer a client stays in treatment, the better he or she does (Simpson and Sells 1982; Hubbard et al. 1989; Simpson and Curry 1997). Twelve months or more of drug abuse treatment may be the optimum length of time to ensure lasting reductions in methamphetamine use. Because drug courts have ongoing contacts with the client to reinforce treatment attendance and participation, a high percentage of participants complete long-term treatment. In fact, more than two-thirds of participants who begin treatment complete it. This represents a six-fold increase in treatment retention over most previous efforts (Marlowe et al. 2003).

Providing Effective Treatment Protocols

Because of the acute and chronic effects of methamphetamine, drug courts provide services for methamphetamine addicts that are more intensive and longer in duration than those received by offenders struggling with other drugs. In addition, case management and case planning are intensive. Treatments plans are based on a sound assessment, individualized to meet the client's specific needs, and designed to be easily understood by the client. Treatment services are structured and supportive. The court addresses co-occurring mental health and other comorbid conditions and implements community reinforcement models coupled with cognitive-behavioral treatment modalities and continuing care.

First, drug courts provide an objective and comprehensive assessment to address all bio-psycho-social domains, including drug use severity; level-of-care placement; drug involvement; medical status; psychiatric status;

employment and financial status, family and social status, and triggers and cognitions; and self-efficacy and motivation to change. Bio-psycho-social assessments are critical to characterizing a client's needs, strengths, and resources along each dimension. Armed with the assessment information, the clinician then develops a clinically competent treatment plan for each individual.

The information gathered by clinicians and other professionals during the assessment process also helps drug court case managers, defense attorneys, and law enforcement and community supervision officers in establishing a baseline and monitoring for changes in the client's behavior and living environment.

Once the treatment plan is completed, drug court clinicians ensure that the client understands the treatment process, the rules and expectations of each program phase, and expectations about his or her participation. Most drug courts that work with a methamphetamine-involved population provide clients with clear, written agreements or contracts that are reviewed with the client at the onset of the program and again after a month of abstinence. This regimen is especially vital for methamphetamine users because of typical cognitive impairments that may be present at the onset of services.

Drug court providers adjust treatment services to address the specific conditions and needs of the methamphetamine user. Early in the program, the clinician helps the participant establish behaviors that will have short-term benefit and long-term utility. Specifically, for the brain to begin to recover from methamphetamine use, the clinician structures sleep, exercise, and eating goals for the client. In addition, the court sets short-term treatment attendance and abstinence goals and rewards the participant when he or she achieves them. The court also establishes support structures such as self-help groups and sponsors, provides drug avoidance strategies, and educates the client about the impact of methamphetamine on the brain and behavior. Together, the court and participant plan ways to identify and manage his or her triggers and cues to relapse. Family participation is enlisted, and early slips are addressed.

Addressing Co-Occurring Mental Disorders

As the client progresses, so does the treatment protocol. Mental health disorders such as major depression, dysthymia, bipolar, antisocial personality disorder, panic disorder, post-traumatic stress disorder, and schizophrenia may coexist with a methamphetamine or substance use disorder. Generally, such co-occurring mental disorders are addressed with one month of abstinence and simultaneously with treatment for methamphetamine and other drugs. Mental health specialists are brought to bear, and medication is prescribed when appropriate. Antidepressants are often used in concert with psychotherapy to reduce depressive symptoms and produce short-term reductions in methamphetamine use and craving.

Community Reinforcement

Another treatment strategy used by drug courts during the treatment of methamphetamine users is community reinforcement. The approach uses individualized treatment to promote lifestyle changes in three key areas: marital therapy, employment and vocational counseling and assistance, and the development of new social networks and recreational practices (Meyers and Smith 1995).

Contingency Management

Drug courts have repeatedly demonstrated the importance of positive reinforcement (that is, rewards that are contingent on positive behavior) as an effective behavioral change strategy. Short-term incentives are immensely important as rewards to methamphetamine users for treatment compliance and abstinence. Rewards need not be tangible to be effective. Praise, for example, when delivered both immediately and continuously for achieving target behavior, is effective (Deci et al. 1999). To that end, drug court judges use public praise, clapping, and handshakes in court to reward compliance. More tangible rewards are also used. Some drug courts provide vouchers that can be redeemed for retail items such as food and transportation or children's books to promote good parenting skills. Such vouchers are contingent on negative urine drug screens or compliance with treatment sessions. Other drug courts provide stars, cookies, or free dental care. The last is particularly helpful because methamphetamine seriously affects gums and teeth.

Drug court treatment programs are subject to higher standards of performance accountability by the judicial system. Due to the collaborative nature of the drug court model and the development of an extended team approach, the accountability most often associated with the client is extended to the team as a whole. This results in a superior level of treatment planning and service integration, which is a critical component of successful outcomes with methamphetamine addicts.

—*Joe Carloni, MSM, Specialty Court Programs, Pensacola, Florida*

Other Treatment Approaches

Finally, drug courts use a full range of other treatment strategies to ensure the best odds for a positive outcome. Cognitive behavioral treatment strategies and carefully prepared treatment manuals such as the Matrix Model,[1] which is specially designed to be used with stimulant addicts, are among the additional approaches used by drug court providers. Relapse prevention modalities systematically teach clients to cope with their cravings and develop refusal and assertiveness skills, coping and problem-solving skills, and strategies to prevent relapse (Marlatt and Gordon 1985). Relaxation strategies such as acupuncture are also used. Finally, to ensure that clients are prepared for long-term recovery, drug courts provide spiritually oriented programs, continuing care/aftercare, and alumni groups.

Addressing Child Protective Cases in Drug Court

An increasing number of households have children present where methamphetamine is used or manufactured. As a consequence, an increasing number of children are considered "drug endangered" because their exposure to methamphetamine puts them at risk of long-term physical and mental damage. In addition, children who are not exposed to a lab but are being raised by methamphetamine-using parents often suffer abuse and neglect. Methamphetamine users, while high, do not sleep for days. Once they stop use and crash, they may sleep for days at a time. During this time, their children are uncared for and unsupervised—often unfed, unbathed, and poorly clothed. Because of the paranoia and violent tendencies that accompany parents' methamphetamine use, children in the home are often irrationally and brutally punished. At a critical time in their development, these children suffer gross abuse and neglect.

In addition, methamphetamine-involved parents frequently exploit gaps in communication between the courts and treatment, child welfare, law enforcement, and other service agencies to better insulate themselves from intervention. Their erratic behavior and elusive lifestyle often make them difficult to find by authorities and have kept systems from being able to provide help.

Family drug courts—also known as family dependency treatment courts—have emerged in response to both the large number of children who are abused or neglected by methamphetamine-using parents and the court's responsibility to enforce intervention in noncriminal family cases. Family drug courts consider children's safety and permanency in addition to the parents' addiction through a collaborative multidisciplinary team approach.

By jointly staffing child protective cases, the discrete disciplines of the family drug court team develop a full understanding of a family's history and dynamics and work together toward the best interest of the child, parent, and extended family. Treatment providers are better informed from the beginning and can make a more accurate and realistic assessment of the parents' needs, taking into consideration community and family resources, strengths, and weaknesses. In a number of communities, the family drug court specializes in the treatment of methamphetamine-addicted women and provides specialized services for co-occurring disorders, trauma-oriented interventions, and parenting skills. The court recognizes the initial limitations of parents and the time they need to regain cognitive functioning before they are ready for an initial visitation with their children and full implementation of their service plans. Parental accountability at all levels is enforced by the court's intensive supervision. Caseworkers who visit the home on a regular basis are trained to recognize the paraphernalia and characteristics of methamphetamine use. As in adult drug courts, participants in family drug courts are required to take random and frequent drug tests and appear weekly before a judge.

In many cases, addicted parents achieve sobriety and are able to provide a safe and fit home for their children. As a result, parents and children are reunited in a timely manner that promotes family healing and stability.

Whether children reside in a home where methamphetamine is cooked or in a home where their caretakers use this deadly drug, children are exposed to toxins and face numerous medical problems, developmental delays, and brain damage. The coordination between law enforcement, child welfare, and medical providers addresses the immediate safety needs for the child, but the long-term safety and permanency needs require ongoing and extensive collaboration. Family dependency treatment courts provide the necessary array of services that support the child's connection to family and provide the parental treatment needs while working toward safe and timely permanence.

—*Rebecca Kessel, Social Work Program director, Buncombe County, North Carolina*

RESEARCH IN ACTION

Below are exemplary drug court practices that effectively address the methamphetamine user.

Butte County, California, Drug Court Program

The Butte County Drug Court is an adult criminal drug court that began operation in June 1995 with support and funding from the U.S. Department of Justice. Methamphetamine has been the drug of choice in Butte County for nearly 30 years. In 2003, 7,072 criminal cases were filed in Butte County that resulted in approximately 1,800 felony probation cases. Of those felony cases, more than 60 percent are methamphetamine involved. Currently, 87 percent of the drug court clients are methamphetamine users. The Butte County Drug Court Program includes frequent and random drug testing, assertive community supervision, and intensive case management. Communication with treatment and the court team is virtually seamless and is conducted in an immediate fashion, or in real time. Response to client behavior is always therapeutic, evidence based, and applied in a manner consistent with the research on behavior modification techniques. This level of accountability is an excellent strategy for addressing methamphetamine addicts. The court and treatment services are structured to maximize motivation and meet the challenges unique to methamphetamine addicts in early recovery. Approximately 500 participants have graduated from the Butte County Drug Court over the past nine years, with an aggregate reconviction rate for any misdemeanor or felony of 14.9 percent.

Orange County, California, Superior Court Drug Court Program

The Orange County Superior Court Drug Court Program began in March 1995 with support and funding from the U.S. Department of Justice in response to a major methamphetamine-involved criminal justice population. Of approximately 11,500 new probation cases each year, 60 percent test positive for methamphetamine. Composed of five drug courts that operate throughout Orange County, the program serves 500 participants each year, of which 73 percent are methamphetamine involved. Additionally, of the new drug court admissions each year, 62 percent are unemployed and 38 percent do not have a high school diploma or GED.

The Orange County Drug Court approach is to place the participants on formal probation and require them to complete a minimum 18-month treatment program. Substance abuse treatment is provided by the Orange County Health Care Agency. The assigned probation officer and health-care therapist form a treatment team and collaboratively provide case management services. The supervision of the participant requires regular reporting to the probation officer, announced and unannounced visits to the participant's home, random searches, and frequent drug testing. Probation also plays a role in keeping the participant engaged in the treatment program. The sheriff's department helps supervise and monitor participants in the southern region of the county.

To successfully complete the program, graduates must test drug free for at least 180 consecutive days, achieve and maintain a stable living arrangement, and achieve gainful, consistent employment or be significantly involved in a vocational or academic program. More than 1,000 offenders have successfully graduated in the past nine years of operation. The drug court has a 72 percent retention rate; 80 percent of the graduates have no rearrest for a drug-related crime and 74 percent have no rearrests at all.

Salt Lake County, Utah, Felony Drug Court Program

The Salt Lake County Felony Drug Court was first planned in 1995 and implemented in 1996 with support and funding from the U.S. Department of Justice. With additional funding from the Substance Abuse and Mental Health Services Administration and local resources, the court serves up to 1,000 active participants at any given time, with the majority of the cases being methamphetamine-related offenses. In fact, 81 percent of drug court participants report methamphetamine as their primary or secondary drug of choice. The drug court seeks to reduce methamphetamine-related crime in Salt Lake County, where approximately 25 percent of the 12,395 cases filed were methamphetamine involved.

The Salt Lake County Drug Court serves both men and women and offers a full spectrum of evidence-based treatment and mental health services.

Supervision and service coordination are provided by specialized case managers. Treatment requirements are intensive, averaging three days per week per client. Participants are afforded other services throughout the program such as anger management and educational and vocational services. Participants are drug tested an average of three times per week and are afforded aftercare and alumni support and assistance upon graduation. In a recent outcome study, only 15.4 percent of graduates were arrested on new drug charges, compared with 64 percent of eligible defendants who did not attend drug court. In addition, 39.3 percent of participants who did not graduate were arrested on new drug-related charges.

Thurston County, Washington, Family Treatment Court

The Thurston County Family Treatment Court Program began operation in March 2000 with the dual aim of treating addicted parents and protecting their children from child abuse and neglect. The program has since received funding from the U.S. Department of Justice and the Washington Governor's Methamphetamine Initiative to address methamphetamine-using participants. Methamphetamine remains the primary drug driving child welfare cases throughout Thurston County. In 2004, 168 cases were filed by the Department of Child and Family services; of those, 70 percent were methamphetamine involved.

The Thurston County Family Treatment Court is specifically designed to reunite families in which methamphetamine abuse resulted in children being placed in foster care. The program provides a strength-based, supportive, yet highly accountable environment to the families served. This is accomplished by weekly court appearances with the family treatment court team, which includes the case manager, treatment provider, mental health therapist, Citizens Against Substance Abuse child representative, defense attorney, assistant attorney general, and a volunteer parenting mentor.

Through frequent drug testing and other accountability measures coupled with community support group meetings, methamphetamine-specific substance abuse and mental health treatment services, and regular court status hearings, participants are ensured the help they need to successfully address their methamphetamine addiction and other co-occurring problems. If a participant is noncompliant, the court immediately responds with treatment services, case management intensification, adjustment to the frequency and level of monitoring during child visitations, suspension from the program, or, as a last resort, termination. To successfully complete the program, participants must complete all treatment requirements, abstain from drugs and alcohol, attain stable housing, consistently illustrate that they can provide a safe, drug-free environment for their child, and be enrolled in vocational or educational programming. From March 2000 to October 2003, the Thurston County Family Treatment Court served 54 adults and 82 children. Of the 82 children, 75 percent have been placed with the birth family or are pending return from foster care to the birth family. Of children who could not be returned to the birth family, 14 percent have been adopted by relatives or foster parents. All of the pregnant women participants have graduated and delivered a total of 13 drug-free babies.

RECOMMENDATIONS

Policy Recommendations for Drug Courts Planning to Target a Methamphetamine-Using Population

To ensure public safety, behavioral accountability, better treatment outcomes, and the overall success of their operations, drug courts that are planning to expand their target population to include methamphetamine users should consider the following recommendations:

1. Drug courts should expand community supervision strategies to include random and unannounced home visits and drug testing. They should also involve probation and law enforcement officers who are highly trained in detecting methamphetamine laboratories and use.

2. Drug courts should increase contact with a methamphetamine-using population by increasing drug court status hearings for the first 90 days of the program. They should implement contingency management strategies coupled with vouchers and other positive reinforcements for short-term achievements and provide the necessary repetitive reinforcements of target behaviors and requirements.

3. Drug courts should ensure that treatment services are longer, evidence based, and relevant to their methamphetamine-using population. They should offer stimulant abuse–specific strategies and use cognitive-behavioral treatment modalities; afford total service coordination and comprehensive case management coupled with simultaneous treatment for co-occurring mental health disorders; provide physical health, comprehensive relapse prevention, community reinforcement, and continuing care and aftercare services before discharge; and maintain monthly telephone contact and provide ongoing alumni with support meetings after discharge.

Recommendations for Policymakers

1. Communities facing an increase in methamphetamine use should mobilize quickly and develop a plan that encompasses the law enforcement, legal, judicial, healthcare, environmental, and retail communities. The establishment of state and local task forces will ensure cross-education and a coordinated strategy for stemming the spread of methamphetamine. Adult and family drug courts should be a key component of any community's response to methamphetamine.

2. Those who use and manufacture methamphetamine put themselves, their neighbors, their family, and especially their children in grave danger. Strategies should be put in place that address the risk at each level and provide education and services to all who may be in danger. This includes educating neighbors, local businesspeople, and other community members on how to detect the signs of methamphetamine manufacturing; what to do with that information; how to detect the signs of methamphetamine abuse; and where to find treatment.

CONCLUSION

Methamphetamine production and use continue to rise and move eastward across the United States, wreaking havoc on communities. Research shows that sustained abstinence from drugs is associated with a 40 to 75 percent reduction in crime (Harrell and Roman 2001). Although drug courts are not the only solution, they are the most effective tool available to restore communities, reduce recidivism, reunite families, and promote abstinence from methamphetamine. Drug courts are successful at sustaining abstinence with methamphetamine-involved offenders because of their added accountability, service coordination, and the precise milieu for evidence-based treatment to be practiced. Drug courts provide the means for a number of systems to work together with a community to ensure public safety, effectively treat methamphetamine addicts, and restore hope to families ravaged by this destructive drug.

NOTE

1. The Matrix Model combines techniques and materials from the cognitive-behavioral therapy literature; it includes information about stimulants' effects, family education, 12-step program participation, and positive reinforcement for behavior change and treatment compliance. The 16-week intensive treatment protocol is available in a detailed treatment manual.

In an eight-site UCLA study of methamphetamine treatment, seven sites were voluntary participants and one site was a drug court. At each site, 75 patients received treatment as usual and 75 patients received treatment with the Matrix Model. In the seven voluntary sites, people treated with Matrix did better than those who received treatment as usual (Rawson and Marinelli-Casey et al. 2004).

In the overall sample and the majority of sites, Matrix participants attended more clinical sessions, stayed in treatment longer, had more methamphetamine-free urine samples while in treatment, and had longer periods of abstinence from methamphetamine use than those who were in the treatment-as-usual group.

However, the study showed that the drug court effects overwhelmed even the Matrix treatment effect. There was little question that the patients treated in the drug court program did better in treatment than non-drug-court patients.

CHAPTER 15

A Creative Partnership among Multiple Systems: The El Paso County, Colorado, Family Treatment Drug Court

Shirley Rhodus, MSW and Julia Roguski, MA

BACKGROUND

In 1994, Colorado implemented the Expedited Permanency Planning (EPP) statute, which requires the state to implement in all counties over a 10-year period expedited permanency for children under the age of six who were removed from parental custody. El Paso County was the third county in Colorado to implement EPP, in early 1996.

Over the course of the next few years, data were tracked to determine what kinds of problems were presenting in these families, and what case outcomes were occurring. It soon became apparent that a major presenting problem causing departmental intervention and removal of children from parental custody was substance abuse by their parents. Although permanency for these young children was being achieved within 12 months of their removal from their parents, as required by the law, only one-third of the children were being reunited with their parent(s) when substance abuse was the presenting problem.

As a result of these dismal reunification outcomes, and after learning about the successes of the San Diego, CA, drug court, the El Paso County Department of Human Services pursued alternative programs to improve its reunification outcomes. It approached Savio House, a private, not-for-profit agency in Denver, CO, which had launched a successful family reunification program for substance-involved families with the Denver County Department of Social Services. A local community collaboration was launched to initiate a drug court in El Paso County. After many months, the efforts were aborted when the department was unable to fund the necessary program components.

However, because of the fragmented response to these cases by all the systems involved, and continued poor reunification outcomes, the department decided to fund Savio House's family preservation program to prevent children of substance-abusing parents from entering out-of-home placement at all. Partners were identified that were necessary to make the joint service management concept work: child welfare, which dedicated one child protective services supervisor and two casework positions, as well as management oversight to the program; Savio House, which dedicated intensive in-home family preservation program staff; Connect Care, the administrative services organization responsible for the management of the substance abuse treatment dollars, and which committed a half-time case manager position and preferred treatment clinicians; and Temporary Assistance for Needy Families (TANF), which funded and transferred an eligibility technician into an entry-level casework position converted by child welfare to target the self-sufficiency needs of the families served.

On September 4, 2001, Savio Direct Link was initiated in El Paso County with no new funding streams. It was determined that these children and families were already being served by the various systems, and by redeploying existing resources into a dedicated joint service management (JSM) team, these families could be served in a different way to achieve better outcomes. JSM partners are jointly responsible for program design and development, continuous quality improvement, case and program outcomes, and collection and reporting of data.

It did not take long for the juvenile court to take notice that the department was no longer asking for custody of these children, but serving them in their own homes or with extended family. After many months of hard work and negotiation, in which systemic problems were addressed head on and trust and cooperation within the treatment team were developed, the juvenile court became the fifth JSM partner. A juvenile court magistrate was assigned to the project with dedicated docket time, attorneys were dedicated to represent the department and the parents, and a guardian ad litem was dedicated to represent the best interests of the children. The Family Treatment Drug Court was launched July 1, 2002.

Meanwhile, the impact of meth within El Paso County was starting to be felt. As children were being taken into custody when meth labs were busted by law enforcement, and as more and more parents were found to be using meth, the JSM partners began taking notice. Although parents were poly-substance abusers, meth more and more became the drug of choice. As parents were being arrested, more children went into kinship care. As family members were being identified, more of them were found to be abusing substances, especially meth. Treatment approaches and parents and caretakers to be served had to be individually identified.

The entrance criteria for Direct Link has remained mostly constant since the program was implemented. Families must be identified and referred by the Child Welfare Intake Division of the department; substance abuse is a primary concern for the child welfare involvement; there is at least one child under the age of 12; there is at least one parent who is willing to participate; and the child(ren) would have been placed in foster care were it not for this intervention. The latter criterion is especially important and is that for which gatekeeping is maintained, because it is foster care dollars that are redirected to pay for the intensive in-home services. Savio Direct Link does serve a small number of families on a voluntary, no-court-involvement basis, but if there is court involvement, the family must be willing to enter the Family Treatment Drug Court.

FAMILY TREATMENT DRUG COURT

Openings f or Savio Direct Link are posted and updated regularly so intake workers know when they can refer families. Families are referred by an intake worker by checking in with one of two gatekeepers: an intake supervisor, who serves on the Quality Improvement Team, or the ongoing supervisor, who manages the Direct Link unit in the department. Then the family is referred to Savio Direct Link, and intensive in-home services begin immediately. Before the initial 72-hour court hearing, called a preliminary protective proceeding (PPP), the county attorney flags the cases that allege parental substance abuse in the dependency and neglect (D and N) petition grounds. Respondent counsel who work in the Family Treatment Drug Court are appointed for the parent(s) at the filing of the D and N. At the PPP, the Family Treatment Drug Court waiver is provided to the family and the pre-trial conference is set within one to two weeks in front of the magistrate who presides over the drug court. At the pretrial conference, the parents either agree to sign a waiver and enter the Family Treatment Drug Court or they return to the regular docket of a different juvenile court magistrate or judge and their children are placed in foster care, as their safety cannot be managed at home without the intensive in-home services of Savio and the oversight of the Family Treatment Drug Court. The Family Treatment Drug Court does not bifurcate the case; the magistrate hears the dependency and neglect peti-tion issues in addition to overseeing the parent's participation and progress in the drug court.

The Family Treatment Drug Court's outcomes were positive and reversed the department's previous outcomes, so that two-thirds of the children remained with parents or reunified with their parents if placement with kin was necessary at the end of the program. However, as there was only capacity to serve 30 families at a time within the program, other children continued entering foster care, and they didn't return home. Anecdotally, child welfare staff was saying that parental use of meth was causing the children to go into care and not home. Terminations of parental rights and adoptions were con-tinuing at a higher rate than wanted by the department.

As a result, a survey of all the termination hearings in 2003 was reviewed in 2004 by department managers in order to determine the primary causes of all of these terminations. It was determined that the primary reason these children were removed from their parents by more than a two to one ratio from the next most prevalent problem was parental substance abuse, the primary drug of choice by far was meth, and the primary reason for the termination of parental rights was a failed substance abuse treatment plan/continued substance abuse. Despite a budget shortfall, a decision was made to increase the capacity of the Direct Link program to 45 families at a time, as good outcomes for families are also more cost efficient for the department.

TREATMENT PHILOSOPHY

There are four phases of treatment in the Family Treatment Drug Court: orientation, achieving sobriety, treatment, and aftercare planning/treatment completion. The four phases were designed to flow with the treatment process for clients, they are behaviorally anchored to make advancement and regression consistent, and all phases are tied into the treatment model.

Orientation Phase: Lasts two to four weeks. Participants are required to:

- Sign the Family Treatment Drug Court waiver;
- Begin providing three poly-substance drug screens per week;
- Have received a copy of the sanctions and rewards sheets;
- Have provided information regarding family/kin;
- Have given their phone numbers to their treatment team;
- Have begun parenting enhancement training;
- Have signed and are following the safety plan;
- Have attended court; and
- Meet with the Savio intensive in-home worker for the required time each week.

Achieving Sobriety Phase: Lasts a minimum of 30 days. Participants are required to:

- Complete the 14–30 day drug-screening assessment (3 times per week);
- Demonstrate 30 consecutive days of:
  - attendance at court
  - clean drug screens
  - attendance at treatment support meetings (defined later in the chapter)
  - meeting with the Savio worker for the required time each week.
- Attend substance abuse treatment intake and start attending recommended treatment;
- Have a treatment plan that has been developed and adopted by the court (dispositional hearing);
- Complete the Colorado Assessment Continuum (CAC);

- Attend and participate in a family group conference and/or a team decision-making (TDM) meetings; and

- Have signed and follow an individual responsibility contract (IRC) if they are TANF recipients.

Treatment Phase: Lasts four to six months. Participants are required to:

- Demonstrate 90 consecutive days of:

  - attendance at court
  - clean drug screens
  - attendance at treatment support meetings
  - meeting with the Savio worker for the required time each week
  - compliance with visitation plan
  - if applicable, following the TANF Individual Responsibility Plan (IRC)

- Have attended 120 consecutive days of attendance at treatment;

- Have completed 10 of 12 parenting enhancement training programs;

- Have attended and participated in a family group conference and/or team decision-making meeting; and

- Have shown improvement on the Colorado Assessment Continuum.

Aftercare Planning and Treatment Completion: Lasts a minimum of 30 days. Participants are required to:

- Demonstrate 30 consecutive days of:

  - attendance at court
  - clean drug screens
  - attendance at treatment support meetings (defined later in the chapter)
  - Meeting with the Savio worker for the required time each week

- Have successfully completed the court-ordered treatment plan;
- Have presented a relapse prevention and aftercare plan to and have accepted by the treatment team;

- Demonstrate an ability to be self-sufficient; and,

- Demonstrate improvement on the Colorado Assessment Continuum and an elimination of safety concerns.

Participants advance to the next phase when they have completed all the requirements for their current phase. Participants regress to the previous phase when they receive three sanctions in a 60-day period. Participants do not regress more than one phase at a time, and they will never be regressed to the orientation phase. The furthest they can regress to is the achieving sobriety phase.

Participants receive sanctions and rewards for compliance with the Family Treatment Drug Court requirements. Each time a participant receives a sanction there is also a treatment response. All sanctionable behaviors are outlined in the Family Treatment Drug Court waiver. By signing the waiver, participants give up their right to due process for those behaviors and the court can sanction them immediately and directly. Violations are cumulative throughout the treatment process, and participants are only sanctioned for the highest sanctionable offense each court hearing. The primary focus of the court is to support clients through their change process and ensure that they are held accountable for their behaviors and are receiving the most appropriate treatment package.

Sanctions occur on a graduated scale, and participants are given a lesser sanction for admitting they have a violation. Additionally, the court sanctions failure to attend treatment and failure to meet with their Savio worker with a jail consequence earlier than positive drug screens. The reasoning behind this policy is that the court recognizes that relapse and/or continued use early on in treatment is expected; however, what is most important is that the participant is attending and engaged in treatment and working with their intensive in-home worker. Failure to appear in court, unless presence is waived, will result in a bench warrant being issued.

Useful community service is used as a sanction before jail time. When participants are sentenced to useful community service, they are required to complete the hours prior to their next court date. Participants are given a list of agencies where they can complete their sentence, and they are also allowed to complete the hours at Savio. If the participant chooses not to complete their community service, they will serve the corresponding number of days in jail.

A goal of the Family Treatment Drug Court is to focus on treatment and recovery of the participants. The treatment team will acknowledge the process of treatment and recovery and will not sanction participants for reasonable and confirmable mitigating circumstance that caused them to have a violation. For example, if a parent was home with a sick child and misses treatment, they will not receive a sanction.

Rewards are also an important type of support the treatment team provides participants. When the rewards system was developed, the treatment team agreed that material/financial rewards are motivating to participants but they should not be the only form of rewards offered. One of the goals of Family Treatment Drug Court is to build the self-esteem of each participant in an effort to increase their likelihood of long-term success. Some rewards are specifically designed to boost participants' self-image and ultimately help them to internalize positive self-talk. For example, as previously noted, even when being sanctioned, participants are commended for what they have done right that week, remembering that no one person has done *everything* wrong. There is a lot of clapping and acknowledgement by the entire treatment team and courtroom for each milestone and accomplishment. This promotes an atmosphere of support, all the while holding participants accountable for their negative actions. Participants receive a certificate of accomplishment signed by each member of the treatment team when they complete a phase. When participants have achieved their first 30 days of sobriety, they receive a flower from the judge. When participants have achieved 90 days of sobriety, they

Table 15.1
Sanctions and Rewards Tables

First Violation	
Positive drug or alcohol screen—admit use prior to result	1 hour community service (CS) or 24 hrs jail
Positive drug or alcohol screen—admit use after result	2 hrs CS or 24 hrs jail
Positive drug or alcohol screen—denial of use	3 hrs CS or 48 hrs jail
Missed or dilute drug or alcohol screen	3 hrs CS or 48 hrs jail
Failure to attend substance abuse treatment	4 hrs CS or 48 hrs jail
Failure to meet with Savio worker	4 hrs CS or 48 hrs jail
Second Violation	
Positive drug or alcohol screen—admit use prior to result	2 hrs CS or 24 hrs jail
Positive drug or alcohol screen—admit use after result	4 hrs CS or 48 hrs jail
Positive drug or alcohol screen—denial of use	6 hrs CS or 72 hrs jail
Missed or dilute drug or alcohol screen	6 hrs CS or 72 hrs jail
Failure to attend substance abuse treatment	Up to 10 days jail (normally starts at 72 hrs)
Failure to meet with Savio worker	Up to 10 days jail (normally starts at 72 hrs)
Third Violation	
Positive drug or alcohol screen—admit use prior to result	8 hrs CS or 48 hrs jail
Positive drug or alcohol screen—admit use after result	12 hrs CS or 72 hrs jail
Positive drug or alcohol screen—denial of use	Up to 10 days jail (normally starts at 72 hrs)
Missed or dilute drug or alcohol screen	Up to 10 days jail (normally starts at 72 hrs)
Failure to attend substance abuse treatment	Up to 10 days jail
Failure to meet with Savio worker	Up to 10 days jail
Subsequent Violations	
All violations	Up to 10 days jail

receive a gift certificate from the treatment team to take their family to dinner or to do some other pro-social, non-substance-involved activity as a family. Again, the emphasis is on recovery and support that will promote long-term success for the family.

TREATMENT SUPPORT MEETINGS

Each family involved with the Family Treatment Drug Court participates in treatment support meetings (similar to child welfare meetings) with the Department of Human Services' social caseworker and supervisor, Savio worker and supervisor, care coordinator (substance abuse treatment coordinator), TANF worker, treatment providers, and extended family and/or kin. During Phase 1 of the program, participants are required to attend treatment support meetings and court appearances weekly. During Phase 2 of the program, participants are required to have a minimum of two contacts per month with the treatment team (treatment support meetings and/or court). Additional treatment support meetings and court appearances are scheduled and required at the discretion of the family and treatment team. During Phase 3, participants are required to attend monthly treatment support meetings and monthly court appearances.

A team approach with mutual ownership works to establish the most efficient and cost-effective services for each family. An emphasis is placed on goal-directed case resolution in a time-limited manner. Staff, along with the family and other members of the treatment team, clearly define the changes necessary to protect the child, achieve and maintain sobriety, and bring case closure. Treatment support meetings focus on strengths and provide concrete plans to address any areas of concern. The treatment team has up-front discussions of time frames and concurrent planning. Families are made aware of legal time frames and are provided with support to successfully complete their treatment plan. Families create a treatment support work plan with the assistance of the treatment team. The work plan details the goals to be accomplished prior to the next treatment support meeting and/or court appearance, time lines for completion, objective steps to complete the goals, and identified strengths the family will use to be successful.

CHILD WELFARE ASSESSMENTS

The Colorado Assessment Continuum (CAC) is used to structure the ongoing evaluation of each case plan. This framework brings consistency and organization to the utilization process, and the assessment package is completed on each participating family. The CAC consists of three tools:

- Safety assessment and plan
- Risk assessment and re-assessment
- North Carolina Family Assessment Scale—Reunification (NCFAS-R)

The results of these assessments guide the treatment team in assessing child safety and risk factors as well as family strengths and needs. Safety concerns are addressed immediately with the family. The CAC is the foundation for the treatment plan and assists in determining when the family has made sufficient progress to be successfully discharged from the program. Results from the CAC are shared with the family and all involved professionals during monthly treatment support meetings and during scheduled team decision-making meetings.

Ongoing assessments by the Savio worker and Department of Human Services social caseworkers occur in the areas of child protection, substance abuse treatment progress, monitoring and supervision, household structure, consistency of delivering consequences and rewards, appropriate housing and cleanliness, ability of parents to meet their children's basic needs, and adequate food, clothing, and shelter. The workers also appraise parenting skills and evidence of age-appropriate child development and establish goals based on observations and assessments. Clients are involved in the assessment process by identifying family strengths and areas in which they need assistance during involvement with the program.

PARENTING SKILLS DEVELOPMENT

The Family Treatment Drug Court offers parenting skills' development in two forms: group and in-home. Both the group and in-home instruction focus on the specific issue of a parent in substance abuse recovery. Each session targets struggles unique to this population, offering parents specialized-skills development and an opportunity to fully explore the challenges they face as a parent recovering from a substance abuse problem. The group is designed to address general parenting skills such as child development, stress management, discipline, and education. The in-home instruction targets the specific areas in which the individual parent needs skill development. Any adult in a parenting role is welcome to attend parenting skills development training. Each parent is required to complete both sections.

- **Parenting Skills Development Group**—A 12-week curriculum that focuses on general parenting skills and offers families the support of a group. Children attend a social skills development group that mirrors the parenting group. This is a curriculum written by Savio staff with the input of parents. Groups are held in the evening hours, and a family-style dinner is provided. This gives parents an opportunity to mingle and give as well as receive support. Transportation and childcare are provided.

- **In-Home Instruction**—Savio staff provides hands-on parenting skills development training to parents from the date of entry. A particular emphasis is placed on household structure, monitoring and supervision, consistency of follow-through of the parent, and child safety. Parents are encouraged to try new parenting techniques and to be creative. Staff offer regular feedback and support. Extended family is included in the training as necessary and for ongoing monitoring. Throughout this learning process, the family and the Savio worker develop an individualized parenting resource manual. As topics are discussed and structure is implemented, the specific plans and information are added to the parenting resource manual. This provides the parents with a concrete reference during and after their involvement with Family Treatment Drug Court.

FAMILY TREATMENT DRUG COURT OUTCOMES

The Family Treatment Drug Court established several outcome measures at the inception of the program. Annually, the outcomes are compiled and the Quality Assurance Committee reviews the outcomes and determines where the program was successful, and if there is an area in which the program was not successful, programmatic changes are implemented to improve service delivery for the upcoming year.

In 2004, 71 families composed of 110 adults and 142 children were served. Twenty-eight of the families composed of 45 adults and 53 children were discharged. The average length of stay for the discharged families was 11.26 months. Of the discharged children, 74 percent were at home, 23 percent in kinship, and 3 percent in joint custody. Two percent were adopted by nonrelatives.

FUNDING ISSUES

These are fiscally challenging times. Agencies must identify programs that have good outcomes for families and be creative and resourceful in funding them. Savio Direct Link prevents children from entering foster care. Direct Link is funded per family and is time limited. Foster care is funded per child and can lead to adoption, which is subsidized for years. These families must be served anyway in our child welfare systems, and substance-abusing parents must be given reasonable efforts for recovery. By redeploying staff and treatment resources to a home-based, placement-prevention program, and by developing collaborative partnerships with equal investment, child welfare agencies can successfully preserve and reunite these families.

CONCLUSION

The message in the outcomes is that this population, including participants who are using meth, is treatable and can safely parent their children when they complete their treatment program. The magic of the program includes the tight treatment team that works together and has developed a strong level of trust resulting in the ability to manage risk and safety factors with the family. Additionally, as with all drug courts, the relationship between the participants and the judicial officer is vital. The participants are in court regularly, every week for a long period of time at the beginning of the process. This regular contact with the judge and the treatment team as a whole develops a strong net around the client and can help to reduce and eliminate some of the drug behaviors. Participants are held accountable immediately for failure to comply with the court orders. This immediate response is essential to their recovery process. Likewise, participants are also supported for their successes immediately. Coming from a strengths-based orientation, even when being sanctioned, participants are also recognized for what they have done right that week, even if it is as small as showing up to court. The goal is to hold them accountable, but even more importantly, to support their recovery process.

For additional resources on drug courts, the following Web sites have drug court information: The National Drug Court Institute: www.ndci.org/; Substance Abuse and Mental Health Association (SAMHSA): www.samhsa.gov; Bureau of Justice Assistance and Office of Justice Programs Drug Courts Program Office: www.ojp.usdoj.gov; and National Council of Juvenile and Family Court Judges: www.ncjfcj.org.

Bibliography

Allcott, J. V., III, Barnhart, R. A., and Mooney, L. A. 1987. Acute lead poisoning in two users of illicit methamphetamine. *JAMA* 258: 510–511.

Amen, D. G. 2004. *Images into Human Behavior: A Brain SPECT Atlas.* Newport, CA: Mind Works Press.

American Academy of Pediatrics, Committee on Drugs. 2001. The transfer of drugs and other chemicals into human milk. *Pediatrics* 108 (3): 776–789.

American Dental Association. 2005. Dental topics A to Z: Methamphetamine use. Updated August 9, 2005. Accessed on line at: www.ada.org/prof/resources/topics/methmouth.asp.

Anglin, M. D., Burke, C., Perrochet, B., Stamper, E., and Dawud-Noursi, S. 2000. History of the methamphetamine problem. *Journal of Psychoactive Drugs* 32: 137–141.

Anglin, M. D., Kalechstein, A., Maglione, M., Annon, J., and Fiorentine, R. 1997. *Epidemiology and Treatment of Methamphetamine Abuse in California: A Regional Report.* Unpublished manuscript, Los Angeles, CA: UCLA, Drug Abuse Research Center.

Anglin, M. D., and Rawson, R. A. 2000. The CSAT Methamphetamine Treatment Project: What are we trying to accomplish? *Journal of Psychoactive Drugs* 32: 209–210.

Baumeister, A. A. 2000. The Tulane electrical brain stimulation program: A historical case study in medical ethics. *Journal of the History of the Neurosciences* 9: 262–279.

Beebe, D. K, and Walley, E. 1995. Smokable methamphetamine ("ice"): An old drug in a different form. *American Family Physician* 51 (2): 449–453.

Belenko, S. R. 1998. Research on drug courts: A critical review. *National Drug Court Institute Review* 1 (1): 1–42.

Belenko, S. R. 2001. Research on drug courts: A critical review 2001 update. *National Drug Court Institute Review,* 3: 117–126.

Blume, S. B., and Zilberman, M. L. 2005. Addictive disorders in women. In Frances, R. J., Miller, S. I., and Mack, A. H. (Eds.), *Clinical Textbook of Addictive Disorders* (3rd ed.) (pp. 437–453). New York: The Guilford Press.

Bond, G. R., Williams, J., Evans, L., Salyers, M., Kim, H. W., Sharpe, H., and Leff, H. S. 2000. *Psychiatric Rehabilitation Fidelity Toolkit.* Cambridge, MA: Human Services Research Institute.

Bonhomme, N., Cador, M., Stinus, L., Le Moal, M., and Spampinato, U. 1995. Short and long-term changes in dopamine and serotonin receptor binding sites in amphetamine-sensitized rats: A quantitative autoradiographic study. *Brain Research* 675: 215–223.

Bonné, J. 2001. Meth's deadly buzz. *MSNBC.COM Special Report.* Accessed on line at: msnbc. msncom/id/3071772.

Bonné, J. 2001a. Meth's deadly buzz: Lab-busting in the Northwest. *MSNBC.COM Special Report.* Accessed on line at: msnbc.msn.com/id/3071775.

Bonné, J. 2004. Hooked in the Haight: Life, death or prison. *MSNBC Interactive.* Accessed on line at: msnbc. msn. com/id/3071769.

Brecht, M-L. 2001. *Update on Methamphetamine Use Trends in California.* Unpublished report. Los Angeles: UCLA Integrated Substance Abuse Program.

Brecht, M. L., Anglin, M. D., and Dylan, M. 2005. Coerced treatment for methamphetamine abuse: Differential patient characteristics and outcomes. *American Journal of Drug and Alcohol Abuse* 31: 337–356.

Brecht, M-L., O'Brien, A., Mayrhauser, C., and Anglin, M. D. 2004. Methamphetamine use behaviors and gender differences. *Addictive Behaviors* 29: 89–106.

Brittain, C., and Hunt, D. E. 2004. *Helping in Child Protective Services* (2nd ed.). New York: Oxford University Press.

Brown, J. M., Hanson, G. R., and Fleckenstein, A. E. 2000. Methamphetamine rapidly decreases vesicular dopamine uptake. *Journal of Neurochemistry* 74 (5): 2221–2223.

Budney, A. J., and Higgins, S. T. 1998. A community reinforcement plus vouchers approach: Treating cocaine addiction. *Therapy Manuals for Drug Addiction.* (NIH Publication No. 98-4309). Rockville, MD: National Institute on Drug Abuse.

Burton, B. T. 1991. Heavy metal and organic contaminants associated with illicit methamphetamine production. In Miller, M. A., and Kozel, N. J. (Eds.), *Methamphetamine Abuse: Epidemiologic Issues and Implications* (pp. 47–59). NIDA Research Monograph Series, Number 115. DHHS Pub. No. (ADM) 91-1836. Rockville, MD: National Institute on Drug Abuse.

Center for Substance Abuse Prevention/National Prevention Network. 2006. *Methamphetamine: A Resource Kit.* Rockville, MD: Substance Abuse and Mental Health Services Administration.

Center for Substance Abuse Research. 2004. *Workplace Drug Tests Patterns Changing.* College Park, MD: University of Maryland. Accessed on line at: www.cesar. umd.edu/cesar/cesarfax/vol13/13-41.pdf

Center for Substance Abuse Treatment. 1997. *Proceedings of the National Consensus Meeting on the Use, Abuse, and Sequelae of Abuse of Methamphetamine with Implications for Prevention, Treatment, and Research.* DHHS Pub. No. (SMA) 96-8013. Rockville, MD: Substance Abuse and Mental Health Services Administration.

Center for Substance Abuse Treatment. 1998. *TIP 27: Comprehensive Case Management for Substance Abuse Treatment (TIP Series No. 27).* Rockville, MD: Substance Abuse and Mental Health Administration.

Center for Substance Abuse Treatment. 1999. *Tip 33: Treatment for Stimulant Use Disorders: Treatment Improvement Protocol (TIP Series No. 33)*. Rockville, MD: Substance Abuse and Mental Health Services Administration.

Centers for Disease Control. 2000. Public health consequences among first responders to emergency events associated with illicit methamphetamine laboratories—selected states 1996–1999. *MMWR Weekly*, 49: 1021–1024.

Centers for Disease Control. 2005. Acute public health consequences of methamphetamine laboratories—16 states, January 2000–June 2004. *MMWR Weekly* 54: 356–359.

Centers for Disease Control. 2005a. *Morbidity and Mortality Weekly Report*. 54 (25). Accessed on line at: www.cdc.gov/tobacco/research_data/economics/mm5425_intro.htm.

Cernerud, L., Eriksson, M., Jonsson, B., Steneroth, G., and Zetterstrom, R. 1996. Amphetamine addiction during pregnancy: 14-year follow-up of growth and school performance. *Acta Pediatrica* 85: 204–208.

Cho, A. K. 1990. Ice: A new dosage form of an old drug. *Science* 249: 631–634.

Colorado Department of Public Health and Environment. 2003. *Cleanup of Clandestine Methamphetamine Labs Guidance Document*. Colorado Department of Public Health and Environment. Hazardous Materials and Waste Management Division. July 2003. Accessed on line at: www.cdphe. state.co.us/hm/methlab.pdf.

Colorado Department of Public Health and Environment. 2005. *Support for Selection of a Cleanup Level for Methamphetamine at Clandestine Drug Laboratories*. Denver, CO: Colorado Department of Public Health and Environment. Accessed on line at: www.cdphe.state.co.us/hm/methlabcleanuplevelsupport.pdf

Colorado Regional Community Policing Institute and Rocky Mountain High-Intensity Drug Trafficking Area. 2003. *Methamphetamine Drug Lab Hazards*. Golden, CO: Colorado Department of Public Safety.

Crawford, C. A., Williams, M. T., Newman, E. R., McDougall, S. A., and Vorhees, C. V. 2003. Methamphetamine exposure during the preweaning period causes prolonged changes in dorsal striatal protein kinase A activity, dopamine Ds-like binding sites, and dopamine content. *Synapse* 48: 131–137.

CSAlert 2004. New trend in ammonia method emerges. *CSAlert* 1: 1,3.

CSAlert 2005. Urine extraction labs. *CSAlert* 2: 1,6.

Davis, W. T., Campbell, L., Tax, J., and Lieber, C. S. 2002. A trial of 'standard' outpatient alcoholism treatment vs. a minimal treatment control. *Journal of Substance Abuse Treatment* 23: 9–19.

Deci, E. L., Koestner, R., and Ryan, R. M.. 1999. A meta-analytic review of experiments examining the effects of extrinsic rewards on intrinsic motivation. *Psychological Bulletin* 125: 627–668.

Department of Justice. 2003. *Information Brief: Methamphetamine Production Methods*. Washington, DC: National Drug Intelligence Center.

Dickinson, J. E., Andres, R. L., and Parisi, V. M. 1994. The ovine fetal sympathoadrenal response to the maternal administration of methamphetamine. *American Journal of Obstetrics and Gynecology* 170: 1452–1457.

Dixon, S. D., and Bejar, R. 1989. Echoencephalographic findings in neonates associated with cocaine and methamphetamine use: Incidence and clinical correlates. *Journal of Pediatrics* 115: 770–778.

Drug Enforcement Administration (DEA). 2004. Drug trafficking in the United States. *DEA Briefs and Background*. Washington, DC: Drug Enforcement Administration. Accessed on line at: www.usdoj.gov/dea/concern/drug_trafficking.html.

Drug Enforcement Administration (DEA). 2004a. *Fact Sheet, U.S. Drug Enforcement Administration.* Washington, DC: Drug Enforcement Administration.

Drug Enforcement Administration (DEA). 2005. *Factsheet: Fast Facts about Meth.* Washington, DC: Drug Enforcement Administration. Accessed on line at: www.usdoj.gov/dea/pubs/pressrel/methfact03.html.

Drug Enforcement Administration (DEA). 2005a. What to do if you encounter a clandestine methamphetamine laboratory. Washington, DC: Drug Enforcement Administration. Accessed on line at: www.usdoj.gov/dea/concern/methlab_whattodo.html. Drug Enforcement Administration (DEA). 2006. *National Drug Assessment 2006.* Washington, DC: Drug Enforcement Administration.

Drug Policy Information Clearinghouse. 2003. Methamphetamine. *Fact Sheet.* Rockville, MD: Office of National Drug Control Policy.

Edwards, D. 2005. Fighting meth in America's heartland: Assessing the impact on law enforcement and child welfare agencies. Congressional testimony to the Subcommittee on Criminal Justice, Drug Policy and Human Resources, U.S. House of Representatives, July 26, 2005.

Edwards, E. M. 2005. CDC: Rising danger of meth labs. Join Together online, April, 18, 2005. Accessed on line at: www.jointogether.org/sa/news/summaries.

Eisley, M. 2004. New meth laws worsen penalties. *Raleigh News and Observer,* December 1, 2004.

Ellinwood, E. H., Jr., Sudilovsky, A., and Nelson, L. M. 1973. Evolving behavior in the clinical and experimental amphetamine (model) psychosis. *American Journal of Psychiatry* 130: 1088–1092.

Elliot, V. S. 2004. Methamphetamine use increasing: Public health officials voice concerns about infants born to addicted mothers. *American Medical News,* July 26, 2004.

El Paso Intelligence Center. 2003. *Children Involved in Methamphetamine Lab–Related Incidents in the United States.* June, 2003. El Paso, TX: El Paso Intelligence Center. Accessed on line at: www.usdoj.gov/programs/epic.htm.

Ericksson, M., Larsson, C., Windbladh, B., and Zetterstrom, R. 1978. The influence of amphetamine addiction on pregnancy and the newborn infant. *Acta Paediatrica Scandinavica* 67 (1): 95–99.

Eriksson, M., Larsson, G., and Zetterström, R. 1981. Amphetamine addiction and pregnancy. II. Pregnancy, delivery and the neonatal period: Socio-medical aspects. *Acta Obstetricia et Gynecologica Scandinavica* 60: 253–259.

Ernst, T., Chang, L., Leonido-Yee, M., and Speck, O. 2000. Evidence for long-term neurotoxicity associated with methamphetamine abuse: A 1H MRS study. *Neurology* 54: 1344–1349.

Erowid. 2006. Meth. Updated March 31, 2006. Accessed on line at: www.erowid.org.

Etten, M. L., Higgins, S. T., Budney, A. J., and Badger, G. J. 1998. Comparison of the frequency and enjoyability of pleasant events in cocaine abusers vs. non-abusers using a standardized behavioral inventory. *Addiction* 93: 1669–1681.

Freese, T. E., Obert, J. Dickow, A., Cohen, J., and Lord, R. H. 2000. Methamphetamine abuse: Issues for special populations. *Journal of Psychoactive Drugs* 32: 177–182.

Furst, S. R., Fallon, S. P, Reznik, G. N., and Shah, P. K. 1990. Myocardial infarction after inhalation of methamphetamine [Letter]. *New England Journal of Medicine* 49: 389–391.

Galloway, G. P., Marinelli-Casey, P., Stalcup, J., Lord, R. H., Christian, D., Cohen, J., Reiber, C., and Vandersloot, D. 2000. Treatment-as-usual in the Methamphetamine Treatment Project. *Journal of Psychoactive Drugs* 32: 165–175.

Gibson, D. R., Leamon, M. H., and Flynn, N. 2002. Epidemiology and public health consequences of methamphetamine use in California's central valley. *Journal of Psychoactive Drugs* 34: 313–319.

Goin, R. 2002. Personal correspondence with HAZWOPPER certification of clandestine methamphetamine laboratory investigations. Thornton, CO: North Metro Task Force.

Golbus, M. S. 1980. Teratology for the obstetrician: Current status. *Obstetrics and Gynecology* 55: 269–277.

Gold, M. S. 1997. Cocaine (and crack): Clinical aspects. In Lowenson, J. H., Ruiz, P., Millman, R. B., and Langrod, J. G. (Eds.), *Substance Abuse: A Comprehensive Textbook* (3rd ed.). Baltimore, MD: Williams and Wilkins.

Gospe, S. 1995. Transient cortical blindness in an infant exposed to methamphetamine. *Annals of Emergency Medicine* 26: 380–382.

Greenwell, L. and Brecht, M. L. 2003. Self-reported health status among treated methamphetamine users. *American Journal of Drug and Alcohol Abuse* 29 (1): 75–104.

Halkitis, P. N., and Martin, F. W. 2005. Sexual behavior patterns of methamphetamine using gay and bisexual men. *Substance Use and Misuse* 40: 703–719.

Hansen, R. L., Struthers, J. M., and Gospe, S. M., Jr. 1993. Visual evoked potentials and visual processing in stimulant drug-exposed infants. *Developmental Medicine and Child Neurology* 35: 798–805.

Harrell, A., and Roman, J. 2001. Reducing drug use and crime among offenders: The impact of graduated sanctions. *Journal of Drug Issues* 31: 207–232.

Heath, R. G. 1963. Electrical self-stimulation of the brain in man. *American Journal of Psychiatry* 120: 571–577.

Heath, R. G. 1972. Pleasure and brain activity in man: Deep and surface electroencephalograms during orgasm. *Journal of Nervous and Mental Disease* 154: 3–18.

Heath, R. G., and Mickle, W. A. 1960. Evaluation of seven years' experience with depth electrode studies in human patients. In Ramey, E. R., and O'Doherty, D. S. (Eds.), *Electrical Studies on the Unanesthetized Brain*. New York: Harper and Brothers.

Heller, A., Bubula, N., Lew, R., Heller, B., and Won, L. 2001. Gender-dependent enhanced adult neurotoxic response to methamphetamine following fetal exposure to the drug. *Journal of Pharmacology and Experimental Therapeutics* 298 (2): 769–779.

Herdy, A. 2002. Methamphetamine's Young Victims: Homes Doubling as Drug Labs Pose Serious Dangers to Kids. *Denver Post*, October 20, 2002.

Herrell, J. M., Taylor, J. A., Gallagher, C., and Dawud-Noursi, S. 2000. A multisite study of the effectiveness of methamphetamine treatment: An initiative of the Center for Substance Abuse Treatment. *Journal of Psychoactive Drugs* 32: 143–147.

Herz, D. C. 2000. *Drugs in the Heartland: Methamphetamine use in Rural Nebraska*. Washington, DC: National Institute of Justice.

Higgins, S. T., Sigmon, S. C., and Budney, A. J. 2002. Psychosocial treatment for cocaine dependence: The community reinforcement plus vouchers approach. In Hofmann, S. G., and Tompson, M. C. (Eds.), *Treating Chronic and Severe Mental Disorders: A Handbook of Empirically Supported Interventions*. New York: Guilford Press.

Hirshfield, S., Remien, R. H., Humberstone, M., Walavalkar, I., and Chiasson, M. A. 2004. Substance use and high-risk sex among men who have sex with men: a national online study in the USA. *AIDS Care* 16: 1036–1048.

Holthouse, D. and Rubin, P. 1997. Methodology—Part I, *New Times*, December 18, 1997. Accessed on line at: www.phoenixnewtimes.com/issues/1997-12-18/feature2.

Holthouse, D., and Rubin, P. 1997a. Methodology—Part II. *New Times*, December 12, 1997. Accessed on line at: www.phoenixnewtimes.com/issues/1997-12-18/feature4.

Hong, R., Matsuyama, E., and Nur, K. 1991. Cardiomyopathy associated with the smoking of crystal methamphetamine. *JAMA* 265 (9): 1152–1154.

Honolulu Advertiser. 2003. Indicators of a worsening problem in Hawai'i, *Honolulu Advertiser*, September 14, 2003. Accessed on line at: www.the.honoluluadvertiser.com/dailypix/2003/sep/14/icebox2. gif

Horton, D. K., Berkowitz, Z., and Kaye, W. E. 2003. The acute health consequences to children exposed to hazardous substances used in illicit methamphetamine production, 1996 to 2001. *Journal of Children's Health* 1: 99–108.

Hser, Y-I., Evans, E., and Huang, Y-C. 2005. Treatment outcomes among women and men methamphetamine abusers in California. *Journal of Substance Abuse Treatment* 28: 77–85.

Hubbard, R. L., Marsden, M. E., Rachal, J. V., Harwood, J. H., Cavanaugh, E. R., and Ginsburg, H. M. 1989. *Drug Abuse Treatment: A National Study of Effectiveness.* Chapel Hill, NC: University of North Carolina Press.

Huber, A., Ling, W., Shoptaw, S., Gulati, V., Brethen, P., and Rawson, R. A. 1997. Integrating treatments for methamphetamine abuse: A psychosocial perspective. *Journal of Addictive Diseases* 16: 41–50.

Huber, A., Lord, R. H., Gulati, V., Marinelli-Casey, P., Rawson, R. A., and Ling, W. 2000. The CSAT Methamphetamine Treatment Program: Research design accommodations for "real world" application. *Journal of Psychoactive Drugs* 32: 149–156.

Inaba, D., and Cohen, W. 1993. *Uppers, Downers, All Arounders* (2nd ed.). Ashland, OR: CNS Productions.

Irwin, K. 1995. Ideology, pregnancy and drugs: Differences between crack-cocaine, heroin and methamphetamine users. *Contemporary Drug Problems* 22: 613–638.

Jaffe, J. H. 1990. Drug addiction and drug abuse. In Gilman A.G., Rall, T. W., Nies, A. S., and Taylor, P. (Eds.), *Goodman and Gilman's The Pharmacological Basis of Therapeutics* (8th ed.) (pp. 539–545). New York: Pergamon.

Jaffe, J. H. 1995. Amphetamine (or amphetamine-like)-related disorders. In Kaplan, H. I., and Sadock B. J. (Eds.), *Comprehensive Textbook of Psychiatry* (6th ed.) (pp. 791–798). Baltimore, MD: Williams and Wilkins.

Joe, K. 1996. The lives and times of Asian-Pacific American women drug users: An ethnographic study of their methamphetamine use. *Journal of Drug Issues* 26 (1): 199–218.

Join Together. 2005. Gay community fights growing meth problem. April 5, 2005. Accessed on line at: www.jointogether.org.

Kamijo, Y., Soma, K., Nishida, M., Namera, A., and Ohwada, T. 2002. Acute liver failure following intravenous methamphetamine. *Veterinarian and Human Toxicology* 44 (4): 216–217.

Kato, M. 1990. Brief history of control, prevention, and treatment of drug dependence in Japan. *Drug Alcohol Dependency* 25 (2): 213–214.

Katsuragawa, Y. 1999. Effect of methamphetamine abuse on the bone quality of the calcaneus. *Forensic Science International* 101: 43–48.

Kim, S. J., Lyoo, I. K., Hwang J., Sung, Y. H., Lee, H. Y., Lee, D. S., Jeong, D-U., and Renshaw, P. F. 2005. Frontal glucose metabolism in abstinent methamphetamine users. *Neuropsychopharmacology* 30 (7): 1383–1391.

Koch Crime Institute. 2003. Prenatal exposure to methamphetamine restricts infant growth. *Drug Abuse.* April 10, 2003. Accessed on line at: www.kci.org/meth_info/sites/NewsRX.htm.

Kolecki, P. 1998. Inadvertent methamphetamine poisoning in pediatric patients. *Pediatric Emergency Care* 14 (6): 385–387.

Kraman, P. 2004. *Drug Abuse in America—Rural Meth.* Lexington, KY: The Council of State Governments.

Lacour, G., and Gregory, A. 2004. Meth is invading Carolinas: Frightening, devastating, spreading. *Charlotte Observer,* March 21, 2004. Accessed on line at: www.charlotte.com.

Lederman, R. P., Lederman, E., Work, B. A., Jr., and McCann, D. S. 1978. The relationship of maternal anxiety, plasma catecholamines and plasma cortisol to progress in labor. *American Journal of Obstetrics and Gynecology* 132: 495–500.

Leinwand, D. 2003. "Meth" moves east. *USA Today,* July 29, 2003.

Leinwand, D. 2005. Counties Say Meth is Top Drug Threat. *USA Today,* July 4, 2005.

Leshner, A. I. 2000. Addressing the medical consequences of drug abuse. *NIDA Notes* 15: 3–4.

Levin, J. N. 1971. Amphetamine ingestion with biliary atresia. *Pediatrics* 79: 130–131.

Lewis, D. C., and Millar, D. G. 2005. *Open letter: To whom it may concern.* July 27, 2005.

Little, B. B., Snell, L. M., Gilstrap, L. C., III. 1988. Methamphetamine use during pregnancy: Outcome and fetal effects. *Obstetrics and Gynecology* 72: 541–544.

London, E. D, Simon, S. L., Berman, S. M., Mandelkern, M. A., Lichtman, A. M., Bramen, J., Shinn, A. K., Miotto, K., Learn, J., Dong, Y., Matochik, J. A., Kurian, V., Newton, T., Woods, R., Rawson, R. A., and Ling, W. 2004. Mood disturbances and regional cerebral metabolic abnormalities in recently abstinent methamphetamine abusers. *Archives of General Psychiatry* 61: 73–84.

Luchansky, B. 2003. *Treatment for Methamphetamine Dependency Is as Effective as Treatment for Any Other Drug.* Olympia, WA: Looking Glass Analytics.

MacKenzie, R. G., and Heischober, B. 1997. Methamphetamine. *Pediatrics in Review* 18 (9): 305–309.

Marlatt, G. A., and Gordon, J. R. 1985. *Relapse Prevention.* New York: Guilford Press.

Marlowe, D. B. 2003. Integrating substance abuse treatment and criminal justice supervision. *NIDA Science and Practice Perspectives* 2: 4–14.

Marlowe, D. B., DeMatteo, D. S., and Festinger, D. S. 2003. A sober assessment of drug courts. *Federal Sentencing Reporter* 16: 153–157.

Marshall, D. R. 2000. *Congressional Testimony to the Senate Judiciary Committee.* July 6, 2000.

Martin, K. R. 2002. Prenatal exposure to methamphetamine increases vulnerability to the drug's neurotoxic effects in adult male mice. *NIDA Notes* 17: 1–3.

Martyny, J., Arbuckle, S., McCammon, C. S., Jr., Esswein, E. J., and Erb, N. 2003. *Chemical Exposures Associated with Clandestine Methamphetamine Laboratories.* Denver, CO. : National Jewish Medical and Research Center.

Mason, A. P. 2004. *Methamphetamine labs.* Presented at the annual conference of the North Carolina Family-Based Services Association, Blowing Rock, NC.

Mathias, R. 2001. Biomedical brain abnormality found in school-age children prenatally exposed to cocaine. *NIDA Notes* 16 (4).

Matsumoto, T., Miyakawa, T., Yabana, T., Iizuka, H., and Kishimoto, H. 2001. A clinical study of comorbid eating disorders in female methamphetamine abusers, third report: In comparison with female alcohol abusers with eating disorders. *Clinical Psychiatry* 43: 651–659.

McLellan, A. T., Kushner, H., Metzger, D., Peters, R., Smith, I., Grissom, G., Pettinati, H., and Argeriou, M. 1992. The fifth edition of the Addiction Severity Index. *Journal of Substance Abuse Treatment* 9: 199–213.

Methamphetamine Interagency Task Force. 2000. *Final Report: Federal Advisory Committee.* Washington, DC: Drug Enforcement Administration.

Methamphetamine Interagency Task Force. 2000a. *Final Report: Part II—Prevention and Education. Federal Advisory Committee.* Washington, DC: Drug Enforcement Administration.

Meyers, R. J., and Smith, J. E. 1995. *Clinical Guide to Alcohol Treatment: The Community Reinforcement Approach.* New York: Guilford Press.

Miller, W. R., and Rollnick, S. 1991. *Motivational Interviewing: Preparing People to Change Addictive Behavior.* New York: Guilford Press.

Mills, K. 1999. Meth of old has morphed into epidemic proportions. *Seattle Post-Intelligencer,* December 13, 1999.

Minkoff, K. 2005. Comprehensive continuous integrated system of care (CCISC): Psychopharmacology practice guidelines for individuals with co-occurring psychiatric and substance abuse disorders (COD). June 10, 2005. Accessed on line at: www.kenminkoff.com/article 1.html.

Minkoff, K., and Cline, C. M. 2004. Changing the world: The design and implementation of comprehensive continuous integrated systems of care for individuals with co-occurring disorders. Psychiatric Clinic of North America. Accessed on line at: www.kenminkoff.com/article2.html.

Missouri Department of Health. 2000. *Guidelines for the Cleanup of Former Methamphetamine Labs.* Missouri Department of Health, Section for Environmental Public Health. September, 2000.

Morgan, P., and Beck, J. 1995. The legacy of the paradox: Hidden contexts of methamphetamine use in the United States. In Klee, H. (Ed.), *Amphetamine Misuse: International Perspectives on Current Trends.* Amsterdam, Netherlands: Harwood Academic Publishers.

Morgan, P., and Joe, K. A. 1996. Citizens and outlaws: The private lives and public lifestyles of women in the illicit drug economy. *Journal of Drug Issues* 26: 125–142.

Moriarty, L. 2005. Personal correspondence regarding drug endangered children's efforts by the North Metro Task Force.

Moses, D. J., Reed, B. G., Mazelis, R., and D'Ambrosio, B. 2003. *Creating trauma services for women with co-occurring disorders.* Accessed on-line at: www.nationaltraumaconsortium.org/documents/CreatingTraumaServices.

Murr, A. 2004. A new menace on the rez. *Newsweek,* September 27, 2004: 30.

Murray, J. B. 1998. Psychophysiological aspects of amphetamine-methamphetamine abuse. *Journal of Psychology* 132 (2): 227–237.

Nagorka, A. R., and Bergeson, P. S. 1998. Infant methamphetamine toxicity posing as scorpion envenomation. *Pediatric Emergency Care* 14: 350–351.

Narconon. 2002. Methamphetamine Information: Abuse Patterns. Accessed on line at: www.narconon.org/druginfo/methamphetamine addiction.

National Association of Counties. 2005. Funding of Methamphetamine Research, Treatment, Enforcement, Cleanup and Education. *NACO Fact Sheet.* February, 2005.

National Association of Counties 2006. The Effect of Meth Abuse on Hospital Emergency Rooms. Washington, DC: National Association of Counties. Accessed on line at: www.naco.org.

National Association of Counties 2006a. The Challenge of Treating Meth Abuse. Washington, DC: National Association of Counties. Accessed on line at: www. naco.org.

National Association of Drug Court Providers. 1997. *Defining Drug Courts: Key Components.* Washington, DC: U.S. Department of Justice.

National Center on Addiction and Substance Abuse at Columbia University. 2000. *No Place to Hide: Substance Abuse in Mid-Size Cities and Rural America.* New York: Columbia University.

National Center on Substance Abuse and Child Welfare (NCSACW). 2004. *Project Overview: In-Depth Technical Assistance to Colorado.* Irvine, CA: National Center on Substance Abuse and Child Welfare.

National Drug Intelligence Center. 2002. Crystal methamphetamine. *Information Bulletin,* August, 2002. Product Number 2002-L0424-005. Johnstown, PA: U.S. Department of Justice.

National Drug Intelligence Center. 2002a. *Children at risk.* Johnstown, PA: National Drug Intelligence Center. Accessed on line at: www.usdoj.gov/ndic/pubs1/ 1466/1466p.pdf.

National Drug Intelligence Center. 2003. *National Drug Threat Assessment 2003.* Johnstown, PA: U.S. Department of Justice.

National Drug Intelligence Center. 2004. *National Drug Threat Assessment 2004.* Johnstown, PA: U.S. Department of Justice.

National Drug Intelligence Center. 2005. *Methamphetamine Drug Threat Assessment.* Johnstown, PA: U.S. Department of Justice.

National Institute of Justice. 2000. *ADAM: 1999 Annual Report on Drug Use Among Adult and Juvenile Arrestees.* Washington, DC: National Institute of Justice. Accessed on line at: www.ncjrs.org/pdffiles1/nij/181426.pdf.

National Institute on Drug Abuse. 1998. *Methamphetamine Abuse and Addiction.* From the National Institute on Drug Abuse Research Report Series, April 1998. NIH Publication Number 98-4210. Bethesda, MD: National Institute on Drug Abuse.

National Institute on Drug Abuse. 2002. *Research Report: Methamphetamine Abuse and Addiction.* Bethesda, MD: National Institute on Drug Abuse.

National Institute on Drug Abuse. 2004. Methamphetamine. *Info Facts.* Bethesda, MD: National Institute on Drug Abuse. Accessed on line at: www.nida.nih. gov/Infofax/methamphetamine.html.

National Institute on Drug Abuse. 2005. *Monitoring the Future: National Results of Adolescent Drug Use.* Bethesda, MD: National Institute on Drug Abuse. Accessed on line at: monitoringthefuture.org/data/.

National Institutes of Health. 2001. Methamphetamine abuse leads to long-lasting changes in the human brain that are linked to impaired coordination and memory. *NIH News,* March 1, 2001. Washington, DC: U.S. Department of Health and Human Services. Accessed on line at: www.nih.gov/news/pr/ mar2001/nida.

National Institutes of Health. 2004. New study suggests methamphetamine withdrawal is associated with brain changes similar to those seen in depression and anxiety. *NIH News* January 5, 2004. Washington, DC: U.S. Department of Health and Human Services.

National Jewish Medical and Research Center. 2004. *Toxic Brew of Chemicals Cooked up in Methamphetamine Labs.* Denver, CO: National Jewish Medical and Research Center. Accessed on line at: www.nationaljewish.org/news/meth.

Nelson, M. M. and Forfar, O. 1971. Associations between drugs administered during pregnancy and congenital abnormalities of the fetus. *British Medical Journal* 1: 523–527.

Nestor, T. A., Tamamoto, W. I., Kam, T. H., and Schultz, T. 1989. Crystal methamphetamine-induced acute pulmonary edema: A case report. *Hawaii Medical Journal* 48: 457–460.

Nestor, T. A., Tamamoto, W. I., Kam, T. H., and Schultz, T. 1989a. Acute pulmonary edema caused by crystalline methamphetamine. *Lancet* 2 (8674): 1277–1278.

New York State Office of Alcoholism and Substance Abuse Services. 2004. *Amphetamines and Methamphetamines.* March 29, 2004. Accessed on line at: www.oasas.state.ny.us/AdMed/drugs/fyimeth.htm.

Newsweek. 2005. The meth epidemic: Inside America's drug crisis. *Newsweek*, August 8, 2005.

Nora, J. J., McNamara, D. G., and Clarke-Fraser, F. 1967. Dexamphetamine sulphate and human malformations. *Lancet* 2: 1021–1022.

Nora, J. J., Vargo, T. A., Nora, A. H., Love, K. E., and McNamara, D. G. 1970. Dexamphetamine: A possible environmental trigger in cardiovascular malformations. *Lancet* 1(7659): 1290–1291.

Nordahl, T. E., Salo, R., Natsuaki, Y., Galloway, G. P., Waters, C., Moore, C. D., Kile, S., and Buonocore, M. H. 2005. Methamphetamine users in sustained abstinence: A proton magnetic resonance spectroscopy study. *Archives of General Psychiatry* 62: 444–452.

North Carolina Department of Health and Human Services. 2005. *Chapter IX: Drug endangered children.* Accessed on line at: info.dhhs.state.nc.us/olm/manuals/dss/csm-65/man/CSs1000.htm.

North Carolina Department of Justice. 2004. *North Carolina Methamphetamine Summit: Final Report.* Raleigh, NC: North Carolina Department of Justice.

North Carolina Division of Social Services and the Family and Children's Resource Program. 2005. Methamphetamine: What child welfare workers should know. *Children's Services Practice Notes* 10: (2) April. Accessed on line at: info.dhhs.state.nc.us/olm/manuals/dss.

North Carolina Division of Social Services and the Family and Children's Resource Program. 2005a. Meth labs and their impact on child welfare practice. *Children's Services Practice Notes* 10: (2) April. Accessed on line at: info.dhhs.state.nc.us/olm/manuals/dss.

North Carolina Division of Social Services and the Family and Children's Resource Program. 2005b. How to recognize a meth lab. *Children's Services Practice Notes* 10: (2) April. Accessed on line at: info.dhhs.state.nc.us/olm/manuals/dss.

North Carolina Division of Social Services and the Family and Children's Resource Program. 2005c. When is it safe to reoccupy a dwelling that has been used to make meth? *Children's Services Practice Notes* 10: (2) April. Accessed on line at: info.dhhs.state.nc.us/olm/manuals/dss.

North Carolina Division of Social Services and the Family and Children's Resource Program. 2005d. Crafting a safe, family-centered response to meth. *Children's Services Practice Notes* 10: (2) April. Accessed on line at: info.dhhs.state.nc.us/ olm/manuals/dss.

Obert, J. L., McCann, M. J., Marinelli-Casey, P., Weiner, A., Minsky, S., Brethen, P., and Rawson, R. A. 2000. The Matrix Model of out-patient stimulant abuse treatment: History and description. *Journal of Psychoactive Drugs* 32: 157–164.

Office of National Drug Control Policy. 2003. *Methamphetamine: Fact Sheet.* Rockville, MD: Drug Policy Information Clearinghouse. Accessed on line at: www.whitehousedrugpolicy.gov/drugfact/methamphetamine.

Office of National Drug Control Policy. 2003a. Office of Drug Control Policy Update 2003. November, 2003. Accessed on line at: www.whitehousedrugpolicy.gov/ publications/policy/ndcs03/table71.html.

Office of National Drug Control Policy. 2005. *Fact Sheet: Methamphetamine.* Updated November 30, 2005. Accessed on line at: www.whitehousedrugpolicy.gov/ publications/factsht/methamph/.

Olds, J. 1973. The discovery of reward systems in the brain. In Valenstein, E. S. (Ed.), *Brain Stimulation and Motivation* (pp. 81–99). Glenview, Il: Scott, Foresman and Company.

Olds J., and Milner. P. 1954. Positive reinforcement produced by electrical stimulation of septal area and other regions of rat brain. *Journal of Comparative and Physiological Psychology* 47: 419–427.

Oro, A. S., and Dixon, S. D. 1987. Perinatal cocaine and methamphetamine exposure: Maternal and neonatal correlates. *Journal of Pediatrics* 111: 571–578.

Peed, C. R. 2004. COPS office attacks the scourge of meth. *Community Links.* November: 1–2.

Pennell, S., Ellett, J., Rienick, C., and Grimes, J. 1999. *Meth Matters; Report on Methamphetamine Users in Five Western Cities.* Washington, DC. : National Institute of Justice. Accessed on line at: ncjrs.org/pdffiles1/176331.pdf.

Plessinger, M. A. 1998. Prenatal exposure to amphetamines: Risks and adverse outcomes in pregnancy. *Obstetrics and Gynecology Clinics of North America* 25: 119–139.

Prochaska, J. O., and DiClemente, C. C. 1992. Stages of change in the modification of problem behavior. In Hersen, M., Eisler, R. M., and Miller, P. M. (eds.), *Progress in Behavior Modification* (pp. 182–218). Sycamore, IL: Sycamore Publishing.

Quest Diagnostics. 2004. *News from Quest Diagnostics.* Teterboro, NJ: Quest Diagnostics.

Quest Diagnostics. 2005. *Amphetamines Drug-Test Positives Are Up Among Safety-Sensitive Workers in the First Half of 2005, According to Quest Diagnostics' Drug Testing Index.* Teterboro, NJ: Quest Diagnostics.

Ramamoorthy, J. D., Ramamoorthy, S., Leibach, F. H., and Ganapathy, V. 1995. Human placental monoamine transporters as targets for amphetamines. *American Journal of Obstetrics and Gynecology* 173: 1782–1787.

Ramer, C. M. 1974. The case history of an infant born to an amphetamine-addicted mother. *Clinical Pediatrics* 13: 596–597.

Rannazzisi, J. T. 2005. *Statement Before the House Judiciary Committee; Subcommittee on Crime, Terrorism, and Homeland Security.* Deputy Chief, Office of Enforcement Operations, Drug Enforcement Administration, September 27, 2005.

Rawson, R. A. 2005. *Methamphetamine Addiction: Cause for Concern—Hope for the Future.* Los Angeles, CA: Department of Psychiatry and Behavioral Sciences, UCLA. Accessed on line at: www.apa.org/ppo/rawson62805.ppt#257.

Rawson, R. A., Anglin, M. D., and Ling, W. 2002. Will the methamphetamine problem go away? *Journal of Addictive Diseases* 21: 5–19.

Rawson, R. A., Gonzales, R., and Brethen, P. 2002. Treatment of methamphetamine use disorders: An update. *Journal of Substance Abuse Treatment* 23: 145–150.

Rawson, R. A., Huber, A., Brethen, P., Obert, J. L., Gulati, V., Shoptaw, S., and Ling, W. 2000. Methamphetamine and cocaine users: differences in characteristics and treatment retention. *Journal of Psychoactive Drugs* 32: 233–238.

Rawson, R. A., Huber, A., Brethen, P., Obert, J., Gulati, V. Shoptaw, S., and Ling, W. 2002. Status of methamphetamine users 2-5 years after outpatient treatment. *Journal of Addictive Diseases* 21: 107–119.

Rawson, R. A., Huber, A., McCann, M., Shoptaw, S., Farabee, D., Reiber, C. and Ling, W. 2002a. A comparison of contingency management and cognitive-behavioral approaches during methadone maintenance treatment for cocaine dependence. *Archives of General Psychiatry* 59: 817–824.

Rawson, R. A., Marinelli-Casey, P. J., and Huber, A. 2002. A multi-site evaluation of treatment of methamphetamine dependence in adults. In Herrell, J., and Straw, R. B. (eds.), *Conducting Multiple Site Evaluations in Real-World Settings* (pp. 73–87). San Francisco: American Evaluation Association.

Rawson, R. A., Marinelli-Casey, P. J., Anglin, M. D., Dickow, A., Frazier, Y., Gallagher, C., Galloway, G. P., Herrell, J., Huber, A., McCann, M. J., Obert, J., Pennell, S., Reiber, C., Vandersloot, D., and Zweben, J. 2004. A multi-site comparison of psychosocial approaches for the treatment of methamphetamine dependence. *Addiction* 99: 708–717.

Rawson, R. A., McCann, M., Huber, A., and Shoptaw, S. 1999. Contingency management and relapse prevention as stimulant abuse treatment interventions. In Higgins, S. T., and Silverman, K. (Eds), *Motivating Behavior Change among Illicit-Drug Abusers: Research on Contingency Management Interventions* (pp. 57–74). Washington, DC: American Psychological Association.

Rawson, R. A., and the Methamphetamine Treatment Project Corporate Authors. 2004. A multi-site comparison of psychosocial approaches for the treatment of methamphetamine dependence. *Addiction* 99: 708–717.

Rawson, R. A., Obert, J. L., McCann, M. J., and Ling, W. 1991. Psychological approaches to the treatment of cocaine dependency. *Journal of Addictive Diseases* 11: 97–119.

Rawson, R. A., Obert, J. L., McCann, M. J., and Scheffey, E. H. 1991a. *The Matrix Manual for the Treatment of Stimulant Abuse* (2nd ed.). Beverly Hills, CA: Matrix Center.

Rawson, R. A., Shoptaw, S., Obert, J., McCann, M., Hasson, A., Marinelli-Casey, P., Brethen, P., and Ling, W. 1995. An intensive out-patient approach for cocaine abuse treatment: The matrix model. *Journal of Substance Abuse Treatment* 12: 117–127.

Ray, S. 2004. Methamphetamine: The "walk-away" drug. *Social Work Today* 4: 30–33.

Ross, T. L. 2001. *Motivation for Treatment Among Women Who Abuse Methamphetamine.* Dissertation Abstracts International: Section B: The Sciences & Engineering, 62 (2-B), 1097.

Rowbotham, M. C. 1993. Cocaine levels and elimination in inpatients and outpatients: Implications for emergency treatment of cocaine complications. In Sorer H. (Ed), *Acute Cocaine Intoxication: Current Methods of Treatment* (pp. 147–155). NIDA Research Monograph Series, Number 123. DHHS Pub No (ADM) 93-3498. Rockville, MD: National Institute on Drug Abuse.

SAMHSA (Substance Abuse and Mental Health Services Administration). 2001. *Prevention Alert: Meth: What's Cooking in Your Neighborhood?* Rockville, MD: SAMHSA.

SAMHSA (Substance Abuse and Mental Health Services Administration). 2001a. *Summary of Findings, 2000 National Household Survey on Drug Abuse.* Rockville, MD: SAMHSA.

SAMHSA (Substance Abuse and Mental Health Services Administration). 2004. *Drug Abuse Warning Network, 2003: Interim National Estimates of Drug-Related Emergency Department Visits.* Rockville, MD: SAMHSA.

SAMHSA (Substance Abuse and Mental Health Services Administration). 2004a. Primary methamphetamine/amphetamine treatment admissions: 1992–2002. *The DASIS Report*, September 17, 2004. Rockville, MD: SAMHSA.

SAMHSA (Substance Abuse and Mental Health Services Administration). 2005. *Treatment Episode Data Set (TEDS) 1993–2003.* Rockville, MD: Office of Applied Studies.

SAMHSA (Substance Abuse and Mental Health Services Administration). 2005a. *National Survey on Drug Use and Health 2004.* Updated October 2, 2005. Rockville, MD: SAMHSA.

SAMHSA (Substance Abuse and Mental Health Services Administration). 2005b. *The NSDUH Report: Methamphetamine Use, Abuse, and Dependence: 2002, 2003, and 2004, In Brief.* Updated September 16, 2005. Rockville, MD: SAMHSA.

SAMHSA (Substance Abuse and Mental Health Services Administration). 2005c. Smoked methamphetamine/amphetamines: 1992–2002. *The DASIS Report*, January 7, 2005. Rockville, MD: SAMHSA.

SAMHSA (Substance Abuse and Mental Health Services Administration). 2006. Trends in methamphetamine/amphetamine admissions to treatment: 1993–2003. *The DASIS Report*, March 15, 2006.

SAS Institute Inc. 1999. *SAS User's Guide: Statistics*, Version 8 edition. Cary, NC: SAS Institute Inc.

Saxen, I., 1975. Associations between oral clefts and drugs taken during pregnancy. *International Journal of Epidemiology* 4: 37–44.

Seiden, L. S. 1991. Neurotoxicity of methamphetamine: Mechanisms of action and issues related to aging. In Miller, M. A., and Kozel, N. J. (Eds.), *Methamphetamine Abuse: Epidemiologic Issues and Implications* (pp. 24–42). NIDA Research Monograph No. 115, DHHS Publication No. ADM 91-1836. Washington, DC: U.S. Government Printing Office.

Seiden L. S., and Sabol, K. E. 1996. Methamphetamine and methylenedioxymethamphetamine neurotoxicity: Possible mechanisms of cell destruction. In Majewska, M. D. (Ed.) *Neurotoxicity and Neuropathology Associated with Cocaine Abuse* (pp. 251–276). NIDA Research Monograph No. 163, NIH Publication No. 96-4019. Washington DC: U.S. Government Printing Office.

Semple, S. J., Patterson, T. L., and Grant, I. 2004. The context of sexual risk behavior among heterosexual methamphetamine users. *Addictive Behaviors* 29: 807–810.

Shah, R. 2006. infants exposed prenatally to methamphetamines: developmental effects and effective interventions. Teleconference Series, National Abandoned Infants Assistance Resource Center, February 21, 2006.

Shaner, J. W. 2002. Caries associated with methamphetamine abuse. *Journal of the Michigan Dental Association.* September 84 (9): 42–47.

Shaw, V. 2004. Drug endangered children. Presented at a Methamphetamine Conference. Asheville, NC: June 3, 2003.

Sherman, W. T. and Gautieri, R. F. 1972. Effect of certain drugs on perfused human placenta. X. Norepinephrine release by bradynin. *Journal of Pharmacological Science* 61: 870–873.

Shoptaw, S., Rawson, R. A., McCann, M. J., and Obert, J. L. 1994. The matrix model of out-patient stimulant abuse treatment: evidence of efficacy. *Journal of Addictive Diseases* 13: 129–141.

Simpson, D. D., and Curry, S. J. (eds.). 1997. Special issue: Drug abuse treatment outcome study (DATOS). *Psychology of Addictive Behaviors* 11 (4).

Simpson, D. D., Joe, G. W., Rowan-Szal, G. and Greener, J. 1995. Client engagement and change during drug abuse treatment. *Journal of Substance Abuse* 7: 117–134.

Simpson, D. D., and Sells, S. B. 1982. Effectiveness of treatment for drug abuse: An overview of the DARP research program. *Advances in alcohol and substance abuse* 2: 7–29.

Šlamberová, R., Charousová, P. and Pometlová, M. 2005. Methamphetamine Administration during Gestation Impairs Maternal Behavior. *Developmental Psychobiology* 46: 57–65.

Smith, L., Yonekura, M. L., Wallace, T., Berman, N., Kuo, J., and Berkowitz, C. 2003. Effects of Prenatal Methamphetamine Exposure on Fetal Growth and Drug Withdrawal Symptoms in Infants Born at Term. *Journal of Developmental Behavior and Pediatrics* 24 (1): 17–23.

Sowder, B., and Beschner, G. (eds.). 1993. Methamphetamine: An illicit drug with high abuse potential. Unpublished report from NIDA contract no. 271-90-0002. Rockville, MD: T. Head and Company.

Specter, M. 2005. Higher risk: Crystal meth, the Internet, and dangerous choices about AIDS. *New Yorker*, May 23, 2005. Accessed on line at: www.newyorker.com/fact/content/articles/0505223fa_fact

Stark, K. 2004. Treatment for methamphetamine dependency is as effective as treatment for any other drug dependency. *Inside Focus* 14: 1, 4.

Stek, A. M., Fisher, B. K., Baker, R. S., Lang, U., Tseng, C. U., and Clark, K. E. 1993. Maternal and fetal cardiovascular responses to methamphetamine in the pregnant sheep. *American Journal of Obstetrics and Gynecology* 169 (4): 888–897.

Stewart, J. L., and Meeker, J. E. 1997. Fetal and infant deaths associated with maternal methamphetamine abuse. *Journal of Analytical Toxicology* 21: 515–517.

Streltzer, J., and Leigh, H. 1977. Amphetamine abstinence psychosis—Does it exist? *Psychiatric Opinion* Jan/Feb: 47–50.

Swan, N. 1996. Response to escalating methamphetamine abuse builds on NIDA-funded research. *NIDA Notes* 11: 1–4.

Swan, N. 2003. New imaging technology confirms earlier PET scan evidence: Methamphetamine abuse linked to human brain damage. *NIDA Notes* 18: 6–7.

Swetlow, K. 2003. Children at clandestine methamphetamine labs: Helping meth's youngest victims. *OVC Bulletin* (June). Accessed on line at: www.ojp.usdoj.gov/ovc/publications/bulletins/children/197590.pdf.

Szuster, R. R. 1990. Methamphetamine in psychiatric emergencies. *Hawaii Medical Journal* 49: 389–91.

Tandy, K. P. 2004. Statement before the U.S. House of Representatives, Committee on Appropriations, Subcommittee for the Departments of Commerce, Justice, State, the Judiciary and Related Agencies, March 24, 2004.

Taylor, N. D. 2004. Understanding methamphetamine addiction: Biopsychosocial effects on parents, children and the community. Lecture presented in Fort Collins, CO, April 2004.

Taylor, N. D. 2006. Myth of Duration Expectations. Training presented by Dr. Nicolas Taylor.

Thomas, D. B. 1995. Cleft palate, mortality and morbidity in infants of substance abusing mothers. *Journal of Paediatric Child Health* 31: 457–460.

Tomiyama, G. 1990. Chronic schizophrenia-like states in methamphetamine psychosis. *Japanese Journal of Psychiatry and Neurology* 44 (3): 531–539.

Uncle Fester. 2002. *Secrets of methamphetamine manufacture: Including recipes for MDA, ecstasy, and other psychedelic amphetamines* (6th ed.). Port Townsend, WA: Loompanics Unlimited.

USA Today. 2005. Counties Say Meth is Top Drug Threat. *USA Today.* Monday, July 4, 2005.

Volkow, N. D., Chang, L., Wang, G-J., Fowler, J. S., Franceschi, D., Sedler, M. J., Gatley, S. J., Hitzemann, R., Ding, Y-S., Wong, C., and Logan, J. 2001. Higher cortical and lower subcortical metabolism in detoxified methamphetamine abusers. *The American Journal of Psychiatry* 158: 383–389.

Volkow, N. D., Chang, L., Wang, G-J., Fowler, J. S., Leonido-Yee, M., Franceschi, D., Selder, M. J., Gatley, S. J., Hitzemann, R., Ding, Yu-Shin, Logan, J., Wong, C. and Miller, E. N. 2001a. Association of dopamine transporter reduction with psychomotor impairment in methamphetamine abusers. *The American Journal of Psychiatry* 158 (3): 377–382.

Volkow, N. D. 2005. Methamphetamine abuse—Testimony before the Senate Subcommittee on Labor, Health and Human Services, Education, and Related Agencies—Committee on Appropriations. April 21, 2005.

Warner, P., Connolly, J. P., Gibran, N. S., Heimback, D. M., and Engrav, L. H. 2003. The methamphetamine burn patient. *Journal of Burn Care and Rehabilitation* 24 (5): 275–278.

Washington Department of Health. 1996. *Guidelines for the Contamination, Reduction, and Sampling at Illegal Drug Manufacturing Sites.* Olympia, WA: Washington State Department of Health, Office of Toxic Substances.

Weil, M., and Karls, J. M. 1985. *Case Management in Human Service Practice.* San Francisco: Jossey-Bass.

Wells, K., and Wright, W. 2004. *Medical Summit.* Presented at Idaho's Second Annual Drug Endangered Children Conference, Post Falls, Idaho. September 14, 2004.

Wetli, C. V. 1993. The Pathology of cocaine: Perspectives from the autopsy table. In Sorer, H. (Ed.), *Acute Cocaine Intoxication: Current Methods of Treatment* (pp. 172–183). NIDA Monograph Series, Number 123. DHHS Pub No (ADM) 93-3498. Rockville, MD: National Institute on Drug Abuse.

Wermuth, L. 2000. Methamphetamine use: Hazards and social influences. *Journal of Drug Education* 30: 423–433.

Williams, M. T., Morford, L. L., Wood, S. L., Wallace, T. L., Fukumura, M., Broening, H. W., and Vorhees, C. V. 2003. Developmental D-methamphetamine treatment selectively induces spatial navigation impairments in reference memory in the Morris water maze while sparing working memory. *Synapse* 48: 138–148.

Williams, M. T., Vorhees, C. V., Boon, F., Saber, A. J., and Cain, D. P. 2002. Methamphetamine exposure from postnatal day 11 to 20 causes impairments in both behavioral strategies and spatial learning in adult rats. *Brain Research* 958: 312–321.

Wolkoff, D. 1997. Methamphetamine Abuse: An Overview for Health Care Professionals. *Hawaii Medical Journal* 56: 34–36, 44.

Woodside, M., and McClam, T. 2002. *Generalist Case Management: A Method of Human Service Delivery.* Belmont, CA: Wadsworth.

Yacoubian, G. S., and Peters, R. J. 2004. Exploring the prevalence and correlates of methamphetamine use: Findings from Sacramento's ADAM program. *Journal of Drug Education* 34: 281–294.

Yui, K., Goto, K., Ikemoto, S., Ishiguro, T., and Kamata, Y. 2000. Increased sensitivity to stress in spontaneous recurrence of methamphetamine psychosis: Noradrenergic hyperactivity with contribution from dopaminergic hyperactivity. *Journal of Clinical Psychopharmacology* 20 (2): 165–174.

Zernike, K. 2006. Potent Mexican meth floods in as states curb domestic variety. *New York Times,* January 23, 2006.

Zickler, P. 2002. Methamphetamine abuse linked to impaired cognitive and motor skills despite recovery of dopamine transporters. *NIDA Notes* 17: 1–3.

Zickler, P. 2004. Long-term abstinence brings partial recovery from methamphetamine damage. *NIDA Notes* 19: 1, 6–7.

Zickler, P. 2005. Methamphetamine, cocaine abusers have different patterns of drug use, suffer cognitive impairments. *NIDA Notes* 16: 1–2.

Zickler, P. 2005a. Thailand conference focuses on methamphetamine research. *NIDA Notes* 16: 1–2.

Zickler, P. 2005b. Ethnic identification and cultural ties may help prevent drug use. *NIDA Notes* 14: 1–3.

Index

About the Editor and Contributors

HERBERT C. COVEY received his Ph.D. in Sociology from the University of Colorado at Boulder. He has published numerous academic articles and has authored or co-authored many books including *African American Slave Medicine: Herb and Non-Herb Treatments* (Lanham, MD: Lexington Press, forthcoming); *Youth Gangs* (Springfield, IL: Charles C. Thomas, forthcoming); *Street Gangs Throughout the World* (Springfield, IL: Charles C. Thomas, 2003); *A History of the Social Perceptions of People with Disabilities* (Springfield, IL: Charles C. Thomas, 1998); *Juvenile Gangs*, 2nd Edition (Springfield, IL: Charles C. Thomas, 1997); *Images of Older People in Western Art and Society* (Westport, CT: Praeger Publishers, 1991); and *Theoretical Frameworks in the Sociology of Education* (Cambridge, MA: Shenkman, 1980). He helped coordinate and has presented at four regional methamphetamine symposiums in 2004 and 2005. His current research involves the relationship between methamphetamine use and criminal behavior.

COLLEEN BRISNEHAN is an environmental protection specialist with the Colorado Department of Public Health and Environment's Hazardous Material and Waste Management Division. She has a BS in Geophysical Engineering. Her responsibilities with the department include oversight of assessment and remediation projects at contaminated hazardous waste sites. Ms. Brisnehan was involved in the development of the department's guidance on the cleanup of methamphetamine labs and coordinated the department's rule-making process to establish methamphetamine lab cleanup regulations. She serves as a technical resource for the department, local health departments, and the general public in the areas of methamphetamine cleanup and sampling. She is involved with Colorado's Alliance for Drug Endangered Children (DEC) and served as a member of the DEC initial response and cleanup subcommittees.

SAMANTHA CAMERON was recently married and is getting her life together. She has been in recovery for quite some time. She has participated in methamphetamine abuse prevention films and often provides testimony on the downside of meth use. She recently was featured in a drug-endangered children video (2005) on methamphetamine.

C. WEST HUDDLESTON III is the director of the National Drug Court Institute (NDCI). Based in the nation's capital, NDCI is the educational, research, and scholarship branch of the National Association of Drug Court Professionals (NADCP), a nonprofit, nongovernmental organization supported by the White House Office of National Drug Control Policy and the Bureau of Justice Assistance, U.S. Department of Justice. Mr. Huddleston is ultimately responsible for the planning and execution of over 75 training events and 50 technical assistance visits throughout the United States and abroad each year. Huddleston is a board-licensed substance abuse counselor with 13 years of clinical experience working with misdemeanor and felony offenders on the county, state, and federal levels. Prior to being named director of NDCI, Mr. Huddleston worked throughout the Tennessee and Oklahoma correctional systems. During this period, he teamed with both states' respective departments of corrections to develop, implement, and operate numerous offender-specific, in-custody mental health and substance abuse treatment programs. Of particular pride to Mr. Huddleston is his team's winning the governor's Team Excellence award for the design and implementation of the first prison therapeutic community and work camp within the Oklahoma Department of Corrections. Huddleston has also served as the director of two community corrections programs and as the interim director of a 125-bed pre-release correctional center. In addition, he co-designed and implemented the first two drug courts in the State of Oklahoma, one of which served as an early mentor court for the U.S. Department of Justice. He has published several articles and monographs on drug courts, in-custody substance abuse treatment, and reentry courts. Mr. Huddleston has served as a special consultant to the National Institute of Justice (NIJ) and Drug Enforcement Administration (DEA) as well as with the Tennessee and Oklahoma Departments of Corrections. He is currently a member of the Substance Abuse Committee of the American Correctional Association and a faculty member of the National Judicial College.

ANGELA MEAD is a child welfare administrator with the Larimer County Department of Human Services. She has her master's degree in social work. She has extensive knowledge and 21 years of experience in child welfare. She is actively involved with the drug-endangered children's effort and created the Larimer County Alliance for Drug Endangered Children. She has been very active in developing community responses to methamphetamine.

KAREN MOONEY is a licensed clinical social worker and a senior-level addictions counselor, and has over 13 years of experience as a child protection caseworker and addictions specialist with emphasis on the impact of substance abuse on parenting and child protection issues. She has worked at Signal Behavioral Health Network, where she was the project director for a CSAT-targeted capacity expansion grant aimed at engagement and retention of underserved women in substance abuse treatment, and then went on to serve as Signal's director of Child Welfare Services. She has served as a consultant to the Child Welfare League of America, on a project to develop an assessment tool to link child protection and substance abuse issues, and currently serves on the Community Expert Panel for the National Center on Substance Abuse and Child Welfare. She has authored chapters in several publications on assessment and treatment of substance abuse among child welfare clients.

LORI MORIARTY, Commander, is considered by many to be a national leader in the response to methamphetamine abuse. Commander Moriarty began her career in law enforcement in 1987. In June 2000 she was assigned as the commander of the North Metro Task Force, a multijurisdictional undercover drug unit in the Adams and Broomfield counties. As the commander of the task force, she has been instrumental in implementing protocols for the safe investigation of meth labs and undercover drug operations. She has appeared on ABC News, *20/20*, Fox National News, MSNBC, Frontline, National Public Radio, Colorado Public Radio, PBS, and local news channels in an effort to educate citizens on the hazards of meth drug labs and drug-endangered children. Under her guidance, the task force combined efforts with local fire departments, paramedics, and Hazmat teams and developed a joint response to these hazardous locations. Commander Moriarty has worked with the Children's Hospital, Kempe Children's Center, National Jewish Hospital and Research Center, the Office of the Child's Representative, and Rocky Mountain HIDTA in addressing the difficult issue of child protection as it relates to drug abuse and meth labs. She is the president and CEO of the nonprofit organization and an executive committee member of the National Alliance for Drug Endangered Children. Commander Moriarty recently received the CASA (Court Appointed Special Advocates) 2004 Friend of Children Award. Her safety stance and public awareness efforts won her regional and national recognition when the president of the United States, Office of the National Drug Control Policy, recognized her in Washington, DC as the 2001 drug commander of the year. She has won numerous other awards including "Peace Officer of the Year" for her efforts.

RICHARD A. RAWSON is one of the most recognized names in the field of addiction treatment. His and his colleagues' work with the Matrix Model at the Matrix Institute for substance abuse treatment is considered to be the most promising in the field. The article by Rawson and his colleagues on psychosocial approaches for the treatment of methamphetamine is a classic evidence-based evaluation of treatment. He has authored or co-authored numerous articles on substance abuse treatment and specifically methamphetamine.

SHIRLEY RHODUS has a master's degree in social work and has worked in public social services for 28 years in Iowa and Colorado, primarily in the areas of child protection, youth in conflict, and permanency planning, as a caseworker, supervisor, and administrator. She is currently the division manager over child welfare intake for the El Paso County, Colorado, Department of Human Services, and previously served as the division manager over ongoing child protective services for eight years. In 2001, she helped implement the Direct Link program to serve substance-involved, child protective services families, which was expanded to include the first family treatment drug court in Colorado in July of 2002.

RHONDA is a noted public speaker on methamphetamine and is moving on with life and enjoying her daughter's recovery. She has been active in public presentations on the effects of methamphetamine on families and lives.

LYNN RIEMER has a bachelor's degree in chemistry and has been a chemist for the North Metro Task Force since November 2001. She is involved in methamphetamine lab response for the Task Force, and decontaminates all children removed from labs. Lynn has provided lab awareness and first responder training to over 8,000 people throughout several western states including Colorado, Wyoming, Montana, New Mexico, and Utah. Before joining the task force, Lynn worked in areas of analytical chemistry, petroleum chemistry, and forensic chemistry for the Drug Enforcement Administration (DEA) in its San Francisco laboratory for five years. She has also been involved in medical research at Children's Hospital in Denver and at the National Institute of Health in Maryland. Lynn currently contracts to provide meth lab awareness and personal safety training to social service providers.

JULIA ROGUSKI has an MA and serves as the child protection coordinator for Savio House. Ms. Roguski has developed an expertise in child protection and in-home counseling with substance-abusing parents. Ms. Roguski is both a licensed professional counselor and a level III certified addictions counselor, providing an important understanding of the co-occurring disorders of mental health and substance abuse. As the El Paso County Family Treatment Drug Court Coordinator since the program's inception, Ms. Roguski, in collaboration with the El Paso County Department of Human Services and the 4th Judicial District, has played an important role in developing the program's services and standards. Ms. Roguski's 15 years of experience as a direct practitioner, addictions counselor, supervisor, and administrator provide important understanding of service delivery and program development.

NICOLAS TAYLOR, Ph.D., is a licensed clinical psychologist and a level III certified addictions counselor. He is the director and primary clinician for Taylor Behavioral Health. He specializes in performing forensic psychological evaluations and delivering psychotherapy and substance abuse counseling services. From 1997–2000 he worked as a substance abuse program coordinator for Midwestern Mental Health Center. He directed the development and management of drug and alcohol treatment services in a five-county region. Through 1998–2000 he facilitated community efforts in three counties to help address the growing use of methamphetamine. This included working with community leaders to establish the formation of drug courts in each of the counties. He was the primary drug treatment counselor for Montrose Drug Court. He is an instructor at Mesa State College, Montrose Campus, teaching courses in Drugs and Human Behavior, Abnormal Psychology, Human Growth and Development, and Social Psychology. He is nationally known for his expertise on meth use and treatment and travels throughout the country speaking on the topic. He has recently been involved in working with Native American tribes in a few western states on methamphetamine use and treatment.

KATHRYN M. WELLS, MD, is currently the medical director of the Denver Family Crisis Center, where she serves as the child abuse and neglect consultant for the Denver Health and Hospital Authority, Denver Department of Human Services, the Denver Police Department, and the Denver District Attorney's Office. She is also an attending physician with the Kemp Child Protection Team at the Children's Hospital in Denver and has an academic appointment as an assistant professor in pediatrics at the University of Colorado Health Sciences Center. She received her B.A. in Biology and Psychology with magna cum laude honors from Carroll College in Helena, Montana, and then attended medical school at Creighton University School of Medicine in Omaha, Nebraska. She received her MD in 1993. She received postgraduate training as a pediatric resident at Creighton University–Nebraska Universities Health Foundation Joint Pediatric Residency Program in Omaha. She has had fellowship training in Denver, Colorado, at the University of Colorado Health Sciences Center, the Kempe Children's Center, and the Children's Hospital in the pediatric subspecialty field of Child Abuse and Neglect. She is often called on as an expert witness in child abuse and neglect cases as well as those involving substance abuse. She travels across the country as a medical expert on the effects of substance abuse on users and the children of users, especially methamphetamine. She is also actively involved in the Colorado Alliance for Drug Endangered Children and has made many presentations on the medical effects of methamphetamine use.

TONYA WHEELER is the president of Advocates for Recovery, a grassroots organization in Colorado dedicated to making recovery from addiction visible to her home state as well as other audiences across the nation as a positive, attainable goal. Tonya works as a certified addictions counselor, level III, for the University of Colorado Hospital at CeDAR (Center for Dependency, Addiction, and Rehabilitation) and has worked in the substance abuse field for over 13 years. She has shared her experiences in her own recovery from addiction to methamphetamine with several audiences across the nation including the Colorado Department of Human Services, KNRC-AM radio in Denver, the National Center on Addiction and Substance Abuse (CASA) in New York City, and numerous other audiences and media.